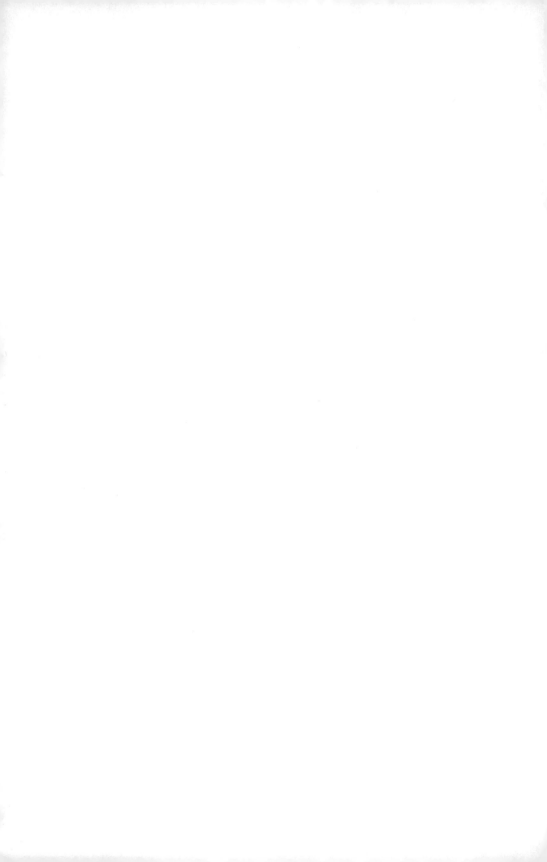

SPLITTING UP

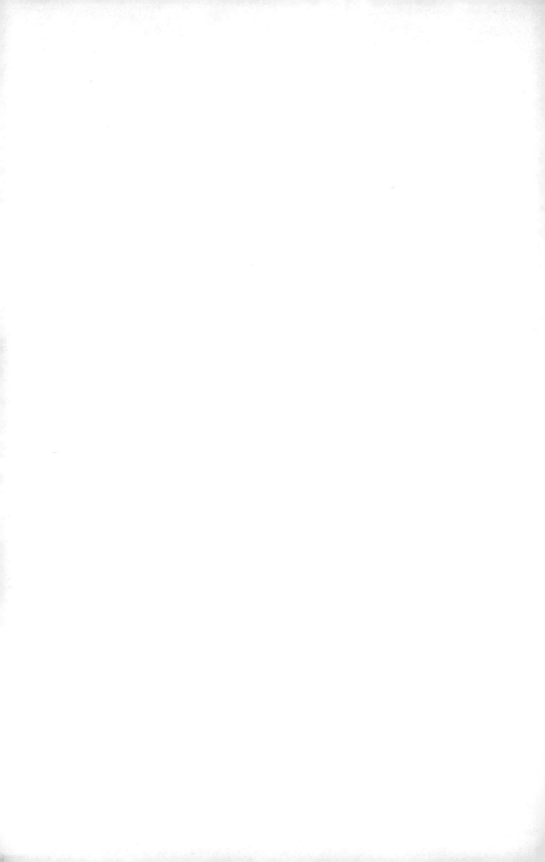

Splitting Up

Enmeshment and Estrangement in the Process of Divorce

ALVIN PAM, PhD
JUDITH PEARSON, PhD

Foreword by James F. Masterson, MD

THE GUILFORD PRESS
New York   London

© 1998 The Guilford Press
A Division of Guilford Publications, Inc.
72 Spring Street, New York, NY 10012
http://www.guilford.com

Printed in the United States of America

This book is printed on acid-free paper.

Last digit is print number: 9 8 7 6 5 4 3 2 1

Library of Congress Cataloging-in-Publication Data

Pam, Alvin.
   Splitting Up : enmeshment and estrangement in the process
of divorce / Alvin Pam, Judith Pearson.
       p.   cm.
   Includes bibliographical references and index.
   ISBN 1-57230-367-0
   1. Divorce—Psychological aspects.   2. Divorced people—
Psychology.   3. Separation (Psychology)   I. Pearson, Judith.
II. Title.
HQ814.P35   1998
306.89—dc21   98-22648
                                                              CIP

*To Mark and Samantha,
Aaron and Simone, and Joshua;
and to all children whose lives
have been touched by divorce*

*To Judy K. F. – embattled housewife
and mother of three, whose reflections
on divorce were the inspiration
for this book*

Foreword

The increase in the rate of divorce (from 40% to 50%) has led to a common assumption that divorce does not have to be painful and frees the person for future better relationships. The authors provide a well-needed antidote to this fantasy in their carefully researched and well-written volume, which stresses that inevitably divorce is painful if the relationship has been meaningful; that divorce often leads to strange, irrational behavior; and that it is better to face these emotions than to deny them.

Drs. Pam and Pearson emphasize the characterological match, which leads to the characterological struggle that results in divorce. They also discuss the relationship system of the pair prior to the breakup, the very nature of which may have made the breakup inevitable.

In their comprehensive coverage of the many issues involved in divorce, the authors present a wealth of information from all perspectives: social, psychological, and psychoanalytic. They elucidate the clinical pictures of both sides of the many paradoxes involved. They elaborate the arguments for each side, deflate many current views as myths and pseudo-situations, and bring a fresh breath of reality by a forthright stand based on common sense and clinical logic. For example, "we will argue that many second-chance unions are doomed to failure because they are born of desperation, not aspiration. Thus, rather than being based on new-found appreciation of the old partner, they tend to be entered into as respites from the strains of separation" (p. 326).

The book is a "must" both for counselors working with couples either contemplating or dealing with divorce, and for the individuals struggling over the issues that arise in such situations.

JAMES F. MASTERSON, MD

Acknowledgments

We would like to express our deep appreciation to all those who lent us their time, expertise, and experiences. And special thanks to Herb Reich, our editor at The Guilford Press.

We extend a final expression of gratitude to our private-practice outpatients and our psychiatric inpatients whose stories are the warp-and-woof of this book.

We have disguised all identifying details of these illustrative cases in order to protect confidentiality.

Contents

SPLITTING UP

Prologue

SOCIAL PERSPECTIVE: VALUES AND HUMAN PASSION

The weaknesses of our society are tied to its strengths.
The flexibility that individualism gives us, for example, is
undermined by the delusions it encourages: that our
fates are not intertwined, that our neighbor's suffering
will not ultimately rub off on us. The traffic jam is a
symbol of what this illusory freedom does to us: a whole
lot of people pretending they're unrelated to one
another and hence frantic with frustration, unable to
move.
　　　　　　　　　　　　—SLATER (1976, p. 168)

Our culture, which until this century insisted that marital vows were
binding, has on a mass scale opened the door to divorce free of social
censure (O'Neil, 1967). Moreover, American society has recently developed new mores that set norms for facile separations. Since the 1960s,
the social climate now more or less expects that we be prepared to
move in and out of intimate unions without getting too "hung up"
about permanent attachments and moral issues; as Shakespeare noted,
"Vows are but breaths, and breath a vapor is" (*Love's Labour's Lost*, Act
IV, Scene I). Our society has now become conditioned to give as much
or more weight to an unhappy partner's need to leave a committed
union as compared with a forsaken mate's anguish about it. The very
bonds of attachment are now often called "possessive" or "addictive."
In order to permit the smooth functioning of a pairbonding–disbanding love cycle, the passions of enmeshment, especially jealousy and
revenge, must be contained so that anyone can leave a committed
relationship and launch fresh sexual–romantic ventures without fear of

1

dire repercussions from a distraught ex-mate or an outraged community.

The contemporary ideal of nontraumatic divorce has become part of a complex social ethos favoring principles of individualism over family commitments. New standards for "healthy" functioning now set tasks for all parties involved in a divorce. The partner who walks out must be able to disengage without being excessively impeded by lingering attachment, guilt, or dread of being on one's own. The mate who loses a still-wanted relationship must be able to readjust, without prolonged mourning or undue resentment. If the parting couple has children, the children too must not become "disturbed," because they still have their two loving (albeit separated) parents, plus access to mental health professionals skilled in helping such children adapt. All told, current views on marital separation presuppose that both adults and children can now be prepared by cognitive technologies that protect them from the shock of divorce, so that breakup need no longer be tragic or traumatic—*as long as the process is properly handled.*

In line with the new view, the conception of divorce itself has been transformed from private failure and public scandal to personal entitlement and civic right. Divorce is now held to fulfill a responsibility to one's self. Much of the popular and professional mental health literature of our day goes a fateful step further by seeking to stretch the psychic capacity of former spouses to take in stride the dissolution of their union. As we shall show, many prominent clinicians are making the case that it is normative for marriages to break up, that protracted or acrimonious separations are psychologically unhealthy, and that despite conflict, parting parents should care for their young in a harmonious manner. Thus, leaders in the mental health field have advanced proposals whereby we could all be "civilized" to the point where dysphoric reactions to breaches of monogamous claims, or even the claims themselves, are eliminated from the modern human psyche.

We are not anti-divorce. We recognize that unhappy marriages cannot be sustained in any productive sense by legal, social, or moral fiat. However, we strongly contest the fantastic promise that termination of committed unions can be so conducted as to occur without major distress for both participants. In contrast, we will contend that such distress bears witness to the importance of the relationship—that what the two spouses have lost was precious to them. We do not advocate pointless suffering, but we are respectful of the grieving function the distress of the parting couple serves. We believe that recovery is made more difficult when these feelings are suppressed rather than worked through.

Further, as psychologists, it is hard for us to see how this culture can dream of dispensing with unwanted, encumbering passion without dispensing with love itself. Even were it possible, human beings who could shed their attachments to mates (and so could take breakup in stride) would not be human. In ridding themselves of any deep involvements and their attendant passions, they would have no cause to love and could not love. Ultrarational organisms, such as Mr. Spock in *Star Trek*, are on a different phylogenetic plane than *Homo sapiens*— higher or lower on the scale depending on whether symbiotic emotions enhance or retard the survival of our species.

But what is really at issue here is not passion itself (which can never really be eradicated from human nature), but *values about passions*. Disputing the American credo that almost any problem can be "fixed," a psychological vision of "human nature" is less sanguine. People are neither so malleable nor so perfectible that conflict with significant others can be averted through sheer application of rationality or technical ingenuity. There are limitations to our ability to tolerate loss. Dependency needs—part of the basic psychological endowment of each of us—set a stamp on how well we love, whom we love, and how we cope with unrequited love. In accord with attachment theory, we assume that human life starts out with an infant held by its mother: this is a template for the innate social mechanism of object seeking. In childhood, bonding to a parent meets this need. In adulthood, attachment originally forged in the family of origin will be reinvested through involvement with a mate. For better or worse, the passions of object seeking are not altogether subject to control by reason or personal will power, nor do these passions subside automatically as soon as a relationship ends. When symbiotic emotions persist and thereby become alien to the self because of cultural pressure, they can be driven underground as "irrational" or even "shameful"—but when this happens, proscribed feelings may emerge elsewhere as symptoms of psychic disorder.

Most divorces occur today because of conflicts that would not have led to divorce only 30 to 40 years ago—a fact that in itself demonstrates the influence of culture on marriage. Yet contemporary culture is ambivalent, caught between receding "traditional" values and the antithetic "progressive" values that superseded them during the "Great Sexual Revolution" of the 1960s. This more recent moral outlook started as a protest against prior bourgeois thinking that stressed family obligation over romantic entitlement, social cohesion over self-actualization, and stability over change. Progressive revamping was a needed corrective for some of the hypocrisies of the past, especially the insistence on maintaining marriages intact even when a couple's love for each other had long since dissipated. We do not spend a lot of time attacking the old values, because their follies have been amply exposed by the social criticism that ushered in the new values. However, now that the pendulum has swung in the opposite direction, society must contend with different and perhaps more dangerous hypocrisies. We shall try to make the case that the progressive approach goes so far as to masquerade as a normative psychology, telling us how we *should* feel. Mostly it tells us what we *should not* feel, regarding passion as something on the order of a neurotic or antisocial impulse whenever symbiotic involvement causes problems for others. Thus, the partner who leaves is expected to disavow any guilt or lingering emotional investment, while the forsaken mate is pushed toward prompt recovery from rejection in love. In this pseudo-psychological climate, people end up wildly out of touch with their most profound affective experience. Certainly, society cannot turn back the clock, returning to til-death-do-us-part monogamous marriage to maintain an institutional structure for symbiotic attachment, but neither can our society trust divorce-on-demand as an institutionalized process to end unwieldy involvements as well as dispense with volatile reactions to object loss.

Our conclusion is that "just leaving" as a prescription for problems of a dissatisfied marital partner, and being "civilized" about breakup as a prescription for the forsaken partner, are simplistic standards. More realistic, it seems to us, is the position that unilateral termination of a committed partnership is innately painful, breeds hostile countermeasures on the part of the forsaken mate, and takes years for both parties to work through. If someone wants to leave badly enough, the price has to be paid. When a would-be dispassionate leaver denies or avoids this price, h/s* can only discover that going one's own way in an interdependent world causes others to do the same, leading inevitably to gridlock.

INDIVIDUAL PERSPECTIVE: EXISTENTIAL CHOICES AND THE PSYCHOLOGY OF REGRET

> [Errors to be addressed by a couple polarized over the issue of divorce:] type I error—marrying . . . for the wrong reasons; type II error—remaining married for the wrong reasons; type III error—divorcing . . . too hastily; type IV error—remarrying too quickly and for the wrong reasons.
> —CROSBY (1989, p. xix)

In this volume we examine the characterological clash between two protagonists in acrimonious divorce, and this was reflected even in our

---

*In order to avoid sexist language, we have used "h/s" for "he or she" and "h/h" for "his or her"; we trust the context will always make clear what is meant.

title search. We wanted a name for the book bespeaking the gravity of this subject matter and capturing the antithetical positions of the parties. When we asked for help, a flood of phone calls came from colleagues eager to contribute. It was not surprising that most of their suggestions projected the same polarization of attitudes usually seen in a parting couple. Titles from either camp were just too partisan to be acceptable.

During much of the composition of the book, we selected as our working title *The Wrong Mistake*. This paradoxical concept derives from a chess joke. A novice loudly bewailed the ruin of a seemingly winning position as the result of having made a move he now perceived was an error. A kibitzer standing at the table quite audibly commented to another onlooker, "He made the wrong mistake!" This parable best conveys our sense of the ironies so often seen in the course of separation, where the "wrong" moves are unknowable for a long time and even a seemingly winning position is fraught with risk.

One discovers only in the future where a given road leads, but one can never anticipate, except in fantasy, the end point of "the road not taken." To complicate matters further, there is the possibility that whatever choice is made at a given time, it may be that eventually "All roads lead to Rome." On his deathbed, psychoanalyst Hans Sachs (1948) wrote:

> [Our biography] is shown to us in the light of growing self-detachment, . . . not only as what it was, or ought to have been, or might have been, but also as what it was bound to be because we were just this sort of a human creature. We admit that it failed to be the fairy tale, heroic epic, or grand tragedy which we planned at different epochs, but we find it a truer expression of our personality than we ever thought. . . . Thus the forerunner of death brings the message of life. (p. 297)

Sachs was applying to himself the Freudian tenet that "character is destiny." This concept recognizes that choices are always the product of personality: no matter how a circumstance is resolved, for better or worse the imprint of one's nature will always be apparent. Standing at the heart of the psychoanalytic worldview, the thesis of characterological destiny emphasizes that only a different psychological makeup would allow us to make different choices, or to resolve the choices we do make in a different way. When all is said and done, a person leads not only the life unconsciously sought all along, but one for which responsibility must ultimately be taken.

It is against the backdrop of these metapsychological premises that we apply the concept of "the wrong mistake" to an examination of the decision to sever or save a committed union, each option constituting an engagement to unknown consequences. In making such a journey into one's future, it is a safe bet that most people in problematic marriages will at some point wonder whether they are trapped in a situation where staying seems to do no more than perpetuate an already dubious course of action, but leaving (especially if children are involved) could pose different and potentially even greater problems. Further, those estranged from their mates still face a decision about whether to stay apart or to reconcile, at times wondering whether the original commitment was an error, but then that separation might have been a worse one, and then again, that reconciliation could be the most egregious error of all! The dilemma now becomes one of deciding what standards or procedures will be useful at the crossroads in order to effect the decision of most benefit and least detriment. There is no "right" choice; the process of living always requires selection among contingencies of competing satisfaction. The plain fact is that we have but one delimited life to lead; Soren Kierkegaard (Mullen, 1981) pointed out a century ago that pursuit of potential experiences must be at the expense of an actual experience—namely, that of engagement.

In the end, *The Wrong Mistake* was relinquished in favor of *Splitting Up: Enmeshment and Estrangement in the Process of Divorce*, because it plainly represents the thematic dialectic inherent in nearly all unfriendly divorces. Further, "splitting up" suggests that the sundering of a committed union is characterized by a self-wrenching and inchoate division. Also, the new title attempts to resonate with the psychodynamic motif of self and object-splitting, so rife in divorce phenomena.

THE PERSPECTIVE OF CHANGE: DIVORCE AND THE WRONG MISTAKE

> This attitude—that nothing is easier than to love—has continued to be the prevalent idea about love in spite of the overwhelming evidence to the contrary. There is hardly an activity, any enterprise, which is started with such tremendous hopes and expectations, and yet, which fails so regularly, as love. If this were the case with any other activity, people would be eager to know the reasons for the failure, and to learn how one could do better—or they would give up the activity. Since the latter is impossible in the case of love, there seems to be only one adequate way to overcome the failure of love—to examine the reasons for . . . failure, and to proceed to study the meaning of love.
>
> —FROMM (1956, pp. 4–5)

In this book we seek to describe typical breakups of committed unions. To ward off possible misunderstanding, we do not restrict our discussion to couples who are legally married or formally divorced—we use the words "married" and "divorce" simply as generic terms. However, we do not address dating relationships which serve to explore the compatibility of a couple before commitment.

It is true that not every marriage breaks up when there are serious problems, but we limit our scope to only those relationships in which parting of the ways does occur. Not every breakup conforms to a pattern in which one mate wants to depart while the other seeks to save the union, but our focus is only on those couples whose breakup is unilaterally imposed by one partner over the protests of the other (which is, after all, the usual situation in divorce). And although not every unilaterally imposed breakup is acrimonious, the vast majority are, so we direct our attention accordingly. As for children, not every parental breakup is hard or unwelcome for them, but most are—hence, we review the plight of youngsters struggling to adapt to families in which there is turmoil over divorce.

If we have a bias, it is one based on clinical experience—to wit, that a couple plus their offspring comprise a *symbiotic system* in which a rift cannot occur without causing psychic wounds and substantial dislocation. Family members do not easily switch their loyalties and identifications, so that there are no real-life solutions whereby the undesirable sequelae of divorce can be manipulated out of social existence. It is almost inevitable for one or both parties to lose control of feelings at times and create difficulties, and this will obviously appear as the "mistake" of somebody in the separation process, but it is the wrong mistake to expect that self, mate, or children will accept the reality of breakup without unruly emotions.

People will continue to fall in and out of love. In the latter case, we recognize that the majority possess considerable resources for adaptation once they have worked through emotional detachment and readjustment. Thus, divorce need not be an occasion for prophecies of doom because most people eventually reorganize their lives after breakup. In addition, we acknowledge validity in the Buddhist Tao that "all compounded things are impermanent, and that all suffering in the world arises from our trying to cling to fixed forms—instead of accepting the world as it moves and changes." Because separation and divorce are manifestations of change, the pain of divorce "largely arises from trying to cling to something that has changed, not accepting the change, or not making other changes accruing from the separation" (Rice & Rice, 1986, p. 195). Yet, despite the fact that life obviously entails adaptation, we still insist that symbiotic forms of attachment are a deep and lasting aspect of the human condition, so adults and children will not go peacefully into that good night of divorce, even if they must.

What we advocate is a considered divorce—by this we mean that it should be recognized that several years are needed for the recovery of all involved, and before that happens many adverse and even tragic events can occur. Once this more or less harsh aspect of breakup is faced, we offer these specific messages to partners who are separating: first, if your committed union ends, expect that you and your mate will be pushed to an extreme by primitive emotions you cannot always master and are not apt to understand at the time; second, once you learn just what consequences are entailed, see whether you and your mate still wish to part; and, finally, if the two of you do part, as soon as you admit your own limitations, watch how the leaving changes.

~ I

The Couple in Separation

Introduction

Divorce is a process that starts long before a final decision is
reached. This process continues through the end of the
marriage, the separation, legal action, and resolutions a couple
must come to about their relationship to each other, their
children, and the larger society. . . . [But] not all separations end
in divorce. . . . The couple [may separate] in order to decide if
they actually want a divorce.
—PRICE AND McKENRY (1988, p. 36)

A love relationship seldom ends when it ends. Instead, the crisis of
breakup can galvanize a couple into the most passionate phase of their
history together. When a separation supervenes, they must sort out
whether to pursue independent destinies or whether to reconcile their
differences. The couple are likely to have many ardent encounters as
this fundamental question is resolved, with each encounter constituting
both a review of their disagreement about the basic relationship as well
as a reenactment of the breakup itself. However, the context of
separation offers fewer constraints to control tempestuous emotions
than existed in the working partnership, and thus acrimony can readily
get out of hand.

Because love relationships do not usually terminate by joint decision, one partner can generally be identified as taking the role of
"rejector" (Baumeister & Wotman, 1992)—that is, the partner who
initiates or instigates the breakup. This partner has the function of
standing forth in the relationship as *destroyer–creator,* unwilling to settle
for a "bad" marriage, directly or indirectly bringing about a dissolution
of the committed union, and serving as a change-agent. In juxtaposition, if there is one party in the role of rejector, there must correspondingly be someone who is "rejected"—the mate devastated by the very
idea of breakup who then struggles to save the union or, at least,

11

chastises the rejector for not letting it be saved. The function usually served by the rejected party within the couple system in crisis is that of *preserver of the family unit*. In this capacity, h/s upholds the inviolability of commitments, the need for stability, and the ongoing interdependence of the couple, even in estrangement. The two protagonists now form opposite sides of a separation tug-of-war. Despite some ambivalence, each maintains a respective course of action convinced that h/h goal represents what will prove, on balance, to be of ultimate benefit to self, mate, and (if such there be) children. This power struggle around breakup can endure for years and is sometimes waged with the utmost ruthlessness.

In typical separations, the rejected party is the carrier of connectedness for the dyad. H/s attempts through assiduous courting to bring the rejector back into the union, or metes out punishment to arrange that the rejector is unhappy apart, or both. These actions ensure that the relationship is not "over" as strategies are put into operation to make the separation untenable. In other words, when a rejector leaves, the rejected party keeps the union alive by dint of symbiotic behaviors that render it as hard as possible to be dismissed, forgotten, or replaced. Accordingly, in the drama of breakup, the "end" of a relationship is turned into an acute middle phase by the rejected party. Meanwhile, the rejector has not even risked losing the ex-mate by leaving, because h/s has the option to return at any time, and hence does not have to *now*. Thus, the true ending of a love relationship is not "breakup" per se, but the letting-go process that must eventually be accomplished in the minds of both partners, particularly by the rejected. If and when the latter disengages (no longer to be enmeshed through such passions as love, grief, jealousy, and revenge), the committed union expires—unless, as sometimes happens, the rejector reacts to that critical juncture by taking up the slack as the new carrier of connectedness and sues for reconciliation.

The foregoing describes the *interpersonal process* of separation, but does not address the *psychodynamics* that drive the principals into a closeness–distance conflict. When we begin dealing with the reason for breakup between mates who were once in love and pledged a committed union, the concept of *characterological match* must be introduced. These are two people who were mutually attracted by their differences, but at some later point could no longer tolerate these differences. Such polarity in respective personalities proves to be a critical factor in their initial commitment to each other as well as in subsequent breakup, including why one party in the marriage turns out to be a "rejector" and the other a "rejected."

Despite a characterological clash around separation, perhaps the acrimony of unilaterally imposed breakups could be avoided if relation-ships were either kept to the casual and transient or if people were prepared to expect and accept that even a committed union will someday end. This brings up the question, "Why can't they be civilized?" Chapter 1 argues that forgoing a lasting union in exchange for a cordial farewell is not a bargain everyone cares to strike. On the contrary, if ex-mates had a relationship of any depth, there will likely be no "friendly" divorce, for when love is dying, attachment needs persist. In addition, rage over the unmet needs the partner used to fulfill overwhelms both parties. Thus, each of the two protagonists undergo a transition in feelings toward the other, and the mutual love in perpetuity that the couple once sought—and thought they found—now tragically turns to animosity and hate. The change from loving a cherished mate to virtually adversarial status during the crisis of breakup represents a fateful and largely unavoidable shift. But no matter how bitter such acrimony may be, this transition from love to hate cannot conveniently be skipped as a mere whistle-stop on the express track to divorce.

Chapter 2 addresses the relationship system formed by the pair-bond prior to the breakup, the very nature of which may have made breakup inevitable. Chapter 3 is devoted to the psychology of the rejector—the person in this role may alternatively be seen as a culture-hero or a menace to family values. Chapter 4 considers the rejected, who must cope with the narcissistic injury of being forsaken but also come to grips with h/h own flaws, which may have led to rejection. Chapter 5 concerns the many ways in which a committed union can end; Each scenario features its own special advantages and drawbacks, but is always in keeping with the relationship system of the parting partners that existed beforehand and will remain in force for a long period afterward.

1

Why Can't They Be Civilized?

It may not start out bitterly. In fact, many a couple undoubtedly intend to be "very civilized" about the whole thing. And some may even manage to do so. But for most people, divorce is about as civilized as a battle with Attila the Hun.

—DE WOLF (1970, p. 27)

TRAUMATIC BREAKUP

The process of marital separation is one of the most stressful events that can occur in a lifetime. In particular, when one party to a committed union becomes dissatisfied and seeks to disband the relationship over the vehement protests of the other, separation strife is bound to ensue. In an atmosphere surcharged with tension, parting of the ways soon becomes a clash of wills. Each protagonist seeks the reciprocal's cooperation—either toward disengagement or toward reconciliation. Their breakup, like their marriage, requires conjoint resolution of contrasting, yet interlocking, needs.

Breakup itself breeds strife between ex-mates, but there are also sequelae to how a couple handles the process of coming apart. A marital crisis can bring out the best and worst behavior in the repertoire of each member of the pairbond; however, it is often the worst that becomes most salient in marital crisis. Actions driven by selfishness, jealousy, or revenge may obtrude into the couple's interactions during and after separation, and alternation of love and hate for one another may be expressed in ardent but confusing encounters. In the turmoil of breakup, separated people frequently exclaim in shock that

15

they never suspected that they could ever act in so primitive, destructive, or uncaring a manner.

Of course, not all breakups are hostile in nature; in some separations both partners operate with restraint and magnanimity. However, nonacrimonious separations generally work out that way because the two parties accept (with some inevitable sadness) that breakup is in their joint interest. In contrast, we draw attention to the much more common phenomenon in which breakup is instituted by one mate's *unilateral decision.* When separation is a matter of dispute between parting partners, they readily become polarized—locked into extreme positions such that conflictual issues are pursued to the bitter end. The ensuing strife in a contested rift, to be seen in financial, legal, child rearing, and other areas of common concern, mounts up to a monumental problem for the couple.

Does it have to be this way? Can't tragic outcomes be avoided if we become more astute in selecting the "right" mate and rapidly leaving the "wrong" mate? If our society has indeed taken the stigma out of divorce, can't people be acculturated to realize that love is time-limited so that if and when separation comes, it need not be so devastating? Does it make sense that in breakup two lovers who once found comfort and promise in each other's arms now savagely tear at each other? Why can't divorce be civilized?

THE DREAM OF DISPASSIONATE DEPARTURE

Taking trauma out of breakup has become crucial in a culture where the dominant sexual–romantic ethos now mandates committed unions be dissolved if either partner so desires. Once the culture is emancipated from traditional assumptions about the sanctity, permanence, and exclusivity of committed unions, the end of a conjugal partnership tends to be presented nowadays as an almost natural eventuality. Divorce can accordingly be treated as less serious than a personal cataclysm, although obviously not casual and entailing considerable readjustment. Analogous to Voltaire's quip that God shaped man's physiognomy so as to permit spectacles to be worn, our current ethos sets forth an assumption that the psychology of modern man is malleable enough to accommodate the exigencies of divorce. Instead of dealing with the psychic impact of breakup on people *as they are,* we will show that many contemporary social scientists and mental health professionals are overoptimistically suggesting that cognitive schemas associated with human attachment can be refashioned so as to make separation from a mate far less onerous.

In line with this trend, the mores of our time now direct that a love relationship should end as much as possible on a "civilized" note. The advantages of a properly conducted separation are seen as valuable enough nowadays to warrant preparations to leave or be left as soon as one takes up with a new mate. Many aspects of currently normative behavior in respect to love, commitment, and marriage (e.g., prenuptial agreements) can be seen as deriving from an implicit credo warning that one must not invest so much in a partner or a committed union as to be vulnerable to wrenching upset or strife if there is an eventual breakup. Granted that certain legal and personal precautions may make separation from a spouse less complex, but such measures cannot be touted as a way to prevent bitter acrimony and reduce the emotional pain of breakup.

In the new divorce-oriented society, it is no longer enough to be acclimated to the contingency that one's marital relationship could be summarily disbanded at any time. Influential voices in the culture have also legislated *psychological reactions* to breakup—imposing values detailing how one "should feel" in accordance with preconceptions posited in the name of "civilization." The operating premise here is that leave-taking can be so orchestrated as to prove relatively swift, decisive, and devoid of commotion. In addition, adverse moral judgments by either party can presumably be curtailed lest they lead to dangerous intolerance and interference. And if children are involved, their care can now theoretically be so structured, preferably through joint custody, as to shelter them from the potentially dire effects of their parents' divorce.

All in all, the new ethos mandates that "overwrought" emotions be held in check so that a spouse's decision to leave is viewed as a personal "right"—a right that ultimately benefits all. *This idyllic picture of how breakup "should" be conducted takes for granted that the process of separation is not inherently traumatic.* If there is trouble, it tends to be imputed to the unenlightened attitude of a protagonist. Proponents of the current ethos thus offer an enticing psychoeducational message: given appropriate preparation for breakup, "irrational" reactions can be shed so that one partner can "just leave" without undue procrastination and the counterpart will rapidly "adjust" in the aftermath of being left.

THE CASE FOR "CIVILIZED" DIVORCE

We will now examine arguments in favor of the feasibility of "civilized" divorce by looking at several published pieces of work that exemplify the main trends. In *The Second Time Around*, Westoff (1977) abhorred the bitterness of breakup. She asked why ex-spouses cannot be civil in their dealings, certainly where children are involved. Her prospectus for divorce was to have a friendship now supplant the failed marriage, or if that proved impossible, for the separated couple to cultivate a meticulous decorum:

> It would be better all around if current partners and ex-partners could, when necessary, be civilized with one another. If people did not expect marriage to be forever, if divorces were more automatic and less traumatic, then perhaps breaking up could be more painless, and a true friendship of former partners would be possible. (p. 49)

> [As for kids with two sets of parents], How sublime it would be if one family had a house by the sea and the other family had a house in the mountains. . . . How really convenient it could be to have four people whose brains can be picked . . . and who can be enjoyed separately and equally. (p. 75)

It is noteworthy that these statements were written in the conditional tense, pointing to a disparity between how actual families behave and Westoff's vision. She maintained that first marriages are essentially on-the-job training for an improved second marriage, when a more "mature" choice can be made. A reader may conclude that everybody should get divorced at least once! According to Westoff, children too are fortunate if their parents split up, remarry, and thus present them with double the number of their original set of parents—only provided that all concerned can get along. Alas, in real life, they usually cannot. The fly in this ointment is the vituperation between ex-spouses (as well as between current and old partners) in the crisscrossed family realignments. Such powerful resentments and rivalries cannot be wished out of existence as if negative reactions were superfluous impediments to the new order of civilized divorce and remarriage. Further, Westoff herself acknowledged that census data clearly showed a higher incidence of divorce in second marriages than in first marriages (Hacker, 1979; Cherlin, 1978) and even higher rates in third marriages (Monahan, 1958), so the "second time around" can hardly be described, as in the saying that inspired her book's title, as "always better." Despite steeper divorce rates for remarriage—a statistic that Glick (1994) has shown still holds—Westoff insisted that breakups could be nice for everyone, and if things were to go awry, it must be that someone was culpable of unsportsmanlike conduct.

A more sophisticated version of the same argument has recently been presented by Ahrons (1994) in *The Good Divorce*. She found in her research that half of divorces in which children are involved are characterized by lasting acrimony or total estrangement; but the other half—the "good divorces"—she considered to be instructive, if for no other reason than they show what can be accomplished if parents are enlightened. Ahrons contended that divorce can be amicable if the couple reconceptualize their "broken family" in more positive terms as a "binuclear family." She urged parting parents to accept the basic right of youngsters to interact with both elders, except in cases of abuse or neglect. She insisted that couples control their separation agreement by not letting lawyers escalate conflicts. As for the relationship between ex-spouses, she recommended that they slow down the process of disengagement to give the rejected party time to assimilate to change and she also advised that both parties need an opportunity to grieve, perhaps by such rituals as returning wedding rings or calling a conference of members of their social network to discuss the end of the marriage.

Although it is clear that Ahrons seeks to promote a collaborative postdivorce relationship between two people who once loved each other, from our skeptical viewpoint it is not obvious why forgoing hostile feelings in separation *ipso facto* amounts to a "good divorce." To be sure, "getting along" presents fewer problems for everyone. But Ahrons—a mental health professional—never examined whether such shifts might be counterproductive surface behavior, conceivably based in certain cases on such dubious motives as denial, covering-over of guilt, exploitative needs, or dependency. Moreover, Ahrons seems unduly concerned about preventing strife between the two parties *because it gives divorce such a bad name!* This sort of public relations approach has been criticized by Arbuthnot: "I . . . seriously doubt there is such a thing as a good divorce. It's making the best of a bad situation, but that's not a very catchy book title" (Edwards, 1995).

A highly popular version of the "civilized divorce" argument was presented in Peele and Brodsky's *Love and Addiction* (1975). They regarded distraught reactions to breakup as pathological behavior that demonstrates an "addiction." In their definition, love is non-needing, whereas "love addicts" cling to a partner to fulfill needs and thus feel bereft if that partner should leave; desperate for "a fix," they make scenes and commit vindictive acts. Peele and Brodsky asserted such "selfish" love is not love at all—a lover should be well-wishing and respectful of the partner's autonomy. In their opinion, feelings ought not change just because the other has departed—that would not be thinking of h/h welfare!

Thus it is possible for two people who have been the most intimate of friends suddenly to turn around and hate each other, because they have been thinking more of themselves than each other all along. Such betrayals are most striking when a lover breaks [an] established relationship in favor of a new partner who better satisfies his or her needs. Only where "love" is . . . self-serving . . . can an external accident destroy the feelings that two people supposedly have for each other. (p. 87)

In this conception of loving as transcending any personal needs, the partner who reacts with grief at being left shows an "addictive" love, while the partner who leaves for another mate but offers friendship afterward ostensibly manifests a "healthy" love. Thus, the "external accident" of a new partner should have no bearing on the feelings of ex-partners for each other; if they were truly "in love," they should continue to care about each other as before, except that one of them has opted to be with someone else! Peele and Brodsky depicted breakup of a committed relationship as a mere incident, upholding a model of attachment calling for enduring altruism instead of passionate involvement.

Still another approach to civilized divorce was presented by Albert Ellis (Bernard, 1986). In "rational-emotive therapy," Ellis therapeutically challenged certain "irrational" ideas, such as that *you are a failure if the marriage failed,* or that *you need this relationship in order to be happy and no other partner can make you as happy again.* For Ellis, it is a self-defeating overreaction to the loss of a loved one when a level of grief and anger exists that gets in the way of a new relationship. Thus, in rational-emotive therapy, a patient mourns briefly and then lays aside "irrational" attitudes generating self-defeating passions so as to be able to be happy soon again. Yet whatever its allure, Ellis's model is unacceptable to many clinicians:

Some people have criticized Ellis . . . for treating human problems superficially . . . [His critics] believe that . . . it is an affront to human dignity to understand human problems in terms of irrationality. [They also question] the overriding importance Ellis places on thinking and its influence over emotion. . . .

In response to these concerns . . . what Ellis is primarily concerned about is not whether [his theory] explains everything about problems in dating, mating, and separating, but the extent to which people's relationships are enhanced by learning to stay rational in the face of their own, and others', irrational behavior. (Bernard, 1986, pp. 124–125)

As we see it, the main problem with Ellis's approach is that the definition of what is "rational" is not always as plain to others as it appears to him. This self-declared clairvoyance then becomes for Ellis a license to tell his patients what to believe, how to feel, and when to recover. The wishful notion that "rational" ideas let one quickly overcome problems that arise from needs for attachment seems to us an irrationality in its own right.

As for exclusive sexual access to a partner in a committed union, Larry and Joan Constantine (1972) criticized the monogamous requirements of conventional marriage as *the* problem in marriage. They considered infidelity to be so "normal" that it need no longer be grounds for divorce, or even the cause of tension between mates; indeed, everybody can be "civilized" about a happenstance in which one of the mates is having an affair with the other's best friend:

> Traditionally, the eternal triangle was resolved either by breaking up the extramarital involvement or by divorce and remarriage. . . . Both alternatives can be especially painful to all parties. . . . An affair with the spouse's best friend is not, in any sense, resolved by either alternative. . . . If the parties can be brought to accept the concept of a triadic marriage as a legitimate and viable alternative, they have opened the possibility of a true resolution. (p. 550)

Here, "true resolution" by setting up a *ménage à trois* would require deconditioning the attitude of one of the marital partners (as well as the lover's) in order to be able to shed all prior sentiment of monogamous prerogatives. The appeal of this approach is that no one will be deprived of anything—the lovers get to keep their affair, and the spouse gets to keep marriage and friend. But what is amicable may not always be psychologically or morally acceptable. Do the Constantines view "civilized" as a standard whereby no one ever gets disturbed and contrary? If this is so, then "civilized" signifies a lack of standards, in effect, an acquiescent stance no matter what another does. What are marital arrangements worth if a couple stays together because no behavior on either side would be an intolerable violation of a commitment? Why is intolerance so intolerable to the Constantines?

We will review in following chapters many more contemporary writers of both professional and trade books who argue that breakups can be managed with civility and who have devised cognitive and other interventions to accomplish this. Their disavowal of unwanted passion will be ultimately justified on the grounds that culture shapes personality and can thereby decree the disappearance of "anachronistic" emotion. In lieu of such typical reactions in breakup as grief, guilt, and jealousy, they seek to impose a purely pragmatic outlook, urging both parties to move expeditiously from a defunct union to recovery with a new partner. In their eyes, a committed union is too inflexible an arrangement to be accepted literally—it stands in the way of individual liberty. In short, theorists from the "Why can't they be civilized?" school tend to demand that people be less emotional, and correspondingly more cerebral, about the loss of a mate. Their goal is more satisfying sexual–romantic lives for everyone, bringing better mental health.

A truly psychological view is quite different. Given that what is called "human nature" is a product not only of culture but also of biological–developmental factors, we doubt whether breakups can be simply transformed by new social fiat from passionate failures to dispassionate successes. What can be accomplished in the current cultural climate, however, is to drive still-lingering forms of attachment more or less underground through shame and denial. Such emotions will not be eliminated, because people have ineradicable needs for attachment from birth on, leading to the formation of love relationships in adulthood (Berman, 1988; Myers, 1989). At an intrapsychic level, a committed relationship psychologically means an implicit contract of mutual love in perpetuity. The perceived revocation of that contract arouses fury. Such fury does infinitely more justice to the significance a lost mate once had in a person's life than would a favorably disposed pragmatism or rationality. A "friendly divorce" is possible only when the love relationship was never or is no longer valued, when the leaving does not hurt. But if the relationship was precious, resistance and resentment will be experienced at its demise. For both parties, a sense of deprivation at the hands of the other will clamor for expression during the course of a separation, generating impulses to protest and punish. In other words, the two people will have a need to fight.

THE PSYCHOLOGICAL FUNCTIONS OF FIGHTING

Our reservations about any proposition affirming the viability of "friendly divorce" can be boiled down to an assessment of the tasks fulfilled by the fighting in a unilaterally imposed breakup.

In our estimation, fighting is needed first and foremost as a forum for the continued emotional enmeshment of the estranged couple— frequently, it is the only connection the ex-spouses can allow. One divorce therapist complained about his clients, "They fornicate in court instead of . . . in bed!" (Kressel & Deutsch, 1977, p. 420). Indeed, the parting couple can, and often do, fight over just about everything, and the dissension binds them together in a common enterprise without either having to admit how much they need the contact the strife concomitantly affords. Larson (1993) stated that "negative intimacy can keep the parties connected even while they act as though apart" (p. 100); she termed this fighting "connection conflict" and saw potential in it for reconciliation.

Second, the fighting is indispensable in order to determine whether reconciliation is indeed possible. The fights clarify positions and clear the air of pent-up grievances. Only thus can the couple see whether they can resolve their most recalcitrant problems.

Third, in terms of moving toward disengagement, the fighting fosters letting go if the couple cannot resolve their problems. The repetitive futility of their conflict is essential in demonstrating that the limitations of the relationship still exist, and perhaps always will exist.

Finally, the fighting arises out of the chilling realization by both partners (though not necessarily at the same time) that the other is no longer willing to meet demands as before; thus, each is now bitterly on h/h own in this world.

In sum, the fighting simultaneously emphasizes the divergence of the couple as they hurtle toward disengagement, binds them as they grope toward reconciliation, and forces them to recognize their existential separateness. Breakup occurs because there is an ongoing struggle within the dyad, it magnifies and clarifies that struggle, and it is often most honestly conducted as a struggle.

Quarrels during separation hardly provide a heartening example of intimacy, but the parting couple thereby bear witness to the fact of suffering for what they are losing. Their battles are at once extension and collapse of their prior partnership; they remain tied through fighting, but in separation their issues concern who each one really is and how nothing can be taken for granted any longer. To be sure, their discourse is marred by tendencies to lay blame, each holding the reciprocal responsible for h/h anguish and thus obscuring respective contributions to the problems of the union. The position of one or the other can turn malevolent and destructive, and the spouses as well as society must set limits on dangerous loss of control, but the passions that keep the conflict raging cannot be regulated. Attachment persists even when one loses the mate one wants, or when one leaves the mate one no longer wants in that role. Such behavior is not "sensible," but until we know how to install into human neurophysiology the emotional hardware needed to treat committed unions as plastic–disposable, so it must be.

THE TRANSFORMATION FROM LOVE TO HATE

The aggression that makes breakup "uncivilized" does not begin with separation. The roots can be traced back to the conflicts of the working marriage, and perhaps before then to whatever wounds were residual from childhood and early adulthood. Naturally, the loss of the committed partnership adds new fuel to the fires of any ancient or current grievances; it becomes indisputably the latest and greatest of all the series of failed expectations. A breakup touches to the core of each person's unconscious demands for love on h/h own conditions. To attribute the acerbity of separation to uncivilized conduct is like asserting that prisons produce crime or that asylums create insanity—the question is begged as to how one got into that particular predicament in the first place. People bring their problems with them into a relationship, experience hurt and disenchantment in the relationship, and in breakup find release for the accumulated complaints about how they have been cheated in life. The once-loved partner becomes the focal point for hatred as a withholder of comforts and supplies to which one feels there is a legitimate claim. For both participants, hatred is often an inherent part of the process of separation. However, it is not the cause of separation but is itself a result of the disappointed illusions and frustrated entitlement of the two parties.

Clifford Sager (Sager & Hunt, 1979) was the original exponent of the idea that every relationship is founded on a psychological "marriage contract." In entering a union, each protagonist usually does not realize that attempts to fill the reciprocal's needs and wishes is based on a covert assumption that one's own needs and wishes will also be fulfilled. Both partners, then, come into the relationship with an unverbalized subjective contract and have tacit expectations that it is a mutually acceptable one. When key aspects of the "contract" are not honored, a disappointed partner may react with depression and rage, ready to provoke marital discord just as though an actual agreement had been broken. Note that Sager was generalizing about all committed unions, not just those that end in breakup. He was pointing out that when internal expectations to be loved are inadequately met, the frustration may engender episodic anger and hatred toward the mate; marriage is thus a love–hate relationship. When a marriage disintegrates, a couple is likely to transition into a hate–love relationship, because their needs to be loved will now go unmet more than ever.

Charny (1972) offered a similar formulation with regard to love and hate in marriage. He contended that even the best of relationships must leave room for an inevitable interweaving of both positive and negative emotions toward the spouse:

> By yielding to the inevitable misery and anger in marriage, just as by yielding to the inevitability of storms as a feature of nature, or the inevitability of sickness in the biological history of man, or to the inevitability of death as the end point of all human life, we may have a somewhat greater opportunity to be happy, or at least to learn not to be thrown quite so much by our unhappiness as we are so long as we hold on to our current make-believe that *we* have gotten stuck with a dirty deal because we are miserable with our spouse. (p. 63)

Charny depicted human beings as ornery creatures—witness the cruelty within our historical record. Marriage cannot hope to be exempt; it is no antidote to human depravity, precisely because two human beings are involved. He went on to advance the sobering contention that because unhappiness is inextricably part of marriage, it is not by itself valid grounds for divorce. Through unhappiness, when we find that the mate on whom we would wish to depend cannot but fail us and drive us to virtual despair, we then have two stark choices: we can work on developing our own autonomy (more realistic expectations, self-sufficiency, etc.) or we can proceed to divorce the miscreant and seek the heralded "right" partner. According to Charny, divorce is not the growth-producing answer; it merely perpetuates or accelerates such damage as the couple are already inflicting on each other, whereas their unhappiness can be most profitably used as a stimulus to personal change leading to subsequent enrichment of the marriage. As can be seen, Charny's conception of marriage combined loving and hating right from the outset as the elemental "stuff" of which it is composed. Despite the married couple's inevitable thwarting of the expectations of one another, Charny proclaimed that mates maximize their chances for optimal development if they struggle nobly and ignobly to live together as best they can.

Charny's conclusions are mainly of academic interest because, in today's world, unhappy spouses will divorce. The weakness in Charny's presentation is, of course, that he does not consider when divorce is necessary and how it too can have growth-producing value in certain instances. But he is correct in stating that people will shortly discover in breakup that they still fight, that their problems are not over, and that love and hate are just different sides of the same coin—namely, *intimate involvement.* The opposite of love is not hate, but indifference. In marriage or divorce, fighting ceases only when mates no longer care about each other.

TWO STYLES OF FIGHTING:
CONNECTIVE VERSUS DISCONNECTIVE ANGER

Although both protagonists join in the combat around breakup, the manner in which each protagonist fights usually exemplifies their contrasting characterological approaches to the symbiotic claims imposed by the committed union. Indeed, it is just this underlying characterological clash, now clearly visible in breakup, that likely was primarily responsible for their marital discord.

We address these personality differences more fully in the next four chapters; for now we focus on one aspect of this pattern, using temporary terms for purposes of this chapter. In situations of strife, one partner tends to fight as a "disconnector" whereas the other's tendency is to fight as a "connector." In respect to the former, when a disconnector is angry, displeasure is vented via *distancing*—that is, by physical or emotional withdrawal or immersion in outside activities that exclude the mate. During the working marriage, demands from the mate for more involvement were often experienced as intolerably "suffocating," inducing movement away from the mate to discourage or even chastise such interference with autonomy by even more withdrawal. This defense was resorted to more and more as breakup approached, but distancing becomes even more pronounced in separation. Because disconnective anger is not always acknowledged as anger, at a conscious level the partner who distances may now feel that "I am merely living my life." Indeed this will be so, but also evident at times may be an unconscious need to inflict hurt on the ex-mate, expressed by refusing to consider the other's needs and making clear that in some crucial ways the other is no longer relevant. Thus, in breakup a disconnector institutes or intensifies behavior h/s regards as being within the purview of personal space and unrelated to the ex—and none of the latter's business to boot. However, these actions will also be transparently provocative and punitive. Although a disconnector often denies any such motivation, many of these actions will exemplify passive–aggressive hostility still carried over from the marriage. An illustration follows.

> A woman asked her husband to leave their home. After breakup they still had intense meetings to discuss outstanding financial and legal problems, as well as the reconciliation the husband very much wanted. As it happened, his birthday fell soon after separation, so she bought him a gift—a cookbook. When she presented it to him, she also chose to show him a manual on sexual technique she had purchased for herself while in the bookshop. He immediately became despondent.

This woman used his birthday to communicate two ideas—his gift conveyed that, as far as she was concerned, he must now fend for himself, and the casual reference to a gift for herself informed him of her intention to do sexually as she pleased without regard for his reactions.

Disconnective anger makes the statement that the bearer is intent on living an independent life and resists recognition of the meaning of any action that manifestly exacts a heavy toll from the still involved ex-mate. Such anger tends to be enacted in a nonchalant show of disengagement that drives the ex-mate into a crashing depression or a vitriolic frenzy. When the ex-mate demands a modicum of consideration, the disconnector can then retort that any criticism is an infringement of autonomy: the disconnector has a right to live h/h life, and the fault lies in the fact that the ex-mate still wants "control." As is apparent, the message is, "Let me alone. Your feelings are not my concern." Such a message does not have to be delivered verbally; it is most effective when it is transmitted in actions, without accompanying words.

Disconnected anger incites, but should not be taken to imply indifference to the ex-mate, as it might seem on first impression. To the contrary, on closer examination it may often reveal subtle and highly disguised symbiotic longings. The disconnector can count on the ex-mate to be goaded by h/h withdrawal of concern and can instigate a fight simply by going about h/h "private business," thereby relying on the other to object and try to interfere. In this vicarious fashion, the disconnector can ride the ex-mate's coattails into relationship-affirming contacts. Larson (1993) described the emotional nexus provided by such incitement in spite of an avowed intention to disengage, offering this insight from her work as a divorce mediator:

> When children are involved, . . . a less involved parent [often] becomes very . . . concerned with his or her "rights." [This assertion] is directed at the spouse and creates grounds to engage each other in connection conflict. In such cases . . . conflict is not about the children but about maintaining connection with the spouse. (pp. 100–101)

The disconnector is largely unaware of these dynamics because h/h thoughts are fastened chiefly on getting apart and managing separately. Hence, the disconnector's emotional ties to the ex-mate remain for the most part repressed, becoming discernible only when the ex-mate no longer reacts to disconnective anger with lectures, entreaties, or reprisals. Only when the ex-mate will not bridge the gap by refusing to be goaded into a fight does the disconnector finally have to realize that the other's struggle for relevance conserved some needed facet of their old linkage for both of them.

In brief, disconnective anger is not only a way to establish autonomy but is often a latent setup to check and see whether the other still cares, without any concomitant admission on the part of the disconnector. We now turn to the response of the reciprocal, which is very different in nature. The connector is someone who perhaps has long felt neglected by the disconnector, and certainly so in breakup, and tends to resort to a compensating "connective anger." In this contrasting but also characterologically driven style of fighting, dire measures to preserve the union are put into effect, designed to make the disconnector pay attention, offer amends, or suffer commensurately with suffering inflicted. To be effective, such actions must be drastic enough to compel the disconnector to stop treating the ex-mate as a person who has served a purpose and can now be consigned to peremptory dismissal. Connective anger is patently symbiotic: its thrust is to bring home the *mutual enmeshment* of the dyad, insisting that neither party can find happiness independently without taking into account the resultant impact on the reciprocal. The mechanism for enforcing this point about intertwined happiness is usually *disruption,* which represents a refusal to cooperate in making the disconnector's demands for autonomy viable. Willison's *Diary of a Divorced Mother* (1980) proudly asserts the would-be connector's right to make trouble:

> I'm happy that there wasn't a single "friendly" thing about my divorce—the words seems to me mutually exclusive, suitable for cataloguing next to "effortless exercise" and "painless torture." . . . If I entered into wedlock as a matter of great import, how could I be expected to pleasantly bid adieu to the man I agreed to cling to unto death? . . . So instead of a friendly divorce we had restraining orders, canceled bank accounts, accusations and counteraccusations. Now that it has all begun to dim into the memory bank of past horrors, I feel that, painful as it was at the time, it was the right way to sever our bond. (pp. 188–189)

As can be surmised, the connector regards disruptive tactics as warranted by the partner's plan to destroy the committed union. A so-called friendly divorce urged by the disconnector is met by frantic noncooperation designed to show that the relationship has value and cannot be dismantled without a struggle. Amity cannot be. Yet nothing the connector tries so hard to do seems able to force a disconnector into renewed approach behavior and, in fact, more likely has the effect of driving the disconnector into even more distancing. Thus, connective and disconnective angers, reflecting the disparate characterological styles of the two protagonists, interlock in a classic separation battle.

DIRTY TRICKS

Connective anger derives from frustrated symbiotic attachment and features a mixture of love and hate. It is the province of those who feel rejected in love, as seen in the following vignette.

> A woman dealt with her reactions toward her decamping partner in a vivid dream: She was driving her car with her partner beside her, but she was speeding so fast that she lost control and crashed into a tree. She was not injured, but her passenger mangled his leg, which later had to be amputated at the hospital. She then took care of him and he afterward said he was lucky to still be with her.

In a psychodynamic interpretation of this dream, we see hostility toward the partner that is largely repressed even in fantasy, inasmuch as she neither plotted nor applauded the accident. But the dream is still her own creation, representing latent wishes coming to the fore in symbolic form. In her scenario, the lover is injured through loss of a body part, but why the leg as the organ that is severed? It seems obvious that its loss would make it impossible for him to leave, and sets the stage as well for the woman to be his permanent caretaker. Moreover, she makes him unattractive to other women and, more subtly, castration impulses are expressed through imposing on him an amputation. Damaged self-esteem is also revealed, for the woman will now settle for an impaired version of the partner she once possessed whole. In this dream, the protagonist has manufactured in imagination a situation in which the errant lover cannot get away, is punished through mutilation for this wish, and must be forever grateful that she takes care of him anyway.

In connective anger, much of the hostility may be indulged on the level of hostile wishes, impulses, and dreams in which no real harm comes to the disconnector. However, as aggressive feelings increase in urgency, we encounter individuals for whom fantasies are not enough and vindictive needs along the lines of the dream described earlier must be fulfilled in action. One such case involved attorney Burton Pugach who hired a thug to throw acid in his ex-fiancée's face in order to disfigure her. She was blinded. After his release from prison, the pair reconciled (Stainback, 1976).

In fact, most connectors do not commit such extreme acts and their vengeful deeds usually fall short of being felonious in the legal sense. They are usually small-scale actions arrived at on the spur of the moment to bring discomfiture, material loss, or guilt to the ex-partner—and thereby afford some consolation to themselves. Weiss (1975) has mentioned typical behaviors:

> The husband or wife may attack each other's property. One woman unscrewed, unsoldered, and disconnected every element in her husband's hi-fi set; she then telephoned him to say that he could move the set to his apartment. Another woman cut one of her husband's suits into small pieces and put it down the incinerator. . . . A man formed the practice of calling his wife in the middle of the night to berate her; among other things, he blamed her for his insomnia. (p. 102)

If there are grounds for jealousy, the would-be connector will pointedly attack paraphernalia associated with h/h ex's new mate. One man ripped his wife's lover's name from her personal telephone directory—although he could not rip the number from her mind. Gifts, photographs, and objets d'art reminding the connector of the rival are decimated. A woman set out on a mission to sink the sailboat upon which her departed husband cruised about with his new girlfriend. Another woman threw a rock through her rival's window. Sometimes wicked attempts are made to sabotage the ex's new relationship. A woman managed to mention to the rival that it was not she but her husband who was delaying completion of the divorce papers. A man informed his children that their mother was seeing Mr. X, whom she planned to be the father to take his place. With tactics such as these, the connector tries to stir up mayhem in the disconnector's new life. Once the deeds are done, there is little risk of the perpetrator's being forgotten.

DeWolf (1970) is a writer with a particular relish for telling dirty trick divorce stories. She related how one separated woman took the car left for her, still registered in her husband's name, and made sure he received a batch of tickets in the mail each morning. Some women picketed their estranged husbands' places of business or turned them in to the Internal Revenue Service for tax evasion. One woman retained residence in her house while her ex-husband sent her monthly checks for the mortgage but never visited his "old" family. To his consternation, the man later discovered the mortgage went unpaid, because the money was used to lease an expensive town house for which he was

also liable, with foreclosure of his former house imminent. An especially ghoulish dirty trick reported by DeWolf is to call the local funeral
director with instructions to pick up a body: "What a shock *that* is to
the 'late lamented' when he or she answers the door" (p. 33)—of course,
the message conveyed here is: "Drop dead!" The following dirty trick
tale is a sample of DeWolf at her sarcastic best:

> One original soul who learned his estranged wife had acquired a
> boyfriend bided his time until he saw the man's car parked, unlocked,
> in front of his wife's house. He then got a friend in the cement business
> to dump a large load of cement through the car window. It hardened,
> naturally. What to do? You can't drive it. You can't tow it. You sort of
> have to leave it there as a monument. (p. 31)

DeWolf was an advocate in her day for easier divorce—the thrust
of her book was that dirty tricks were played to block divorce in order
to extract a more favorable financial settlement. We believe her
interpretation overemphasizes mercenary motivation and focuses too
narrowly on the divorce settlement rather than on the overriding
characterological struggle. However, where the settlement is concerned, we agree that often a spurned connector's anger is calculated—
not necessarily to achieve a good settlement but rather to ensure that
the disconnecting partner receives a bad settlement. In turn, the
disconnector frequently wants to use h/h money for a new life and
begrudges resources going to the ex-mate. As they fight over a separation agreement, legal conflicts over property division, alimony, and
child support simply become incorporated into their strife like everything else.

JUST WHAT IS "CIVILIZED" ANYWAY?

The couple dynamic in breakup is often depicted as "barbaric" because
there is so much unbridled malice emanating from two hitherto
"normal" people who were once in love. We have noted that the
preceding marriage already contained some more or less restrained
aspects of this rage, but separation imposes its own norms which now
sanction unrestrained callous disregard and vengeful reprisal. As alienation progresses, the respective ex-spouses cultivate philosophies of
personal survival that may mandate quashing the resistance of the
partner–adversary. In such cases, malevolence mounts to a pitch
comparable only to that seen in actual warfare. Even a couple's
children, their most sacred commonality, can be hurt in the cross fire.

The machinations of some couples locked in separation strife refute the illusion that psychologically intact folk in modern society do not vent (or even have) base emotional reactions.

The concept of "civilization" sets standards of conduct, but this need not necessarily be construed to require composed, genteel, and altruistic behavior at all times. Of course, such traits are socially desirable, and mankind has historically striven to evolve and inculcate *empathic identification* as the key to socialization (Mussen & Eisenberg-Berg, 1977). According to the Golden Rule, we learn to modulate natural pursuit of self-interest by sympathy and moral stricture based on picturing ourselves in the position of those with whom we interact. This not only sets a limit on how far we should go in manipulating others to our ends, but also helps to make understandable their reactions to our claims. Yet deportment along well-mannered, philanthropic lines would be inappropriate in the face of mistreatment from another, which instead calls for disapproval, protest, and finally countermeasures. The meaning of "civilization" is twisted when it mandates a forbearance that is tantamount to lack of conviction or emotional depth.

Moreover, emotions per se cannot be "civilized." They can be balanced by empathic considerations, but they exert formidable pressures on the ego in determining an individual's response to a situation. Sometimes emotions cause terrible internal conflict or take twisted turns, but they cannot be engineered out of the human psyche. It would be nice if we could all be unfailingly courteous and considerate, but such behavior is beyond our resources, as well as unbefitting when a serious offense has been inflicted by another. Even when one tries to "turn the other cheek," this can be viewed as a subtle way to retaliate by inflicting guilt on an oppressor rather than as a forgiving attitude.

From a mental health perspective, the limit of human tolerance is the crux of the following several cases. A woman, mother of two adolescents, was admitted for her first psychiatric hospitalization at the age of 39. Her husband visited solicitously every day. As background information was gathered, it was ascertained that she had an intact marriage, although—for a long time unknown to her—her husband had fathered another child in what was still an ongoing affair. One day shortly before she was hospitalized, the husband actually brought this youngster home to "meet" his wife—that is, to make her aware of the existence of this child and, therefore, of his relationship to the other woman. The wife responded calmly because she did not want to hurt the feelings of the child. She served milk and cookies. In this controlled manner, the bizarre visit went off without incident. That evening, she "inexplicably" (to quote her husband) slashed and threw out some furniture he had just purchased for the home and then went mute and immobile so that she had to be hospitalized. This wife was "civilized" until she cracked up.

The second case raises the issue of courtesy in separation. A jilted wife called her ex-husband's apartment, where he was living with the woman for whom he had left his family. This woman answered the telephone, said the man was not at home, and politely offered to take a message. The wife replied that she would not speak with her and started to hang up. The woman angrily stated that she thought it rude to refuse to relate to her on the phone inasmuch as she lived there. For the wife, that was just the problem! She hung up. When the wife told this story to her circle of friends afterward, they all chided her for her conduct toward the woman. Thus, we have a situation in which the woman extended courtesy and was met with rudeness; she could not comprehend why the wife was not civil. Yet the woman could hardly maintain that the jilted wife should treat her like any other person, as if this were an ordinary social interaction. Perhaps true civility in their exchange was for the woman not to insist on being addressed with proper decorum, but rather to recognize with compassion the pain she had caused another human being. The demand for "civilized" comportment from a jilted spouse by a rival is essentially narcissistic. Only when there is an egregious absence of empathy can automatic goodwill be expected, as if entitlement to courtesy and consideration still obtains from those whom one has seriously injured.

Although it may seem far afield from our topic, we believe the last case best answers the question of just what is "civilized." Psychiatrist Frantz Fanon worked in a state clinic during the revolution in Algeria against French colonial rule. A Third World person himself (a black man from Martinique), he became a secret member of the resistance movement. In his book, *The Wretched of the Earth* (pp. 267–270), Fanon tells about his work with a police officer who came to the clinic seeking treatment because he had begun battering his wife and children following his assignment from France to Algeria to augment police forces during the uprising. Fanon soon learned that his new patient's duty was "interrogation" (torture) of suspected Algerian insurgents. The policeman wanted his psychiatrist to help him gain control over his violent domestic eruptions, but he did not complain about his duty other than to say that he was very busy. Fanon pondered how to proceed and made an unusual decision from a therapeutic viewpoint: he declined to treat the patient. Countertransference issues may be assumed to have played a part in this decision (Fanon himself could have fallen into this man's hands if his underground activities were discovered), but he did not deal with this aspect in his writing. Rather, his focus was on ethics: the violence the policeman displaced from his professional duty to his family seemed to Fanon a way of getting in touch with his guilt, for it was only sadism *at home* that was unacceptable to the patient's conscience. Fanon's conclusion was that this man's unwanted symptom was the only piece of humanity remaining to him. To remove the symptom through psychiatric intervention was to enable the man to continue to perform his torture of prisoners with equanimity, thus rendering him a person who could be acclimated to monstrous misuse of his authority. Fanon also realized it was not within his power to remove the symptom unless the man first resigned his post, but the patient immediately rejected this recommendation. In our understanding of this fascinating but all-too-brief narrative by Fanon, if the police officer *had not* gone awry or lost control in some manner, he would already have been "uncivilized" beyond redemption. The logic here is that in dealing with hurtful human behavior, on whichever side of the interaction, emotional discord and irrational behavior may bespeak a higher level of mental health than does unreflective adaptation. Fanon seems to be saying that it is sometimes best to leave a psychiatric symptom untreated as a means to regain self-respect by not being callous enough to be well-adjusted in a heinous situation!

Contrary to Fanon's wisdom, social demands are now being made for cordiality and accommodation from those in separation trauma. Such demands amount to imposing denial of dysphoric passion, as if anguish and rage are inappropriate and in any case should never be vented. Like war, breakup is an inherently brutal business; many socially reprehensible actions and reactions may be unleashed, although these must be considered as occurring within a conflictual context where adults and children will unavoidably be hurt (Medved, 1989). In general, it is not necessarily "uncivilized" for human strife to occur, but what makes divorce seem so is the popular illusion that spouses should part company, at the minimum in a civil manner and at best on friendly terms. But this visionary position ignores the reality that, by definition, divorce is not about mutual consideration. Put simply, *good friends don't divorce.*

∾ 2

Dynamics of the Couple System

There is evidence that mates are selected for their ability to confirm attachment-related expectations, even if these expectations are negative.

—HAZAN AND SHAVER (1994a, p. 16)

THE SOCIOLOGY OF MATE SELECTION

Research has shown that choice of a mate does not occur at random. Sociologists long ago established that "birds of a feather flock together" (Burgess & Wallin, 1953) by investigating such extrinsic factors as "homogamy" (having similar backgrounds in ethnicity, class, religion, etc.) and "propinquity" (prospective mates cross paths by moving in the same social circles). Parents arrange for their children to encounter potential "appropriate" partners by choosing their neighborhood, school, and church, as well as by inculcating preference for someone from a socially-compatible "pool of eligibles" (Goode, 1959). Homogamy thereby promotes pairbonding affinities that maintain the structure and stratification of society. It should be noted that these findings apply only to marriage, not to casual sexual contacts or to affairs, which may readily occur outside social legitimacy.

But research along demographic lines cannot elucidate who in the pool of eligibles will be chosen as a marital–family partner. Another explanatory principle, more psychological in nature, must operate secondary to the social filtering of homogamy. Winch's (1958) concept of "need complementarity" rounds out a two-stage process in mate selection: after meeting, a couple is romantically compatible only if contrasting temperaments mesh, or "opposites attract." Winch's

35

hypothesis has received considerable empirical confirmation—for example, in the dominant–submissive match (Murstein, 1976) and in the obsessive–hysteric marriage (Bergner, 1977).

FAMILY SYSTEMS THEORY AND MATE SELECTION

In family therapy, systems theory postulates that interactions of a couple are governed by a homeostatic process in which change in one partner induces accommodations by the other in order to preserve an existing equilibrium (Jackson, 1965). Children too will be fitted into this schema, extending, complicating, and stressing the system, but the marriage goes on true to its own dynamics (Boszormenyi-Nagy & Framo, 1965). Family therapists also contend that mutually complementary patterns of defensive organization will generate striking overt trait differences, but that a couple are usually on about the same developmental level (Solomon, 1989). Thus, Napier and Whitaker (1978) stated that however opposite conjugal partners may seem in personality style, they are virtual "psychological twins" because both members of the dyad rely on the reciprocal to supply some "missing piece" of the self and the extent of problems in each are matched in some latent form by those of the other:

> They are truly mates. The partners may look very different psychologically. An alcoholic's wife, for example, may appear . . . very mature in comparison with the childish dependency and impulsiveness of her husband. But scratch the surface, and chances are she will reveal herself to be just as insecure . . . as he is; she, however, is someone who gets her feeling of security by taking care of someone else. She has carefully concealed her insecurity by playing the role of helper. (p. 117)

But valuable as the findings of sociological and family systems theory are, such general principles do not fully explain the vicissitudes of love over time. To account for variations in such patterns, a psychodynamic formulation is needed.

THE PSYCHODYNAMICS OF MATE SELECTION

Symbiosis

In psychoanalytic theory, a couple is more than the sum of its two partners. To be sure, two people conduct a real relationship, but this leaves out the psychological "contract" in the mind of each, largely unverbalized, about what devotion and services should be provided (Sager & Hunt, 1979). Such implicit expectations can give rise to serious marital problems; as Strean (1980) noted, "The fate of an unhappy marriage is decided long before the marriage occurs. The human psyche is formed in early childhood and the result is enshrined in the person without his conscious knowledge" (pp. 203–204). Yet even successful marriages are fraught with neurotic demands based on "infantile prototypes of behavior" (Arlow, 1980). The standard psychoanalytic view is that pairbonding typically begins with a "reunion fantasy" in which each mate sees in the other the undoing of mother–child separation (Bak, 1973; Bergmann, 1980; Kernberg, 1995). This premise can be traced to Freud, who said: "The sucking of the child at the breast of the mother [is] the model of every love relation. The finding of the object is indeed a re-finding" (Hitschmann, 1952, p. 423). Thus, falling in love is assumed to start with the magical belief that it is within the province of the new object to recreate the primal experience of total loving care. Even if childhood was unhappy, a romance may still seem a "rebirth," in that things should now come right because the partner is seen as the antithesis of the "bad" parent; Bergmann (1971) called this "counter-selection," but noting that such matches usually fail because cognizance is taken only of certain differences rather than the full personality of the mate.

In addition to reunion fantasy, forming a pairbond involves a sense of completion as a person. An enmeshed attachment begins from the moment two people first fall in love (Solomon, 1989), regarding their romance as a union capable of overcoming earthly obstacles to bliss together, surmounting prior personal problems, and transcending their limited individuality. In Western society, where the idea that romantic love is needed for marriage has now become culturally prescriptive (Beigel, 1951), falling in love endows the new pairbond with emotional cohesion. For each partner it is a symbiotic experience in which there is an unconscious basing of expectations, entitlement, and transcendence on the personage of the new partner as a valued extension of the self. Thus, romance always involves fusion with the object, or more precisely, with what the object represents. Bak (1973) quoted Kosztolany, a Hungarian poet, who wrote, "Sometimes I don't know whether you are I, or I am you," and later, "Thou, I" as a composite noun, as well as E. E. Cummings who expressed his ecstasy in a single line: "For love are in you am in i are in we" (p. 6). As seen in these literary examples, a lover incorporates the other into h/h conceptualization of a future that largely determines perceptions of who the other "is" and h/h function in that lover's life. This contract with the introjected mate in one's own psyche operates within the context of the actual marriage, and its fulfillment determines the perceived quality of the relationship. Inevitably, problems occur in regard to intimacy, for which two truly separate partners are required (Boesky, 1980).

Idealization

The phenomenon of transference brings us to love a *certain* somebody, not just anyone who fills a need. Because sought-after qualities are imputed to this person, a suitable love object tends to be idealized; Freudians cite George Bernard Shaw: "Being in love means greatly exaggerating the difference between one woman and another" (Hitschmann, 1952, p. 421). Kernberg (1995) has added that sexual aspects of the partner are also given special status in love relationships, so that "idealization of the body of the other . . . is an essential aspect of erotic desire" (p. 25). The psychoanalytic viewpoint is that idealization based on unconscious associations to an archetype of the "good" pre-oedipal mother constitutes the Cupid's arrow that goes to the heart of romantic love.

Nor are psychoanalysts the only ones to note the indispensable role of idealization in love relationships. Greenfield (1965), a sociologist, declared marriage would be too discouraging to try without romantic illusions. The French novelist Stendhal (1822–1957) called idealization of a love object "crystallization"—a term he coined after seeing a bough that had fallen into a salt mine be retrieved encrusted with iridescence. By analogy, Stendhal held that lovers impute luster to their more or less unattainable romantic objects until, through later familiarity, they realize that the perfection formerly seen was only in the eye of the beholder. Alfred Binet, inventor of the intelligence test, explained idealization in love as a generalized form of sexual fetishism: what is loved in the other is an aesthetically pleasing body part or trait, which is why extraordinary attractions and puzzling marriages occur, so that "a person with many assets [can be] mismated with someone quite lacking in merits" (Grant, 1976, p. 92). Recognizing idealization in love, but attacking it as a basis for marriage, the Catholic philosopher DeRougemont (1956) criticized romantic passion as a death instinct—a dissolution of the self by seeking immersion in the beatified object; although love can lead to marriage, it can also destroy marriage inasmuch as a wild pursuit of the romantic often occurs at the expense of social stability and spiritual values.

Like DeRougemont, psychoanalysis finds a downside to romantic idealization. Freud maintained that overvaluation of a love object had troubling implications for the future of the relationship. If love for the partner is rife with unconscious associations from the pre-oedipal and oedipal periods, then after initial ecstasy has subsided, the partner is bound to evoke negative feelings based not on h/h own flaws but on transferential projections toward a partner now invested with parental attributes, good and bad (Strean, 1980). Hence, conflicts more properly pertaining to childhood than to the actual partner have to be worked out now as they never were before.

In sum, a real relationship may be far less important to the genesis of romantic love than idealization based on projective associations. Both lovers bring this ideational baggage to the experience of being with the actual partner, and the aggregate is, from then on, the committed union each one has crafted. It follows that *there is no such thing as "a" marriage–there are only "his" and "her" marriages superimposed on a real relationship.*

Dependency Needs

What the professional literature now refers to as "attachment" largely coincides with what clinicians used to call "dependency needs," although the older term is less socially desirable and thus tends to be disavowed by lovers as an aspect of emotional investment in a partner (Pam, Plutchik, & Conte, 1975). In psychoanalytic theory it is assumed that needs for dependency are formed in the mother–child dyad and transposed later to adult love relationships via transferential processes in which nurturing expectations are carried over to the present, as well as the impulse to repeat traumatic early experiences. Such impulses result in reenactment of these experiences with the current partner in futile attempts to repair previous ego damage (Kernberg, 1995). Kernberg added that through projective identification, "each partner tends to induce in the other the characteristics of the past oedipal and/or pre-oedipal object with whom he or she experienced conflicts" (p. 82), with the partner set up to comply, willingly or not cast in the role of a problematic parent. However, long before such induced collusion becomes a fixed feature of the relationship, mate selection is already based on the perceived availability of a partner to play h/h assigned complementary role (Ottenheimer, 1968). In sum, psychoanalytic doctrine holds that dependency needs determine mate selection along collusive lines of reciprocity, set up repetitions of childhood traumas, and entail transference-based conflicts with the providing/depriving love object. All told, dependency needs can both make and break a love relationship.

A lay exposition of such couple dynamics comes from Memmi (1979/1984), a French political scientist specializing in relations between imperialist countries and their colonies; in *Dependence,* he applied his knowledge of international affairs to close personal relationships. Memmi maintained that love cannot exist without dependence because "no one ever becomes completely adult" (p. 54) and "no one can ever be totally independent" (p. 151). Despite the cost to self-esteem, people tend to turn to a mate to satisfy areas where the self is incomplete or needy, with that mate seen as indispensable and irreplaceable.

Memmi noted that dependence is never a satisfactory or stable relationship over time, as the same feelings that initially bind two people may later drive them apart. This can occur because once someone has been chosen as a potential provider, h/s is expected to be transformed into an actual one, but "there is always a margin between what is asked and what is offered, between the hopes, which are unlimited, and the response, which is necessarily limited" (p. 48). Hence, a greatly unbalanced relationship fails if the dependent's needs are unmet or h/s begins to resent the dependent role, or if the provider feels drained over time, so that the mates eventually constitute—in his eloquent phrase—an "inharmonious duet."

ATTACHMENT RESEARCH AND MATE SELECTION

Bowlby (1979) conducted research on maternal deprivation and described a sequence of three emotional reactions that typically follow separation of a child from its primary caretaker: protest, despair, and detachment. By regarding object-seeking behavior as an innate biological propensity, Bowlby broke with the Freudian view that adult relationships were attempts to recapture the early union with one's mother, instead coming to view attachment needs "as a pervasive and fundamental aspect of human motivation from birth to death. . . . The child's need for the mother is thus regarded as merely one manifestation, rather than the cause, of an underlying need for social attachment" (Baumeister & Wotman, 1992, p. 33).

In follow-up investigations of Bowlby's work, Ainsworth, Blehar, Waters, and Wall (1978) observed three distinct patterns of infant attachment to a caretaker: anxious–ambivalent (about 15% of cases), anxious–avoidant (about 25%), and secure (about 60%); Main and Solomon (1990) added disorganized–disoriented (less than 5%) as a fourth category. The process of secure attachment to a primary caretaker takes about 2 to 3 years and is characterized by the young child's demonstrated motivation to maintain proximity with (or resist separation from) the caretaker, viewing the caretaker as a safe haven for comfort and support and using the caretaker as a secure base from which to engage in exploratory behavior. Note that other than secure attachment, three of the patterns have pathological implications as future "internal working models" for relationships; however, research has indicated that some change is later possible under favorable environmental conditions (Hazan & Shaver, 1994a).

The next step in attachment research has been to determine whether different attachment styles of early life are extended into close adult relationships. Hazan and Shaver (1994a) considered pairbonding to be based on three "systems": choice of a partner starts with *sexual mating*, moves on to whether *caregiving* needs are met, and culminates in *attachment*, which is composed of the same behaviors as the infant–mother dyad—namely, proximity maintenance, safe haven, and secure base. In terms of subsequent course, after an intense initial attraction, a close relationship can enter into crisis because "unfortunately, people in the throes of romantic passion may give relatively little thought whether the people to whom they are attracted will make reliable long-term providers of care and support—which in time will come to dominate their feelings about the relationship" (p. 14). Once the attachment system is disrupted, the triadic sequence Bowlby observed in children occurs: protest, despair, and detachment. Nevertheless, even a disrupted union can survive in some form because of the prolonging attachment factor.

As for attachment styles, using questionnaires about current relationships and early childhood bonding experiences, Hazan and Shaver found that ability to sustain a love relationship seemed to follow earlier patterns. Thus, anxious–ambivalent children were generally found to become adults obsessively preoccupied with their partner's responsiveness and inclined to view their partners either as reluctant to commit or as inadequate caregivers; this group had a high rate of relationship dissolution, but even when involved in a relationship they tended to be anxious, lonely, and jealous. In contrast, avoidant children were generally found to develop into adults who preserved felt security by avoidance of intimate social contact and by compensatory engagement in activities. They tended to use work to reduce social interaction, were prone to engage in uncommitted sexual relations, used alcohol or other substances to reduce tension, manifested discomfort with self-disclosure, and were pessimistic about marriage. Like the anxious–ambivalent group, they too were liable to a high rate of relationship dissolution. These results indicated that the two childhood insecure-attachment groups were far less able to maintain an adult love relationship than those subjects who had been securely attached in childhood.

The continuity of early attachment styles into adult life was also demonstrated by Simpson (1990). In a survey of undergraduate dating couples, he found that those who had been securely attached in childhood had greater current relationship interdependence and satisfaction than either ambivalent or avoidant types. Further, if the relationship ended, the avoidant group (especially males) had significantly less postseparation distress than other attachment groups, which in itself may suggest that they could not attach.

Attachment research has also addressed need-complementarity in love relationships. Belsky and Cassidy (1994) cited one study in which, from a sample of 250 dating college students, "not a single dismissing–dismissing or preoccupied–preoccupied pairing occurred, whereas dismissing–preoccupied pairing occurred at a significantly disproportionate rate" (p. 28). They speculated that "partner appeal" rests on a need to have relational expectations validated:

> Thus, the dismissing person, whose devaluation of attachment and closeness derived from a history of rejection . . . fundamentally expects . . . rejection, which is exactly what he or she will receive from a partner with exaggerated needs for closeness when the dismissing individual fails to provide . . . the support desired. Similarly, what makes the dismissing individual appealing to the preoccupied person is that the dismissing individual virtually ensures that the preoccupied individual will end up feeling abandoned, thereby confirming exactly what the preoccupied individual has been led to expect on the basis of his or her past relationship experience. (pp. 28–29)

Dealing with criticism that current attachment literature is based on a theory about three (or maybe four) types of babies, Hazan and Shaver responded that it is a normative theory that takes account of individual differences. But major methodological limits of this research have been pointed out. Noller and Feeney (1994) were troubled by "preconceived typologies" drawn from infant studies and then extended to adult love relationships. Crowell and Waters (1994) argued that infant observational studies and adult questionnaires about childhood attachment are not equivalent; Hendrick and Hendrick (1994) complained that longitudinal data are sorely lacking; and Bartholomew (1994) wanted verification of complementary attachment patterns to be based on data gathered prior to pair-bonding. Lewis (1994) wondered how a study could determine an attachment "pattern" based only on the infant–mother dyad, ignoring significant others such as father, siblings, grandparents, and so forth, and Duck (1994) held that attachment theory ignored social structure. Weiss (1994) regarded the adult love experience as very different from an infant–mother bond and concluded that the main value of attachment theory in an adult setting is its account of reactions to marital breakup.

Granting the merit of many of these points, Hazan and Shaver (1994b) still thought that the attachment literature had succeeded in showing how dispositional factors (attachment style) interacted with contextual factors (the actual behavior of the partners) to determine the outcome of a close relationship. They asked, "Does anyone who has ever come into contact with human infants really believe that the way they are treated by people on whom they are utterly dependent for survival has no implications for their subsequent development or view of the world?" (p. 72)

FROM ROMANTIC TO CONJUGAL LOVE

In long-term love relationships, psychoanalytic theory posits change over time. In the initial phase of *romantic love,* there is fusion with an idealized object and a temporary denial of conflicts and ambivalences residual from childhood. Although romantic bonding is a type of "transference acting-out" (Masterson, 1981), it can still be productive and lead to a lasting committed relationship. As Kernberg (1995) stated:

> Unconsciously an equilibrium is established by means of which the partners complement each other's dominant pathogenic object relations of the past, and this tends to cement the relationship in new, unpredictable ways. Descriptively, we find that many couples in their intimacy interact in many small, "crazy" ways. This "private madness" . . . occurs in the context of a relationship that may well have been the most exciting and satisfactory and fulfilling one that both partners could dream of. (p. 83)

Kernberg found that he could not predict the outcome of a particular love relationship on the basis of psychopathology in character structure; sometimes different types of psychopathology led to a congenial match, but at other times were a source of incompatibility. Masterson (personal communication, 1995) concurred: "They don't necessarily have to be healthy—they just have to fit."

After the initial bonding, however, "if the selection of the spouse is based on the dominant wish to correct infantile traumata and is much less concerned with the reality qualities of the partner, the marriage is threatened" (Ottenheimer, 1968, p. 69). Previous problems are soon brought into the marriage and become issues between the couple; then the partner is likely to be seen as disappointing in certain respects because, as a separate person, h/s may not meet expectations, especially in regard to caretaking. The romantic idealization of the partner has paved a way into marriage, but once there, each partner has to come to grips with who h/s is and who the other person is. The success of the match now turns on the real relationship, because earlier estimations have by now been shown to be discordant with the actuality of the partner.

How do two people deal with the disillusionment of discovering that they have paired up with partners more different and difficult than they ever imagined? It is crucial that there be open and frank communication about the ensuing problems, with empathic sensitivity to what the other is feeling—which may be very much at variance with what one assumes the other to feel. Gottman (1994) correctly predicted marital breakup in 94% of a sample of married couples, basing his forecasts on whether each couple did the communicative work that is so essential to the real relationship in taking up the slack for failures in the wished-for idealization. If such essential interpersonal collaboration occurs, *conjugal love* founded on mutual solidarity and appreciation emerges from all the joys and hardships the couple have conjointly experienced as a functional unit. When conjugal love can compensate for the waning of romantic passion, the partners tend to handle individuation issues within the structure of the marriage, respecting boundaries and making accommodations for each other's needs and aspirations. In this fashion, the idealizing transference toward the mate will be modified in the course of living together to enable the marriage to remain cohesive through a series of compromises and adaptations.

However, if the real relationship proves to be unworkable because unacceptable character flaws have been brought to light in the partner, a mate may finally walk away after concluding that the marriage cannot go on once the dreams affixed to this partner are shattered. The validity of h/h transferential criteria for an ideal partner may even be questioned—it is often necessary to learn to love less blindly next time if one is to choose more wisely.

In contrast, in some cases the marriage will be sacrificed to preserve a partner's idealizing transference, avoiding the painful necessity of relinquishing cherished expectations and entitlements. A partner operating in this way assumes that relational problems can be solved by means of changing mates, progressively perceiving the current mate as an unappealing object to be shunted aside. The marital trouble here may have little to do with actual neglectful behavior by the partner; the trouble lies instead in excessive romantic demands that lead to a view of the partner as deficient. For anyone seeking to retain an idealizing transference at all costs, a good real relationship is not seen as a good-enough relationship, which inevitably makes it a bad relationship.

Thus, in marriages in which conjugal love provides a lasting cohesion, similar to the initial cohesion provided by romantic love, idealization does not so distort as to be hopelessly misaligned with the mate's actuality—the partner must be seen in the main as a discrete person, not as a mere instrument serving the emotional needs of the self. In troubled marriages, either the course of the real relationship has called into serious doubt aspects of the original idealizing transference, or the initial symbiotic attraction has blurred self–other boundaries to a point where the partner is perceived as having "betrayed" an implicit contract and thus must be replaced. When all is said and done, however, the idealizing transferences of both partners in any marriage are an omnipresent factor. What this means in practice is that each partner forever experiences conflict in regard to psychic integration of h/h mate, so that the sense of entitlement to sexual–romantic fulfillment has to be constantly weighed against dependent and interdependent needs more or less met by the mate. When both transferential longings and security needs are directed toward the same person, the conflict essentially resolves in a synthesis, although one must keep in mind that no mate ever perfectly fills both bills over time.

THE INHARMONIOUS DUET

In regard to committed unions that undergo marital crisis or breakup, many investigators have described in similar terms a polarity in management of distance regulation by each member of the dyad. A representative sampling of different wording for the same basic polarity is provided in the following chart:

Partner A	Partner B	Source
Pursuer	Distancer	Fogarty (1976)
Limerent	Non-limerent	Tennov (1979)
Partner	Uncoupling initiator	Vaughan (1986)
Would-be lover	Rejector	Baumeister and Wotman (1992)
Centripetal mate	Centrifugal mate	Jurich (1989)
Left	Leaver	Everett and Everett (1994)
Type I: Fear of abandonment	Type II: Fear of engulfment	Napier (1978)

This list combines two conceptual categories, one referring to *relative role* within a troubled relationship, the other concerning *personality dynamics*—in other words, mixing together state versus trait distinctions. Thus, whereas "leaver" describes the position of the partner who calls the relationship to a halt, this term applies to a situation in a given relationship and makes no reference to character structure. Such taxonomy has the advantage of being objectively descriptive and value neutral. It also allows for the fact that a partner who takes the leaver role in one relationship may reverse roles in another; indeed, Baumeister and Wotman (1992) have shown that most people have been on both sides of unrequited love equations: "Just as we all have had our hearts broken at one time or another, we are also all heartbreakers" (p. 6).

However, another conceptual schema appears on the list, one suggesting that psychological dimensions underlie breakup of a long-term committed union, no matter which partner takes the role of leaver. In this approach, the discrimination as to *who* leaves is seen as far less important than *why* someone leaves. Just which one walks out the door or puts the other out may have historical meaning for the couple but is essentially a technicality that does not necessarily indicate which partner was more committed to the marriage, is more devastated by breakup, or will be more intent on reconciliation. The relevant issue now becomes which mate is the *emotional* leaver and which is the *emotionally* left. Vaughan (1986) had to consider psychological factors in determining which partner is the true "initiator" of breakup, despite her wish to adhere strictly to a social role paradigm in her "uncoupling" research:

> Although partners sometimes act in ways that cause others to attribute the responsibility for separation to them (and, indeed, partners often lay this unwelcome burden at their own feet), they do not assume the role of initiator as I have defined it: the person who first begins a transition out of the relationship. The partner's actions are precipitated by the initiator's display of discontent and occur, for the most part, without benefit of a social transition similar to the initiator's, which would prepare the partner for the physical break. (p. 122)

Moreover, the positions of the two mates in breakup usually correlate with respective personality attributes. Anticipating recent developments in attachment theory, Napier's (1978) system of classifying personality variables in marriage presupposed that differences over distance regulation were the crux of conjugal tension, at times leading to divorce. Similar to the anxious–ambivalent attachment group, his Type I (fear of abandonment) partners were defined as those "who seek 'oneness' in marriage with little sense of conscious anxiety about loss of identity" (p. 6). Thus, maximum closeness with the partner is a prime relationship goal, with an emphasis on "we" rather than "I" experiences, and distance is experienced as threatening. Napier (1988) later added that most emotional pursuers are sexual pursuers as well.

In juxtaposition, similar to the anxious–avoidant attachment group, Napier's Type II (fear of engulfment) partners were defined as those who "strive for a sense of personal freedom and autonomy, and for a clear definition of the self-boundary within marriage" (p. 6). Such partners feel angry and defensive about perceived threats to outside control of their lives, with two principal dimensions to their sense of danger: fear of being contained or trapped within a relationship, and fear of being intruded upon or criticized by a needy and often disapproving spouse.

Napier contended that these two characterological styles unite to make many troubled marriages function the way they do. Although both spouses perceive that the chief source of "danger" in life comes from their partner, they still need each other to distill an identity. Further, they covertly meet ego-dystonic needs through being in precisely *this* marriage—on the Type I side, avoidance of intimacy by marrying a person leery of closeness, and on the Type II side, having dependency needs met by marrying a determined caretaker. Napier believed that shifts can occur in which positions are temporarily exchanged, but "the overt patterns regarding interpersonal distance which became evident early in the marriage are associated with the personality structures of the partners and *are* relatively stable" (p. 8). When a marital crisis occurs, Napier observed that it is usually the Type II partner who provokes it. He believed both patterns result from childhood experiences in the family of origin. Type I partners tend to come from families in which they were insecure, often because parental involvement was too unstable or they had been prematurely placed in a caretaking role as a condition of adult approval, whereas Type II partners tend to come from families in which they were overcontrolled or infantilized.

Based on attachment theory, Bartholomew (1990) investigated relationships in which avoidance of intimacy is a feature. She too saw the "working model" of attachment in children as a forerunner to patterns later repeated in marriage. Thus, she described how children who show "compulsive self-reliance" have a tendency to become emotionally detached adults who deny their dependency needs, whereas anxious–ambivalent children, resulting from parental inconsistency, tend to become adults enmeshed in their marriages. Bartholomew concluded that there are two main forms of avoidance of intimacy, quite similar to Napier's Type I and Type II: *fearful,* marked by a conscious desire for social contact, which is undermined by a sense of being undeserving of love and support; and *dismissing,* characterized by a defensive denial of attachment needs so as not to compromise autonomy.

Although Bartholomew did not address the pairbonding affinity of these two styles of avoidance of intimacy, Larson (1993), a divorce mediator, saw the matching of these two styles as typical of most of her client couples. However, Larson stressed their joint struggle for a solution rather than their antithetical attachment styles. Within her frame, divorce is part of a closeness–distance cycle, in which extreme acts force distance, eventually to be followed by some sort of rapprochement. Thus, the relationship becomes "an ongoing negotiation between two individuals for emotional closeness and distance, with emotional divorces occurring cyclically throughout the marriage. The question couples must work out is how close is too close (engulfing) and how far is so distant that there is no relationship?" (p. 98) Bartholomew held that mates can enter and leave a marriage as a way to deal with separation–individuation conflicts of childhood, noting that in some cases,

> the act of divorcing may be the only way the dependency or emotional oneness can be interrupted so that the individuals are out of the emotional field of the relationship and can experience a sense of their own autonomy and individuality . . . perhaps for the first time in their lives. Divorcing then may be said to represent the push for individuation that the family of origin never provided. (p. 99)

She concluded that once these issues are confronted, even the most acrimonious divorces have surprising reconciliation potential.

Despite some differences, the aforementioned three theorists arrive at consensus in regard to the notion that the closeness–distance drama in a divorcing couple is usually represented by a partner at either pole, but with each sharing in latent fashion what the other overtly expresses. In terms of complementary needs, they seem drawn to each other but later encounter severe interpersonal strife. Both mates tend to manifest equivalent problems in intimacy but—given their conflicting attachment styles—each may soon demonize the frustrating other. As Napier quipped, "People tend to marry their worst nightmares" (Solomon, 1989, p. 24). Respective attachment patterns are assumed to be formed in childhood and to be relatively enduring throughout life, but some modification can occur in the working partnership of the marital relationship.

CHARACTEROLOGICAL CLASH IN BREAKUPS
OF COMMITTED UNIONS

Although every breakup is *sui generis* and some will not fit one or another paradigm of stock characters clashing in divorce, the professional literature universally depicts a polarity in the closeness–distance struggle between parting partners that must be incorporated into any study of this subject. A descriptive nomenclature is needed that conveys each party's attachment style within the committed union. From now on, we will designate the mate who has typically manifested connective behavior in order to ward off fear of abandonment as a *symbiant,* and we will call a *countersymbiant* (Rachlin, Milton, & Pam, 1977) the partner who has chosen involvement with an enmeshing other but typically employs disconnective behavior to defend against engulfment. These terms are intended to be flexible enough to apply at the conceptual level of either "role" or "character." Thus, on the one hand, they may be used to denote respective roles in a current union, without regard to relative position in committed relationships at other times with other partners. For example, in a new pairbond between partners who in antecedent unions were both symbiants or both countersymbiants, it is relative who will now have which role should their second marriage become problematic.

At the same time, our terms are also meant to be suggestive of personality traits that influence choice of a partner, operate in the critical-distance regulation of a marriage, and determine disparate behaviors of parting partners in breakup. When pairbonds in a committed union enter into crisis at separation, it is standard for there to be a familiar but intensified struggle in regard to closeness–distance boundaries. This struggle tends to follow characterological lines, placing the two mates on opposite sides of the issue as to what form their future relationship should take. Thus, if one party goes to an extreme in one direction, the other party will go to an extreme in the opposite direction, so that in general *the more a symbiant is observed to be clinging and masochistic, the more a countersymbiant will be observed to be distancing and narcissistic.* Like the chicken-and-egg problem, it is never clear which aspect came first and who is reacting to whom (cartoon, p. 50). But it is often quite clear that the relatively enduring attachment styles of the two parties are now fully exposed. An emotional "match" that at one time brought the couple together will still continue apace for a long while after breakup. Consider a symbiant example: a spouse whose history involved desperately trying to preserve the marriage will very likely cleave to this same pattern in breakup, attempting to induce or coerce a return of the countersymbiant as a means to forestall the

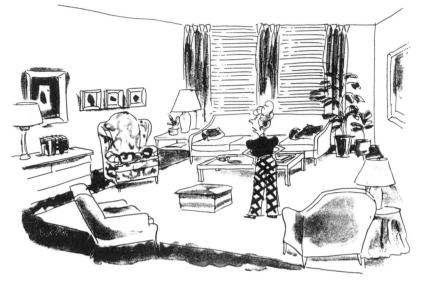

"Raymond! Stop being evasive!"

aloneness and separateness inherent in accepting that the marriage has ended. A countersymbiant example is a spouse who may have entered the union with implicit needs to be cared for, but resents the mate's dominance and encroachments on autonomy. As a needed defense, distancing is increasingly utilized, followed by rapprochement because h/s is not yet ready to give up the mate. Eventually, h/s leaves or is thrown out of the marriage, but the former expectation to be taken care of may still recur in separation, leading to sporadic contacts with the ex-mate for emotional or material supplies or both. These sorts of respective postseparation patterns exist because changing the domestic arrangement between two partners—from living together to living apart—does not alter their characters.

THE IRONIC FACTOR IN BREAKUP

Initially, a symbiant–countersymbiant match seems as tenable as any other, providing each partner with a suitable arena to compensate for problems in relating, because each one's excess on one side of the homeostatic intimacy balance expresses the latent needs of the other.

However, there is a point of imbalance that leads to tilt—this occurs when strife over closeness–distance boundaries becomes so intolerable for one of the partners that the marriage collapses. If this happens, the couple do not come apart any more accidentally than they came together, for their pairbonding already contained the seeds of sub-sequent estrangement; paradoxically, they will part for much the same reasons as they came together.

Dreikurs (1968) observed this perverse dynamic, giving many examples from his clinical practice: "A girl falls in love with an unselfish man and then complains he never thinks of himself and his family, only of others" and "A boy feels attracted to a girl who tells him what to do and is protective; but after a few years of marriage he cannot tolerate her dominance" (p. 493). He concluded that a partner may at first be considered kind and later weak, or seen as strong and then domineer-ing, depending on change in the perceiver. "We do not like a person for his virtues or dislike him for his faults. When we like him, we emphasize his good points, and when we reject him, we use his weaknesses as an excuse" (p. 493).

Aaron Beck, a cognitive therapist, also has described how the same qualities in a mate that were once exotically exciting can become, in marriage, annoyingly foreign. He cited how an easy-going manner can later be seen as "flakiness" or what was "bubbling enthusiasm" is now "overemotional and destructive" (Kayser, 1993, p. 33). These traits have become obnoxious—a strange, uncongenial way of being, so unworthy of the earlier appreciation of the partner. The couple watch the breakdown of their relationship in stunned horror, each believing it would never have happened if only the other were not a person h/s can hardly stand at times but more like the person h/s was supposed to be. "Why can't a woman be more like a man?" sighed Professor Higgins in *My Fair Lady,* the musical adaptation of Shaw's *Pygmalion* (1969).

Yet given these dynamics, a breakup can rarely be the end for such couples. The often underemphasized factor that constitutes the nub of the postseparation relationship is that a symbiant and countersymbiant need each other too much to readily disengage; they frequently stay enmeshed despite no longer being under one roof. Their ambivalence at ending represents a new attempt on their part at establishing a collusive compromise in regard to respective closeness–distance de-mands. During the separation tug-of-war that starts as soon as breakup is imminent and does not end until both partners let go, the symbiant attempts to reform and recapture the ex-partner (with whatever mis-givings), whereas the countersymbiant tries to break free of this control (with whatever trepidation). In this new–old struggle, each is well convinced that h/h course is for the betterment of both. It remains only to convince the other.

HOW THE PAIRBOND SYSTEM ALLOCATES RESPONSIBILITY

Beyond a characterological struggle between two protagonists, there is also a philosophic–moral clash as each justifies h/h own position in terms of abstract principles and values. Starting from different perspectives, each party develops a distinct explanation of why their committed union failed. Such divergence reflects the respective willingness of each partner to assume responsibility, taking upon the self some measure of guilt and assigning to the other some measure of blame. Because guilt and blame stand in inverse relation, and human nature being what it is, the two accounts are bound to interpret the same basic facts in disparate ways. Each is apt to frame a story of the breakup in a way protective of self-esteem by making the other the primary cause of the trouble.

Moreover, each partner speaks a different language in terms of moral outlook, espousing a point of view that both serves as self-vindication and expresses h/h personality. Gilligan (1982) drew a dichotomy between a justice-based and a care-based ethic that illustrates this difference in moral outlook. Justice-based, the countersymbiant sees the relationship as comprising two sovereign individuals with "rights," and in so doing ignores the couple's interdependence. Care-based, the symbiant holds that the marriage subsumes the individual identities of the members, and in so doing ignores that the parties are unique people. Given such polarity, there can be no clarifying dialogue about what went wrong. Instead, the bitterest moments in separation occur when the two protagonists are in the mood to pursue whose fault it all is, overlooking that they were—and still are—in a relationship of their mutual making.

To listen to countersymbiants who leave a marriage, the tale could be simply told: it was an unhappy relationship and so h/s left. This bare plot may then be embellished to the effect that h/s wanted to find an "identity," pursue "true love" with someone else, or had been "immature" or "weak" when h/s married. There may also be complaints about feeling uninvolved, infantilized, or suffocated within the union, prevented from leading a self-actualized life. Implicit in this presentation will be *externalization of responsibility, putting the onus on the mate (or "the marriage") for h/h personal unhappiness.* The mate is usually cast in a dominating role, setting the tone for a "bad" relationship, whereas the countersymbiant tends to appear as an innocent wayfarer, victimized while passing through the mate's domestic territory. Many countersymbiants thus evade responsibility for what went awry in the union, perhaps not seeing that they were in a bad relationship because they too were in it!

As for the symbiant, h/s learns with the passage of time to repudiate any scapegoat position taken to justify the other's dubious behavior. Indeed, a symbiant soon pays the countersymbiant back in the same coin: where fault is concerned, the countersymbiant is alleged to be devoid of those qualities necessary for commitment to a family unit, which is now seen as the main problem in the ruined marriage. The symbiant soon arrogates the function of conscience for the couple, charging that the countersymbiant has reneged on obligations and deserves castigation. In such fashion, the symbiant meets faultfinding with moralizing. The couple's interactions have degenerated into a "blamefest" in which both persons can now interrupt each other's litany of complaints with sarcastic or truculent rejoinders about their own perceived maltreatment.

For the countersymbiant, the strife of a blamefest is usually not nearly so upsetting as it is for the symbiant. Every fight merely recapitulates the fundamental issues of the original breakup and ends up validating anew the decision to separate. Moreover, the symbiant's sanctimonious diatribes help the countersymbiant to distance, because h/s can back up h/h stance vis-à-vis the breakup by playing the same trump card in every fight—that is, by leaving. The countersymbiant's absence is a far more forceful statement than anything the symbiant can say about why the partner should not have abandoned h/h in the past, or in the present fight.

The symbiant's lack of traction is visible in the spinning of argumentative wheels, as h/s futilely rails at the countersymbiant by "laying guilt trips." Although the symbiant's presentation of h/h case may be articulate and cogent, it is woefully short on behavioral clout and the message can easily be ignored. The moral censure—actually a plea that the countersymbiant apologize and reform—is the last hurrah of a symbiant; it is connective anger toward an unrequiting lover who just refuses to be the familiar, still fervently needed mate of yore. Thus, in the mutual onslaughts of a blamefest, the disputation of the symbiant may in some cases be superior, but (until the symbiant learns to let go) the distancing of the countersymbiant ultimately wins the debate.

OSCAR WILDE'S *DE PROFUNDIS*: A MODEL CASE OF CHARACTEROLOGICAL MATCH

We will now attempt to present in some detail an illustrative case that pulls together the themes of this chapter—namely, that breakup highlights the same interpersonal dynamics that originally drew the pair-bond together, and that arguments over the meaning and justification of breakup also reflect such personality differences.

As noted in the section on how the pairbond allocate their mutual responsibility for breakup, the universal starting point for a symbiant's moralizing is the lament that h/s has been supremely betrayed by the beloved—the tragedy is that the inestimable gift of love has been bestowed on an unworthy partner. Oscar Wilde's *De Profundis* (1905/1977) is a literary exemplification of this genre. Bak (1973) regarded the work as "one of the most heart-rending documents of love, portraying as it does . . . submission to the whim of the loved person [as well as a] tragic attempt to free love from ambivalence and to extinguish self-interest to the point of moral suicide" (p. 5). As an extreme example of symbiant–countersymbiant dynamics in a failed love relationship, *De Profundis* makes the characterological struggle stand out all the more clearly.

Wilde's tract was written from prison to his paramour, Lord Alfred Douglas. The text bitterly reproached Douglas for abuse of virtually unconditional love and for setting in train the events that culminated in Wilde's going to prison for 2 years on a morals charge after unsuccessfully bringing a libel suit against Douglas's father, the Marquis of Queensbury, for having publicly accused him of homosexual practices. Although the troubled Wilde–Douglas relationship was indeed a homosexual one, for our purposes it should be noted that its dynamics around attachment are similar to those encountered in equally troubled heterosexual unions.

De Profundis spells out in exhausting detail Wilde's case for how unappreciated and exploited he has been; it is the sort of recriminating recitation expressed by nearly every rejected lover:

> You have to go to London on business, but promise to return in the afternoon. In London, you meet a friend, and do not come back till late the next day, by which time I am in a terrible fever, and the doctor finds I have caught the influenza from you [that I just nursed you through]. . . . Saturday night, you have left me completely unattended and alone since morning, I asked you to come back after dinner. . . . I wait until eleven o'clock and you never appear. . . . At three in the morning, unable to sleep . . . I found you [downstairs]. . . . You accused me of selfishness in expecting you to be with me when I was ill, of standing between you and your amusements. . . . I went back upstairs in disgust. (pp. 114–115)

And what is the windup of Wilde's grievance that he watched over his partner when sick but was neglected himself when sick? On the morning after the aforementioned incident, he confronted Lord Douglas: "[I wanted to hear] what excuses you had to make, and in what way you were going to ask for the forgiveness that you knew in your heart was invariably waiting for you, no matter what you did; your absolute trust that I would always forgive you being the thing in you that I always liked best, perhaps the best thing in you to like!" (p. 115). This is an utterly revealing pronouncement on the part of the long-suffering and much put-upon Oscar Wilde. By the ritual of absolving Lord Douglas at the first sign of conscience or compassion, he was thereby sanctioning his own torment. For all his complaints and exhortations, Wilde keenly looked forward to "making up" as soon as his partner had been chastised and was "remorseful." Of course, Wilde was implicitly inviting Douglas to manipulate him—even instructing him how to do it—which may be, in turn, a way of manipulating Douglas to preserve the relationship as it existed. Theirs was a highly collusive system.

Lord Douglas's reply in the morning-after scene was equally informative: "When you are not on your pedestal, you are not interesting. The next time you are ill, I shall go away at once!" (p. 117) Douglas refused to feel guilt or pity and retreated as soon as any emotional demands were directed his way. Even Wilde's most valid criticisms had negligible impact, because Douglas was impervious to the sermons of a half-stern, half-indulgent moralist. Flagrant maltreatment by his partner did not make Wilde do the necessary: set limits that the lover must honor or else forfeit a continued relationship. Instead, Wilde rushed in to scold Douglas, smooth things over, and pardon his faults. He had placed his life at the disposal of a coddled Douglas and was doubtless insufficiently self-protective in their dealings, which ultimately caused both his romantic and legal downfall.

The conclusion of *De Profundis* epitomizes overinvolvement with the beloved at the expense of self: "You came to me to learn the pleasure of life and the pleasure of art. Perhaps I am chosen to teach you something much more wonderful—the meaning of sorrow and its beauty" (pp. 210–211). As if transcending his own ego, Wilde presented his personal suffering as a work of art; in beholding this aesthetic grief, Douglas must at last feel guilty for what he had wrought. Thus, despite manifold reasons to dismiss his lover, Wilde committed "moral suicide" by looking upon his plight as an object lesson to elevate and transfigure the character of his paramour. We can surmise that Wilde's unconscious needs were being fulfilled in this relationship through the following sequence: devotion and sacrifice on behalf of an adored love object, abuse of this love by the profligate partner, efforts to show the young aristocrat the error of his ways, passionate reunions in which past sins were absolved, each amnesty leading to a replay of the cycle, and the final betrayal and martyrdom of the great artist, leading to a prison-enforced estrangement. Surely this was a masochistic love presented as altruism, but revealing an immense, blind grandiosity.

In contrast to the emphasis on "giving" claimed by Wilde, his counterpart in the relationship, Lord Douglas, was widely known to his contemporaries as fickle, unfaithful, hedonistic, amoral, and opportunistic. Nevertheless, despite selfish exploitation of anyone to whom he had access, Douglas could always come back to Wilde assured that a few words of solace, or intimations of improvement, would suffice to pull his caretaker right back into his customary role. He respected his mentor–lover when the latter was providing, but only then, for he did not want to be bothered whenever Wilde's neediness led to insistence that Douglas curtail his activities and attend instead to his partner. Wilde appeared to exist for Douglas insofar as he supplied Douglas's wants, but Wilde's demands for reciprocity were regarded as impositions to be refused. He seemed even to resent his partner for *having* problems. For Douglas, Wilde should ideally have been an all-sufficient parental figure—so strong as to have no needs of his own.

The match was exact. The older man wanted to be a selfless caretaker whose happiness consisted in cultivating the well-being of his beloved, but there was also a powerful need to control and transform his partner. Meanwhile, the younger man did want to be educated, pampered, and sheltered by Wilde. Yet the interlocking system constructed by the two lovers had an insidious time bomb ticking toward breakup, though even then each party still played the same role as before. Thus, the incarcerated Wilde persisted in moralizing to his wayward partner, dedicating his own disgrace to the edification of Douglas, who thus became both cause and beneficiary of Wilde's tribulations. In this fashion, the beloved Douglas remained central in Wilde's life, Wilde never could extricate himself from this fascination, and it is apparent that Wilde never ceased to love his fantasy of the redeemed Douglas, but not Douglas himself. From jail, his reproach to Douglas was, "How could you let this love die?" as if the real Douglas was forcing Wilde to kill off the internalized Douglas in his mind. Here is a perfect instance of a symbiant who pursues a flesh-and-blood person but in reality is chasing the illusory lover of his dreams. In addition, by choosing a man like Douglas as a mate, the distancing underside of Wilde's dynamics is seen in his fruitless attachment to a virtually phantom partner, indicating that his own problems with intimacy were equivalent to those of Douglas.

As for Lord Douglas, he too continued ingrained patterns of behavior after separation. He soon sold off all his letters and memorabilia from Wilde to defray gambling expenses. He also tried to get hold of the original manuscript of *De Profundis* after the author's death (he argued it was written to and about him) in hope of extracting a profit from its sale! Further, he sued a biographer of Wilde's for libel, but the court found no misrepresentation that would be grounds to award damages. Even after his lover's death, it seems Douglas still expected Wilde to provide for him.

Technically, Wilde and Douglas never separated so much as they unconsciously contrived to be separated by the criminal justice apparatus. But Wilde was clearly the rejected partner of the two; he would not have left his mate and was, in effect, abandoned by Douglas in the workings of his arrest. In a review of the history of their union, it is clear that it was headed for calamity from the start because the same forces that drew them together (their respective ways of loving) would in the end drive them apart. Lord Douglas never did become the worthy recipient of Wilde's incessant tutelage, always remaining an unregenerate in search of new pleasures and people to pay for them. He did not see any necessity to be grateful for the services lavished upon him—Douglas thought of these as his due. But he could be scornful whenever Wilde, for some reason, failed to make provision. Through withholding, Lord Douglas could then readily extract from his lover far more than his share of loving, though it was never enough to satisfy his narcissistic needs.

Nor did Wilde ever become an ideal need supplier, despite his almost boundless masochism, for he occasionally would ask, "What about me?" At those times, Wilde would become disenchanted with his mate and, narcissistic in his own way, try to reform him back into the image of the admiring apprentice with whom he originally fell in love. As a psychological document, *De Profundis* speaks of the frustrations of a symbiotic love mandating that the mate must be the introject one needs, while not accepting the mate as an actual person. A clinician reviewing the situation could not possibly take Wilde's account of the affair at face value. It would be simplistic to diagnose Douglas as a person with a "character disorder" who took advantage of a too loving partner. This one-sided view would be biased, overlooking Wilde's "enabling" in the relationship and seeing only Douglas's "badness." As already mentioned, the behavior of each principal in the dyad is not a sheer response, but rather an input into their common union. Did not Wilde pick Douglas as a partner? Did he not invite or reward precisely those interactions he most bewailed? Could Wilde reality test his partner properly, and did he ever address Douglas's need to be accepted as himself, not as the "raw material" of the Lord Douglas Wilde envisioned? Did Wilde have problems with intimacy to be blamed on Douglas—how could he not know on some level that he could never get close to him? Would Wilde have conducted himself differently were he to have reconciled with Douglas? And if he gave Douglas up, would his next love affair simply have repeated former folly?

In the following three chapters, we will take a closer look at the psychological workings of the two protagonists in the midst of the acrimony so often attending a marital breakup. We will start with the countersymbiant because, in Vaughan's (1986) definition, it is this partner who is the "initiator" of separation.

ᔐ 3

The Countersymbiant Partner

The Panther—Jardin des Plantes, Paris

His sight from ever gazing through the bars
Has grown so blunt that it sees nothing more.
It seems to him that thousands of bars are
Before him, and behind them nothing merely.

The easy motion of his supple stride,
Which turns about the very smallest circle,
Is like a dance of strength about a center
In which a mighty will stands stupefied. . . .
—RILKE (1903/1940, pp. 64–65)

COUNTERSYMBIOTIC ASPIRATIONS

Rilke's panther stares through the bars of his cage into a similar cage and beyond to other cages in the zoo. Enclosed in this world, what are the reveries of the panther? Does he impute some special promise to the adjoining cage, not realizing that if he were there he would simply be staring into his own cage? Does he recognize that every cage is congruent, and so be resigned to his cage? Were he able to prowl at will, the panther would discover that the zoo consists of a series of cages; padding through, he would conclude that the zoo itself is an extended cage. And beyond, does this panther have any idea that exit from the zoo, for which he yearns, risks placing him in a worse plight?

Rilke's panther is a metaphor for the quandary of aspiring to liberation. Realizable or not, the dream must be dreamt. So it is with a countersymbiant who feels trapped within an unhappy marriage and yearns to leave—h/s feels confined and ponders some way out in hope of achieving a more fulfilling existence. In a sense, what would happen next is unimportant, for escape would be a behavioral statement about present disillusion. In refusing to settle for what *is,* h/s remains faithful to an ideal of what a committed union *should be.* Because the marital partnership is judged to fall short of such ideals, getting out is regarded as a matter of integrity. It is a question of standing up for one's vision of life and love.

THE STIFLING MARRIAGE

At the point of instituting a breakup, the countersymbiant's relief, if not jubilation, is much less striking than the suffering of the forsaken symbiant. Yet the scope of the countersymbiant's sorrow over time may be comparable in that much of this grief was experienced *prior* to separation as h/s mourned the shattering of marital expectations, endured emotional isolation, and felt forced to decide on a coming breakup (Kayser, 1993). During this period, h/s has come to view existence within the marriage as a spiritual death. Nearly always, options are considered and reconsidered until, at last, it is clear that going on is just psychologically impossible. Yet, in order to leave, the countersymbiant has to violate solemn commitments, hurt spouse and children, deal with economic stress, submit to social disapproval, and adapt to changes in life style. These factors serve as inhibitors; they are apt to be onerous enough to paralyze any marital rupture before it starts or just as it starts. Marriages are not easy to leave. Kitson (1992) found that unhappy spouses took an average of 4 years to dissolve their unions, with a range between 1 and 29 years. In addition, the fear of being on one's own must be overcome (Lubetkin & Oumano, 1991). All told, leaving usually requires the impetus of an all-encompassing desperation. One woman said that to remain in her marriage was "to live without hope." Another complained that her desolation had be-come "too dangerous"—she departed only after an abortive suicide attempt. A man engaged in an affair said he could not go on "living a lie" and maintain any self-respect. Another man beat his wife in uncontrollable rages, finally walking out because he could not continue to resent "entrapment" in this manner.

In short, countersymbiants may feel susceptible to disastrous reactions or to sapping of essential vitality if they try to stay within the stifling marriage. A comment frequently heard in retrospect is that they do not know how they managed to carry on for as long as they did. Meanwhile, their symbiant spouses were often relatively contented within the very same marriage, perhaps only dimly aware of the disaffiliation of the partner with whom they had lived for years. For countersymbiants, such dissonance in itself confirms just how little the spouse noticed, understood, or really cared about them. Hence, countersymbiants experience the "love" of the spouse as a burden inasmuch as they have derived little happiness from it and yet are tied into the marriage by it. Moreover, a symbiant spouse—however complacent ordinarily—will work to save the relationship if any threat of dissolution appears, making departure still harder. The seeming contradiction between being loved by the symbiant and yet feeling unhappy and even deprived within the marriage is usually understood as follows: the unhappy partner does not feel loved for h/h "self" but rather for h/h "functions" within the dyad. There is a sense of "just being there"—a kind of human prop—to meet the needs and expectations of the symbiant, assigned to perform sex-role tasks that keep the marital relationship more or less on course. To the countersymbiant, it seems that the union is supposed to endure no matter how h/s feels.

Despite growing disaffection, a countersymbiant generally attempts many accommodations to stay in the relationship, only to be repeatedly thrown back into the same conflict. Even after what seems like "trying everything," the marriage may still feel like a living tomb, holding the unhappy partner captive to stultifying routines, as well as required to make great sacrifices at the expense of deferring personal needs. Eventually, a countersymbiant decides that leaving is the sole recourse. Breakup results from a despairing recognition that the present relationship is not, or never was, the romantic union into which h/s contracted. This account of the demise of a marriage is the experiential truth of nearly all partners who decide to dissolve a committed partnership.

THE PREDOMINANT COUNTERSYMBIANT TYPE: THE IDENTITY-SEEKING REJECTOR

In leaving a marriage, those who take the role of "rejector" will often assert that they have been shortchanged, taken for granted, or maltreated over many years. They tend to report feeling needed rather than loved by the spouse. Despite efforts to bring about change, they have concluded that the marriage cannot be very different from what it is. The resolve to leave only crystallizes after bitter comparisons are made between the life that is led and what could and should be once free of marital entanglement. Given this view, the one who ends the relationship maintains that such leaving is *reactive*: the spouse has prompted that fate and richly deserves it. The appellation "rejector" will not seem accurate or fair.

Although it may be true that the spouse contributed in many respects to the countersymbiant's unhappiness in the marriage, we nevertheless believe that the term "rejector" is appropriate when applied to a partner who *unilaterally and unconditionally* dissolves a committed union in order *to seek more satisfying new fortunes elsewhere*. Baumeister and Wotman (1992) also think "rejector" is an appropriate designation. They point out that although the term has been taken to imply "a kind of villain's role" (p. 48) because it describes someone so often viewed only through the unsympathetic eyes of a would-be lover, it is not inherently invidious. Moreover, a relative lack of popular literature also fosters stereotyping, so "the figure of the rejector remains an enigma" (p. 3).

The word "rejector" applies particularly well when departure occurs in the midst of an identity crisis in which separation from a mate is a necessary component of establishing a new life style. In such cases, breakup is needed because the marriage no longer fits in with the leaver's changing aspirations, personal entitlement, and self-image; disengagement must occur in order to shed the dependent "old" self (for whom the marriage may have been suitable) and make room for an autonomous "new" self (for whom more congenial opportunities will soon be—or are already—at hand). Accordingly, nothing the symbiant can now do will make any difference: breakup is not tied to a specific issue or to a definite fault of the mate, in which case separation could presumably be reversed were the symbiant to make adjustments. It is ironic that the symbiant mate, however devoted a spouse in the past, is now seen as an obstacle to loving and being loved, and even as an enemy for refusing to grant the opportunity to seek outside fulfillment.

We call this type of leaver, who departs more in the spirit of "liberation" than of "tragedy", an *identity-seeking rejector,* or more simply, a *rejector.* As we shall show, h/s is generally a countersymbiant by character—an emotional distancer—and markedly so during the crisis attendant to separation. As an example of such a psychological stance, consider the statement of a disaffiliated wife to her husband as she quit the marital therapy he insisted they needed to avert breakup: "There are just some private areas of me I just won't reveal to anyone. . . . That's the way I feel . . . and you'll have to accept it" (Martin, 1975, p. 98).

In contrast to the the identity-seeking rejector, we will discuss later in this chapter a vastly different pattern of leaving, which may involve the appearance of a person's being a rejector but is, in effect, a form of being rejected. We will show that this sort of leaver—whom we call an *involuntary rejector*—is typically a symbiant who finally chooses, in despair, to give up on a committed union in which there are major marital transgressions or other hurtful behaviors, while a countersymbiant partner—whom we call an *insidious provoker*—wants the relationship to remain as is, in effect driving the spouse out.

ANTECEDENTS TO BREAKUP:
THE CONFLICTED SELF AND THE DOUBLE LIFE

Rejection starts with an intrapsychic phase: a partner who has become disenchanted will initially keep such feelings secret, only later to be communicated to the mate. As Vaughan (1986) stated, "This secret is different from other secrets partners keep from each other [since it] is about the relationship. . . . Thus, uncoupling begins as a quiet, unilateral process" (p. 13). Vaughan pointed out that this sort of secret creates a power imbalance because it gives its owner control over the flow of information. In a problematic relationship, the secret area tends to grow, moving from a sense of marital alienation to the creation of a social world from which the mate is deliberately excluded and about which h/s knows little or nothing. As conjugal ties weaken owing to the bracketing out of a key dimension of the disaffiliated partner's life from the mate, the former prepares for separation, while the latter can at best only surmise what is happening and is unprepared for uncoupling. In the meantime, until the nascent rejector is prepared to leave, some kind of adaptation is needed to stay in the committed union for as long as h/s stays. In short, during that period when it seems necessary to still stay with the mate, coping patterns are evolved that will maintain the existing marriage and yet protect the secret domain.

In the most common form of such coping, a rejector establishes a double life in order to tolerate h/h conjugal situation, so that a private, nonmarried sector is created to balance the sacrifices made in the name of the marriage. *Outwardly,* the rejector is a member of a pairbond: h/s upholds the partnership and cooperates in the conduct of a family unit. In such fashion, the rejector behaves more or less as expected by the social network, reaping the rewards associated with this persona. *Inwardly,* however, the functional partner in a marriage presented to the world at large is just a facade: psychologically, the fact of being in this relationship is cause for resentment. From the rejector's point of view, emotional balance can be restored only by going beyond the confines of this marriage, via some activity inconsistent with its terms and thus to be furtively conducted, although perhaps at serious cost to moral integrity, peace of mind, or attention to duties. The evolution of such a compartmentalizing adaptation is an unmistakable sign of serious marital distress. On the one hand, the clandestine outside outlet expresses and compensates for emotional estrangement from the mate—in this segment of h/h life, a rejector is already divorced. On the other hand, concealing the alienation speaks to ambivalence around any dangerous impulse to abandon the marriage; the union can be preserved intact, provided that the nature and meaning of the outside pattern remains screened from the mate's awareness. The rejector's "other side" is reserved for sharing only with bosom buddies privy to the person behind the mask, receiving their tacit support for this sort of accommodation to a "bad" marriage. Still, the rejector must always return home to face the disapproving mate, fearing condemnation of h/h "bad" self were the mate to find out about the hidden facet. As can be seen, the rejector assumes that the mate will refuse to accept the compartmentalized pattern were it to be discovered. If and when that day of reckoning ever comes, this expectation about the mate's reaction may well prove accurate, although it can turn out to be more a projection of the rejector's own shame onto the anticipated attitude of the mate.

In the double life, conflicted personality traits are split: one side (the conventional, responsible, "public" self) is brought home to a somewhat feared mate, while the other side (the zestful, rebellious, "real" self) is given expression only outside the home. The clandestine side always has to do with some aspect of the self whose existence threatens the marriage's viability. Most often, the issue is *forbidden sexuality*. Such impulses may be dealt with by repeated casual, opportunistic contacts—for example, at the extreme, the "madonna–whore complex" wherein men with conflicts about sexuality look upon their wives (mothers of their children) as too "pure" to be sullied by their lustful needs and so take their sexual desires to prostitutes or "loose women" who can deal with this dark aspect of themselves (Lief, 1974). In contrast, forbidden sexuality may be expressed in an illicit affair, often passionate and long-term. Whatever its specific form, the surreptitious sexual liaisons of a double life are seen as incompatible with the image of married respectability the rejector wishes to cultivate. In psychodynamic terms, disconnective hostility to the mate is acted out via sexual transgressions; yet both the adultery and its concealment make it possible to cover over enough of the hostility to preserve the working marriage. The mate's compliance in the double life through gullibility, indifference, or even acquiescence, may make it seem evident to the rejector that the mate is as emotionally disengaged from the marriage as h/s is. Lack of discovery in itself, and certainly failure to do anything about known infidelity, becomes a post hoc rationalization for this behavior, which tends to obviate guilt. Nevertheless, the rejector is still vulnerable to racking guilt feelings. H/s is jeopardizing the intactness of the family unit, engaging in deception and hypocrisy, and violating ethical rules governing married life. Ultimately, the rejector becomes cognizant of both internal and external pressures to give up either the marriage or the double life, whether h/s does so or not.

If there is an intense extramarital affair, in most cases a rejector gets more flagrant in conducting it over time. From this we can infer a conscious or unconscious need to let the problems of the marriage come to the surface. It may even seem a mercy to be "caught" and thereby bring a long overdue crisis to a head. After a "dumb mistake," when the deceits of the past are finally exposed to a shocked mate, the rejector can craft the marital breach that was often "an underlying wish all along" (Vaughan, 1986, p. 91). Indeed, the rejector could already have made provisions that enable h/h to readily leave or be thrown out. However, with exposure of the double life, the rejector too can be in for a shock, having to admit desires not only to keep the marriage as is, but also to keep the double life as is. The rejector will then plead (stall) for time to give up an outside affair, or bargain for permission to conduct it on an open basis, or promise to give it up without ever intending to do so. But no matter what the rejector does, the transformational act of discovery lays bare the flaws of the union. Once the secret is out, the marriage can never be the same again.

The double life allows the best of two worlds. The rejector retains the benefits of the marriage as well as the freedom of the single state. But the price is high: guilt, a schismatic existence, and the self-concept of a duplicitous, conniving person. Although some rejectors profess virtually no remorse for deceit or deny that hardships are being imposed on their mates, it is more typical for them to experience acute discomfort concerning the strategy being used to survive. If the intrapsychic tension becomes too great, change is called for—and that may mean mobilization to leave the marriage.

AFTER BREAKUP: THE REJECTOR'S LOVE ENTITLEMENT QUEST

It's been done. In all probability, the leave-taking was not nice, definitive, or totally honest. But, at last, the dreaded scene has been consummated: the mate now knows the real situation, the announcement of breakup leads to irrevocable consequences, and—for better or worse—the rejector is out of the committed union.

In the period looming just ahead, the rejector has a new life to fashion, which is encapsulated in the motif Shakespeare described in *Love's Labour's Lost* (1598/1937): "Let us lose our oaths to find ourselves, Or else we lose ourselves to keep our oaths" (p. 208). However, this new identity, like the old one, often turns out to be, at least temporarily, a double life. The lesser component is the work of emotional disengagement from the former mate and disposing of the defunct marriage legally and otherwise. An aspect of this task that can cause a degree of shame has to do with dependency patterns the rejector still has not overcome, leading to sporadic episodes of returning to the ex for support, sex, or material wants. Meanwhile, the more engrossing theme in the rejector's immediate future is likely to be some enactment of what we have called the "love entitlement quest."

The love entitlement quest is the previously unattainable or forbidden objective on behalf of which the foregoing marriage was destroyed. It is most commonly expressed in the situation where the rejector has lined up, before breakup, a fresh relationship to supplant the repudiated marriage—a comparatively dreary former mate is exchanged for a revitalizing new one. In another variation, the rejector needs a lover as an emotional support to break free of the marriage but the new person is not seriously seen as a future mate, having instead the function of smoothing the way through an ordeal that cannot be faced alone. Other rejectors immediately pursue multiple sexual contacts following breakup, finally allowing themselves to gratify sexual impulses without having to account to anyone. There are also those who refrain from any third party involvement until their marriages are safely terminated. Their love entitlement quest resides in the conviction that an ardent new mate awaits once they have disposed of the encumbering spouse.

Breakup can also signal an opportunity to pursue other forms of passion, such as an artistic endeavor, a social–political cause, or a personal predilection that was hindered by the person's being committed to a mate. In short, with the marriage safely out of the way, during the course of a love entitlement quest the rejector will feel intoxicated by some lover, sexual pattern, or engagement that makes the previous existence seem stultifying in comparison.

In many instances the rejector leaves as a free spirit. To whatever extent h/s had previously been a stable and settled family person, in the act of breaking out of the family constellation the rejector may now throw caution to the winds and disregard practical considerations. Thus, financial limitations may no longer impede as before—the rejector can simply appropriate, misspend, or finagle money with which to start anew apart from the mate. Indeed, often the most reliable early sign of an impending move toward breakup is the handling of money; nascent rejectors frequently have episodes of impulsive expenditure, express great vexation at any restraints imposed by the mate, and argue for pleasure over budget. Before separation this attitude is probably an initial eruption of rage owing to felt deprivation by the mate; the rejector's response progressively hardens to: "If you don't give it to me, I must take it!" If such self-aggrandizement evolved within the context of strict fiscal discipline imposed by the mate, financial recklessness will surely increase once the person is out from under this control.

Likewise, geography may no longer be a limiting factor at the moment of separation—the rejector may trek off to any locale that holds romantic promise. Quite often the announcement of breakup occurs just prior to, during, or just after a sudden trip, which is used by the rejector as a *rite de passage* to wrench free of the relationship (Vaughan, 1989). Indeed, in the period just preceding separation, the rejector tends to evolve a telltale pattern of frenzied activity that not only acclimates the mate to absences without causing too much wonder, but also makes it possible to spend less time with the mate because the rejector no longer feels "at home" at home. Rejectors themselves, at the brink of formulating their decision to split, often speak of their lives as "crowded", "hectic", or "running," so that by the time a conjugal rift is precipitated, the art of how to be busy being busy has been mastered. However, after breakup, this same restlessness can readily translate into an unfettered wanderlust that temporarily reaches mammoth proportions.

As a free spirit, the rejector similarly appears to transcend pledges, obligations, position, reputation, pragmatics—all the elements that previously combined to connect that person to a circumscribed time and place. Having dared to emerge from h/h customary role as a married partner, the rejector has suddenly transformed into someone emancipated from previous identity, who now may cast away built-up equity earned by years of investment in work and family.

To illustrate how the love entitlement quest can be conducted when a rejector is a newly hatched free spirit, we present several vignettes. One gentleman gave up the practice of law, left wife and children, and sold off all property in order to join a commune, giving this new "family" all his remaining money. A mother of two suddenly flew to Europe and called her astonished husband from there to inform him that she would no longer function as "a beast of burden" for their family; she intended in future "to go it alone." A psychologist not only deserted his family without warning or forwarding address to go to another state in the company of a lover, but he also left in the lurch his caseload of patients who had no idea of what had become of their therapist.

Going to such extremes, these rejectors proclaimed in word and deed that it was time to live for themselves and exited in a manner that virtually precluded their ever being able to return. To be sure, such departures seemed irresponsible, foolish, and self-destructive to their social circle left behind. Thus, rejectors who go this far appear to burn their bridges to the former life in a determination to live for *now*, no matter what the ultimate cost.

MARITAL CRISIS OR IDENTITY CRISIS?

The rejector views h/h behavior, including some self-admitted follies and inconsistencies, as the outcome of a marital crisis that follows its own logic of desperation: it is not easy to get out of an unhappy marriage. In fact, *it is so hard that one may just have to ignore the problems and do it anyway*—the motif of the free spirit. The rejector worries that if h/s hesitates too long to make the break, some untoward event, even death, may intervene to prevent once and for all escape from marital incarceration.

Once the rejector leaves, the extent and pace of change can at times become totally overwhelming and disorganizing. It is more or less inevitable that the rejector—the change agent—now must face h/h own reactions to future shock. After breakup, h/s still tends to miss many of the solid, relatively serene aspects of the way of life that was renounced in order to rush into unknown terrain. The separation correspondingly takes on a driven quality, wherein the fearsomeness of each new experience living apart may impel a brief but reassuring visit back to the old situation.

The rejector often asserts that h/h turmoil, ambivalence, and trepidation are products of the demise of the marriage, fixating on the idea that h/s is only passing through a period of readjustment. Concomitantly, the mate is apt to be blamed for keeping the marital crisis going. But the rejector often suffers from tunnel vision. H/s is so intent on emerging sexual–romantic aspirations, so long throttled, neglected, and forbidden in a confining marriage, that scant attention may be paid to the possibility that a major psychic upheaval far exceeding a marital crisis is in process.

Note that in the rapid unfolding of a love entitlement quest, the rejector often puts h/h whole life up for revamping. There will certainly be a change in sexual partners or patterns, but attitudes toward parenting, career, leisure, values, and even sense of self are equally subject to psychological transformation. The key factor is that in the rejector's fantasy, h/s can finally do whatever h/s wants once the marriage is over: *that is why the marriage is over.* Although the actual faults of the mate definitely push the rejector toward leaving, the rejector departs at this point because h/s has been swamped by an intrapsychic tidal wave impacting adaptation at a critical moment in developmental history. Heretofore, the mate may have been appreciated, but after the rejector's internal shift, the mate stands in the way of unfinished business with a side of the self that until now has had to lay dormant.

There appears to be a link between the decision to leave a marriage and specific life phases; a female rejector may typically leave her marriage in her early 30s, whereas a male counterpart may do so in his 40s. Both sexes are often aware that waning youth influences the timing of their decision. They leave while they are still sexually competitive, or perhaps even at the height of their allure, so that a new mate can be attracted who would not have considered them before. The precipitation of the identity crisis may also have to do with a recognition that life is not forever; recovery from a dangerous illness or the sudden demise of a friend or relative is in some instances the trigger to this insight. Other common precipitants may be the acquisition of much higher status or wealth, or the death of a controlling parent. In any event, sometime at about the mid-life point, a vastly different conception of "me" comes into being that leads the rejector to pose hitherto unthinkable questions and reach daring answers. Self-fulfillment now takes on previously suppressed importance, encased as that person was in social roles and conventional thinking.

Sheehy (1976) described the developmental dynamics for women, whereby an adjustment fostered over many arduous years is in mid-life suddenly deemed inappropriate in the eyes of a "new" self:

> It is frightening to step onto the treacherous footbridge leading to the second half of life. [There is also] grieving to be done because an old self is dying. By taking in our suppressed and even unwanted parts, we prepare for . . . reintegration of an identity that is ours alone—not some artificial form put together to please the culture or our mates. . . . Women sense this inner cross-roads earlier than men. . . . The time pinch often prompts a woman to stop and take an all-points survey at age 35. Whatever options she has already played out, she feels a "my last chance" urgency to review those options she has set aside and those that aging and biology will close off in the *now foreseeable future.* For all her qualms and confusion about where to start looking for a new future, she usually enjoys an exhilaration of release. . . . There are so many firsts ahead. (p. 36)

As for the male, Mayer (1978) has sympathetically portrayed an equivalent crisis when a man in his 40s begins to question his commitments: "Forced to abandon some youthful dreams and illusions, the choices a man made earlier allowed him to live out certain parts of himself while others were excluded. Now these parts that were never fully used, that were ignored or repressed, begin to clamor for attention" (p. 36). Such unmet yearnings, which impel the mid-life male to break up his home (often for a relationship with a younger woman), are characterized by Mayer as the outcome of "growth" or "maturity." Whereas Sheehy pointed to a search for integrated identity as the driving force for mid-life change, Mayer asserted that healthy self-actualization is the primary motivation:

> It is only those over forty who really know who they are, what they want, and how to get it. . . . Maturity . . . means possessing the courage and confidence to redesign one's life, and one's marriage, to suit personal proclivities. Society be damned. (pp. 233–234)

Mayer's tone in this passage conveys the defiant mood of many mid-life males as they renounce the status quo ante and, refusing to settle, move toward an unsettled future. She placed the option of divorce within the context of an identity crisis in which "me" will finally get its due, after long sacrifice for the sake of "we." She imputed jettison of the marriage to normal development; the man's hard-earned "maturity" stands in contradistinction to the stunting conformity that remaining in the marriage may have represented.

But Mayer's viewpoint raises disquieting issues. Can a return to earlier dreams be held up as "maturity"—or is this regression? Is it self-actualization when one's life is peremptorily revamped to "suit personal proclivities"? And if "society be damned," what is the rejector's responsibility to wife and children? Such questions usher in consideration of characterological factors in an identity-seeking rejector's decision to dissolve a family unit and set out on h/h own version of a love entitlement quest.

CHARACTER ISSUES IN THE IDENTITY-SEEKING REJECTOR

We have seen that the rejector experiences unmet expectations as to what h/h marriage should be and that the mate may be left because dreams long deferred must at last be honored. In contrast to Mayer, who endorsed the rejector's self-proclaimed emancipation, Saul (1950) pointed to *excessive needs to be loved* as the cause of disillusionment and the disruption visited upon the family unit:

> Much of mankind's sufferings arise not from loving, but from infantile demands for love in some form. . . . Too strong needs to be loved [may] conflict with our cultural standards of self-reliant individualism [so that injured] self-esteem generates intense and unremitting rage [out of feelings of inferiority]. Rage is engendered by failure to satisfy excessive needs to be loved which are predestined to failure because the adult cannot satisfy needs which belong to childhood. (p. 412)

Note that where Mayer said "maturity," Saul said "infantile." In our view, both have a point. As noted in the previous chapter, the identity crisis of rejectors often emanates from a growing sense of having been unduly reliant on a mate for approval, direction, or support. They have been attracted to someone who willingly serves as a template for endowment with parental attributes, but eventually in this process rejectors have recoiled at their own self-images as "immature" or "submissive," regretting and rescinding their original involvement. Consider this passage from Martin (1975), whose wife explained why she left him:

> I think I had a poor relationship with Mother. She was a perfectionist. . . . [As a daughter] I could never satisfy her. If I did something well, Mother would say I could do it better. She never gave me affirmation. . . . What I think . . . is that I saw the same perfectionist in you and married you to get the affirmation from you that I never got from Mother. . . . Anyway, I think that a few years ago I began to say subconsciously, "Fuck you, Mother," and that's when we began to have trouble, or *I* began to have trouble. I didn't need, or wasn't getting affirmation from you either. I think I married you for the wrong reasons. (p. 167)

Thus, many rejectors who have "outgrown" their marriage show in breakup that they have developed a reaction formation to their own dependency traits. Given a perception that one had been "weak" by virtue of attachment needs, which then led to engulfment by a relatively "strong" caretaker, cultivation of a more acceptable self-image may impel a marital rupture, while the rebelled-against parentified mate becomes a displacement object who can now be dominated and punished (as one could not do with one's parents). But such denial of one's own dependency is hardly maturity. Soon after renouncing the security of the marriage, the rejector will find out just how integral these needs are, for one does not get rid of dependency by getting rid of the object on whom one depends! Many rejectors learn the limits of their ability to overcome dependency needs only after they push as far as they can on their own and see what happens. As for what will likely happen, we return to the metaphor of the panther: (1) From inside the marriage looking out, the rejector yearns to escape the marital cage; but (2) once outside the cage, h/s will find that in the effort to transcend personal limits, the universal need for secure attachment reemerges in some idiosyncratic form. In our view, maturity requires coming to terms with legitimate attachment needs, which sternly constrain how much autonomy one can optimally handle.

Another point is that where Mayer spoke of possessing courage and confidence to redesign one's sexual–romantic life, Saul spoke of hostility and cruelty, in that the rejector's focus is fixed not on what h/s has received from the mate, but on what h/s was supposed to receive—but did not. Saul argued that when a rejector refers to "love," h/s is really talking about "being loved," based on grandiose expectations and insatiable cravings. He also foresaw likely failure in mid-life striving for gratifications missed in young adulthood; such grasping for the past–future at the expense of present commitments only brings one back to the starting point—feeling unloved in a thwarting world. Although Saul did not express himself in diagnostic language, his position amounts to a clinical finding of narcissistic pathology in the rejector.

Such narcissistic tendencies are often most clearly seen in a rejector's postseparation relationship with the ex-mate. Until rejectors are sure they can survive on their own, most tend to rely on their ex-mates in certain respects, trying to retain the latter's emotional involvement after breakup. Although in many instances such exploitation is merely transient and situational, in other cases intractable narcissistic character traits are in operation that were manifested in long-standing egocentric behavior prior to the breakup and will persist indefinitely afterward. At this level of personality disorder, the rejector designates the still-needed but unwanted mate as "loved in some way." Such holding onto an ex well beyond the crisis of breakup appears to be based not on uncertainty about the wisdom of breakup, but rather on wanting a caretaking object to provide rescue should a new love disappoint, or to purvey material support, or to serve as a comfort station for emergency sexual–romantic supplies. Indeed, narcissistic rejectors may find it impossible to ever let the former mate disengage—instead, sporadic "dangling" and double messages may systematically extract security, services, and forgiveness from a still involved but otherwise abandoned mate. Thus, narcissistic rejectors expect forsaken mates to accept them as they now are, including the fact that they can no longer accept their mates as they are.

It can be difficult for a forsaken mate to know just what it is that a narcissistic rejector truly desires, so complex and ambiguous are the cues sent out. For example, a man told the "dominating" ex-wife he had left behind how unhappy he was with the woman for whom he had left her; he implored his ex to come to his new apartment, chase off the other woman, and take him "home." It seems this man wanted to use each woman in turn to save him from an overwhelming relationship with the other, without commitment to either. He clearly felt more secure when he set the two females to fight over him. In a second example, a mother of two put her husband out; she soon asked her estranged husband for several hundred dollars over and above the usual child support to pay for household expenses. He complied, hoping to improve chances for eventual reconciliation. The next week she announced she was going on a Caribbean trip with some friends— including the man with whom she was having an affair. The already jealous husband was irate, feeling she had asked for this money to underwrite a trip with his rival. She did not admit to having duped him, arguing instead that he should be relieved to hear that she paid her own way in lieu of having her lover pay. Vignettes such as these suggest that the ex-mate is still seen as a parental resource whose concern should be everlasting and unconditional. The rejector's dealings with an ex may well express a measure of residual attachment, but h/h motives at times can also readily revolve around grandiose expectations and selfish manipulations.

Another clinical sign of narcissistic traits in the identity-seeking rejector is difficulty with emotional reciprocation. The rejector feels engulfed by the mate in the working marriage, and certainly so at the time of breakup. Tennov (1979) noted that the word "suffocating" was repeatedly used by those who did not return the passions of their "limerent" (in love) partners. In general, she found that nonlimerents could not bear the claims made on them for frequent contact, exclusive sexuality, and intimacy; Tennov quoted a student's paper to present the nonlimerent's viewpoint:

> First, let us inquire whether the state of passion is objectively good or beautiful. The answer will be evident to anyone who has been an object of it ... [but did not] love in return. Nothing is more tedious or oppressive; for the one who has eyes for none but us has lost the world and, having nothing to talk about, can only repeat a handful of tiresome phrases ... because they are shorn of the medium in which our interests are engaged. From our situation within the spacious world,

the other's obsession appears hermetically sealed, a stifling closet. Moreover, it debilitates us, making us clumsy; for the eyes forever upon us make us hyperaware of our own simple acts—like walking—which we do best without thought. (Tennov, 1979, p. 137)

Tennov's nonlimerent respondents insisted on asserting their independence whenever a partner made emotional demands, but resumed the relationship as soon as things quieted down. Some of her nonlimerent subjects had acquired considerable expertise in fending off closeness, sometimes dealing with several fervent suitors at a time. One woman regarded the involvement of men she dated as an affront, complaining, "They would call and wonder what I was doing when I really had something to do that was important to me and had nothing to do with them. . . . They simply have to learn that if they want my companionship at all, they must let me breathe." Another woman added, about the men who had fallen in love with her, "They are always being 'hurt' and it's impossible to predict what will hurt them. I'll have a good time at a party only to be hit on the way home with something like, 'Why did you ignore me all evening?' Really, it's exasperating!" (p. 139). Granted that suitors can sometimes impose, or be oversensitive about a lapse of attention, or be paranoid about innocent solo activities, but these two women did not seem at all empathic to the feelings of the men they were dating. They seemed to want "private space" that left their suitors feeling neglected or mistrustful. Is it sheer coincidence they had chosen to be with men who were not easily put off and not with men as emotionally aloof as they were?

Although Tennov's cases concern premarital dating among undergraduates, one still gleans from her material how certain nonlimerents can stay snugly in a relationship so long as intimacy or commitment is not sought; when such demands are made, these nonlimerents hurriedly depart, usually puzzled as to why the partner would ruin an otherwise excellent match. Nonlimerents of this type receive a pledge of love, then proclaim it restrictive and participate in the relationship afterward only when expedient. Their attitude toward intimacy is contradictory: on one hand, the nonlimerents in question seek out limerent partners; on the other hand, the limerents' demands for mutual involvement are then seen as bothersome and a signal to distance. Such an inability to tolerate closeness, while setting up receipt of abundant emotional supplies from an ardently pursuing partner, seems to indicate in this group of young people a characterological predisposition toward rejectorhood. The proof of this pudding lies in how they will fare when—and if—they do make a sexual–romantic commitment.

OTHER TYPES OF BREAKUP

Not all breakups come about as a result of the situation in which an identity-seeking rejector opts to terminate the committed union despite the entreaties of an anguished mate. We differentiate two other modal configurations for breakup. First, there is *mutual rejection*, obtaining when a relationship is an unhappy one for both partners, and, for all practical purposes, it is incidental as to which one initiates the split. Hurt pride will probably be evident in the one who is technically "being left," but after grieving for a short while, h/s will realize that neither member of the pairbond has much interest in a protracted struggle to work things out. The history of such a marriage is usually stormy, and the wisest course seems to be giving up for the sake of both. Although sorrow always attends the ending of a significant relationship, separation is not subsequently viewed by the parties as particularly "tragic." The leave-taking is frequently done with a minimum of acrimony, with an aftermath that ordinarily involves little contact. To be sure, there are borderline cases in which one cannot be quite sure whether a breakup is authentically mutual or at the behest of one partner, but, in general, if such a distinction is made, it is academic.

Second, there is the complicated situation in which the leaver—an *involuntary rejector*—is equally or more in pain about the breakup than the partner who ostensibly wants the union to be maintained. Here, the "left" partner has engaged in behavior that renders it impossible for the mate to remain in the committed union despite every intention to do so, thereby impelling that mate toward "rejecting." The mate of an alcoholic can represent a model of this type of reactive rejection: the person who formally leaves the marriage and files for divorce does so with a sense of having been reluctantly wedged out by an intractable partner who gave no real choice. A key feature of this type of excruciating departure by an involuntary rejector is that h/s would return if there were genuine change in the mate; the involuntary rejector moves firmly and decisively away only when convinced that the mate is unable or unwilling to alter destructive patterns. In the case of a male alcoholic, he will not want to lose his wife, but as a rule he will not stop drinking either, and finally his wife will conclude that he values drinking more than the marriage. *She* feels rejected—her marriage has left her. Meanwhile, the alcoholic often insists that he loves his wife; he counts on her to provide a home for him, and he goes to great lengths to keep her in his life—short of lasting abstinence. When she walks out, or puts him out, he is apt to be bitter and vindictive. In the same vein, Vaughan (1986, p. 93) mentions other specific behaviors likely to cause the mate to enforce a breakup; these include assault, adultery, and sexually withholding or demeaning attitudes toward the mate.

Paradoxically, involuntary rejection generally occurs as a result of connective anger. The inner experience is that departure is the only remaining way to show the partner how serious certain derelictions are, which sets the last possible stage to save the union. A history of multiple separations is not uncommon, with reconciliations occurring whenever the partner promises to reform. If no real change is forthcoming, the involuntary rejector eventually walks out with an unmistakable resolve never again to invest effort to make that particular relationship work. The leaving is done in an atmosphere of defeat. Mourning reactions are often profound, just as if the involuntary rejector had been forsaken in a classical rejection. Indeed, in such cases, it is plain that an involuntary rejector reacts like a symbiant, not a countersymbiant.

The reciprocal, the one who is left, can be at either of two poles. H/s may be someone who more or less *consciously* hopes the relationship will end, showing little sign of loss if this happens, but who needs the partner to take responsibility for the breakup. The following case illustrates this pattern, wherein a husband is thrown out of a marriage he never would have left of his own accord, but whose behavior after breakup was that of a person undoubtedly relieved to be out of the relationship.

A man built a flourishing business with his wife's help. Ten years and three children later, the husband introduced his wife to his principal financial backer and his wife; the two couples became the best of friends. Five more years had passed when the wife, M, became convinced that her husband and the woman who was her "best friend" were lovers. She had seen them looking intently at each other, several times touching, and once kissing. M then received an anonymous phone call, warning her that they were having an affair. All efforts to confront her husband were met with stout denial. She even went so far as to call her friend's husband for confirmation, only to be told that she must be crazy to suspect such things. One night, after her husband called to say that he would be working late, she followed her friend and watched her enter a restaurant—to meet her (M's) husband! She stormed away and angrily faced him with this information the next day. Yet her husband still denied that he had met this woman for anything other than conversation, explaining that because he knew how mistrustful his wife would be, he could not tell her where he was really going. The wife finally hired a detective, who documented a long-term affair. On the day she presented him the written report, her husband calmly replied that he did not know any married men of his ethnicity who did not have a girlfriend on the side. Incensed at his reaction at this crucial moment, she gave him 3 hours to pack and get out. She immediately filed for divorce. A week later, however, she was distraught and attempted suicide by overdose. Her husband showed disconnective anger—for instance, he never visited her in the hospital and refused to pay for medical treatment. His lover now broke up with *her* husband and moved in with him. At no point after breakup did the man display any interest in reconciliation, but he did insist on visiting the old house at all hours, without calling, to see the children. He asked to be invited to Christmas dinner, which his ex-wife declined to do on the grounds that she would not be invited to spend New Year's Eve with him (again, connective anger). At last report, she was talking about extracting "street justice" as her sole remaining vengeance.

In our view, such cases as this are theoretically important. They demonstrate how the partner who did not make the decision to leave sometimes readily transfigures into a recognizable "rejector" once out of the marriage—an *insidious provoker* in relation to the involuntary rejector, or in other words, a countersymbiant. In the preceding illustration, the husband showed scant grief over the breakup and used his wife's outrage to provoke a severing of their bonds. He swiftly replaced her and did not seem to care whether she lived or died. While he contended that he did not want the marriage to end, his flagrant behavior with his lover meant discovery sooner or later, almost as if he feared *not* being discovered. The wife was the one who could not bear the prospect of life unmarried to him, yet she instituted the breakup. Once the separation was an irrevocable fact, she continued to be bound to her husband through hatred just as much as she was during the marriage through love.

Alternatively, one might see a left partner who insists that the relationship be conducted along lines clearly impossible for the mate but who nevertheless seeks to make the mate stay in the marriage as if the derelictions did not exist or have magically disappeared. In this reaction, the so-called left partner is a second kind of insidious provoker who ushers the mate into walkout—but this time the work of extrusion is done *unconsciously,* with vehement denials that breakup is what was wanted, indignation when it happens, and sometimes dire threats to compel return, which are manifestly counterproductive. The aforementioned example of a "rejected" and sorely aggrieved male alcoholic can serve as a prototype for this sort of situation. Vaughan (1986) has listed many forms of marital "rule violations" in which a partner has to conclude that "a person who cares would not act this way" (p. 93) and thus becomes someone who looks like an initiator.

SUMMING UP

In considering the characterological struggle of acrimonious separation, we have theorized that in most cases a countersymbiant in identity
crisis seeks individuation outside marriage as the only way to deal with
an engulfing mate, leaving when h/s is daring, desperate, or reckless
enough to stand on h/h own. Further, it appears that this identity crisis
involves a need to overcome dependency that has become so ego-
dystonic as to make it imperative to establish autonomy by escalating
already existing distancing traits. In the process, narcissistic traits may
be manifest in that: (1) the breakup often appears driven by personal
entitlement and an excessive need to be loved; (2) the breakup is for
the countersymbiant's personal benefit at the expense of significant
others; and (3) there is frequently exploitation of a distraught ex-mate
after breakup.

In the next most common pattern of breakup, an insidious
provoker's emotional distancing, narcissistic demands, and refusal to
change pushes a parentified spouse into an agonizing departure. In
effect, the countersymbiant drives the symbiant spouse out, more or
less forcing the latter into the role of involuntary rejector.

We shall say more in Chapter 5 about those who wittingly (identity-seeking rejectors) or semiwittingly or unwittingly (the two variants
of insidious provokers) end their marriages. But first we must address
the psychodynamics and character limitations of the other protagonist
in acrimonious separation—the symbiant mate.

~ 4

The Symbiant Mate

It's very hard when you're as much in love as I am. Have mercy
on me. I don't mind that you don't care for me. After all you
can't help it. I only want you to let me love you.
                                        —MAUGHAM (1915, pp. 296–297)

Lovesickness is . . . that condition which ensues when a lover
who is separated . . . languishes, mopes, and pines for the
beloved. The lovesick mind becomes distracted from other
duties . . . and is preoccupied instead with an hypertrophy of
desire and longing. . . . There is no sense of well-being except in
the presence of the lover, who thus . . . wields inordinate power.
                                        —MONEY (1980, p. xiii)

THE WORLD OF THE LOVELORN SYMBIANT

In the throes of unrequited love, the French author Stendhal claimed
that had he been shot, he would have thanked his assassin before he
expired (Josephson, 1946). Despite this levity, Stendhal was conveying
the agony of rejection in love. The pain is not only about object loss;
Rice and Rice (1986) pointed out that "the coming apart of a marital
relationship requires . . . reckoning with the loss of being valued by an
[idealized] other. Felt narcissistic injury is . . . the result" (p. 112). Thus,
lovelorn symbiants suffer palpable loss and, in addition, their internalized conception of worth and position in the world is thrown into
severe disarray. Their sense of self loses continuity. Unable to adjust
to such profound change, an unrequited symbiant feels only integrated
when in the presence of the beloved and will go to incredible lengths
to stay connected, often contrary to what pride and proper reality
testing would dictate. This is a time of crisis, and it will not pass swiftly.

The traumatic reactions seen in the aftermath of rejection in love have been attributed to the activation of primal fears in regard to separation from an essential object, originally the mother figure (Masterson, 1981; Seinfeld, 1996). After loss of the love partner, behavior commonly occurs that recapitulates infant reactions observed in primate and human maternal deprivation studies, most notably an incapacitating dysphoria, disorganization, and self-soothing rituals. A bereft symbiant may not want to see anyone (except the wished-for partner); conversely, h/s may latch onto any interlocutor who will listen to long hours of lament. Symptoms of clinical depression are standard, including fixation on the lost object, weeping, eating and sleep disturbance, susceptibility to illness, and social maladjustment. During the acute phase of loss, concentration at work may also be affected, especially where solitary functions are concerned. Similarly, parenting skills may be impaired. Even the ability to provide routine self-care suffers.

But as serious as these disruptions are, even worse are the emotional storms vis-à-vis the estranged partner. A forsaken symbiant loves and hates, tending to dwell on fantasies in which separation is either undone or—in contrast—is avenged by harming h/h self or the beloved. Few symbiants actually enact such impulses to inflict injury or death, but it would be an egregious error to say that most of them let their partners "just leave." Research drawn from the literature on attachment theory demonstrates that the response to separation from a beloved is initially *protest behavior,* in which "individuals report feeling agitated, anxious, preoccupied with thoughts of the lost partner, coupled with a compulsion to search for him or her, as though trying to undo the loss even if it is consciously known to be irreversible" (Hazan & Shaver, 1994a, p. 14). Driven by separation anxiety, forsaken symbiants often discover unsuspected capacities for clinging and vindictive reactions, which later cause horror at how dignity and self-control could have been so compromised during the process of breakup. Thus, rejection tends to call out regressive behaviors—primitive aspects of the self one never wanted to know were there.

INTRODUCING THE HYPERGIVER

In Chapter 2 we presented the view that pairbonding is not random; it is based on need complementarity so that each partner selects a particular mate in order to express latent internalized templates of relationship. Chapter 3 addressed the psychology of the countersymbiant, tracing dynamics that result in distancing behavior to counter ego-dystonic dependency needs within the marriage and to provide narcissistic enhancement outside the marriage. The present chapter now deals with the dynamics of the symbiant: a complementary pattern wherein the road to relationship consists in binding the other through *indispensable caretaking*. Current attachment theory postulates that this interactive style begins in early childhood during anxious–ambivalent attachment to a caregiver, establishing a predisposition in adulthood to be the mate most concerned about loss and therefore most invested in preserving a committed union. As Hazan and Shaver (1994a) stated, "The proximal goal of all attachment behavior is to achieve a felt state of security. In the case of anxious–ambivalent attachment, this is attempted and at times accomplished by devoting immense mental energy and behavioral effort to keeping others close by and engaged" (p. 15). Thus, attachment theory holds that insecure, preoccupied attachment becomes a compensatory characterological trait manifested in overinvolved relations with significant others; this pattern has its inception in the family of origin, extends to social functioning in general, and becomes most salient during adulthood in intimate relationships. An illustration of such dynamics is provided by a woman who said about her husband, "I can't believe it, when I see how I have related to Stan all these years. It's like an instant video replay of taking care of my mother. I don't know how I did it—everything in my childhood was about making her feel better, and in adulthood, I'm still at it with him."

In short, the defining characteristic of symbiant mates in committed unions is that they display a "need to be needed" from early on and use caretaking as a strategy to ward off or repair any threat of relational dissolution. At the upper ranges of this proclivity in personality development, a mate may be so invested in preserving an intimate partnership that h/s can be characterized as a *hypergiver*. In lieu of engaging in projects that promote self-actualization, the hypergiver is much more prone to defer private goals in favor of making sacrifices for the larger marital or family unit. Basing h/h security on this cognitive model, a hypergiver may indeed have redoubtable talents to foster and stabilize the lives of others, working assiduously to keep things on track for the unit as a whole, and thereby often being an invaluable agent in any social system in which h/s partakes. However, stalwart devotion as a way to become essential to others is not pure altruism: hidden needs to control can constitute an underside to the hypergiving orientation, so that even though hypergivers may be impressively involved in caretaking functions and often are the mainstay of their families, they are also meeting their own unacknowledged dependency needs through vicarious identification with the objects to whom they are dedicated. Taking care of others makes them feel taken care of themselves. Should loss of the object occur, their true level of neediness will quickly become apparent, as well as the masochistic extremes to which they will go to maintain or restore their love investment.

Writing from an object relations perspective, Seinfeld (1996) interpreted overinvestment in a love partner as a sign of inner emptiness, because there is so little sense of self independent of this object. If the partner does not cooperate by playing the role assigned, despair and desperation lead to attempts to pull the partner back into the role. No matter how disaffiliated the partner, intrapsychic incorporation of the other remains intact for a long time, making the symbiant a virtual love slave. Seinfeld held that "the object is . . . internalized as a defensive effort to deal with the unsatisfactory [partner]. Thus, internalization . . . is an effort to omnipotently control and possess the other. However, the result is that the individual attempting to possess the object ends up being possessed by it" (p. 6). We see an exemplification of this perverse dynamic in Maugham's novel *Of Human Bondage* (1915/1963). Philip, the well-educated central character, unaccountably worships a crass and cold working-class woman, begging her to stay with him on any terms she chooses, as seen in his pathetic plea: "I only want you to let me love you," quoted at the beginning of this chapter.

We should make clear that we are not stereotyping forsaken lovers as irrevocable hypergiver character types. Just as not all countersymbiants go to the extreme of character pathology to warrant a clinical diagnosis of narcissism, not all symbiants have been so selflessly devoted to preserving their marriages as they might claim. However, in our clinical experience, hypergiving patterns are most prominent and most often found in the mates of partners with pronounced narcissistic traits. Four very different cases of hypergiving are now presented, in which a symbiant did everything possible to hold onto a partner but was ultimately unsuccessful, eventually facing a wrenching separation. In each example, concern for the partner's welfare during the course of the relationship seemed to take precedence over the symbiant's own needs.

A woman, N, deferred her own education and proudly worked to pay her husband's way through medical school, only to be left upon his graduation. He had become involved with a woman from his class who, he stated, "fit in better" with his new professional status. N felt that she had been used by her husband to achieve his goals and then "dumped." The woman brought a civil lawsuit that sought a share of her ex-husband's anticipated future income as a physician. Although she did win a large lump sum alimony payment in court, afterward she remained bitter as well as very mistrustful of men.

The "enabling" wife of an alcoholic, a mother of three, was driven out of a 15-year marriage after much abuse, despite efforts to be patient and tolerant where her man's drinking problem was concerned (which included joining him at bars in hope of controlling his consumption). She justified what she did on the grounds that she loved him and believed he would eventually overcome his vice, and also that the children needed a father image in the home. Several near-breakups occurred after incidents in which she swore she could no longer stand his alcoholic bouts, which resulted in demeaning and often violent assaults on her. But he would then make promises to "change things," so she would relent and give him another chance. Yet, aside from some brief improvements, the marital situation only worsened over time. In the end, the wife had to admit that staying with this man in order to hold her family together went beyond the dictates of good sense and self-interest. She was no longer young, had no education or job skills to manage on her own, and her children had lost respect for her because she continued to live with her husband no matter what he did.

A man was so intent on making his wife happy that he gave her nearly everything she wanted, even though he could not afford their lavish life style, the many vacations she took with or without him, and her pursuit of education instead of working. He exhausted his credit and took a second and then a third job, but he still could not keep up with their bills. He finally told his wife that although they were in the same marriage, they were in different economies; whereas she could purchase on credit whatever she wished, he seldom had money for personal needs and worried incessantly about keeping up with payments. She soon left the marriage, stating that in view of their latest conversation about money, she now had to learn to fend for herself (which would be very hard), yet expecting that he would pay off the bulk of their outstanding debt.

A woman's affair with a married man went on for 10 years while she waited for the time when his children would be old enough for the man to divorce so that he could marry her. Despite repeated pledges to leave his wife, the man seldom called after his last child graduated from high school, citing new business concerns that made him currently unable to find time for her. She was patient at first, trying as usual to be understanding and to accept his problems. When he did call, she indicated that his absences were all right and that he need not worry about her. But when even these accommodations did not produce any significant time spent together, she became angry, pointing out to him the many years she had already waited, relinquishing any committed relationship that was exclusively her own. His behavioral response to her tirade was to increase his distancing behavior even further, and she finally had to give up the relationship. What made her most upset was the realization that she was alone now, but not much more so than she had been all along while waiting for and catering to him, living on hopes and promises.

In the preceding cases, symbiants made great sacrifices on behalf of their partners, so as to prepare the way to a better future for the couple. However, they were humiliated later for having invested in a partner who offered comparatively little reciprocity and ultimately delivered a de facto rejection. The heartbreak of these symbiants was overwhelming in each instance, highlighting the fact that they had centered their lives on the caretaking of their particular love object and went to the limits of commitment to foster and save this relationship. They seemed to operate on the assumption that their efforts on behalf of the working partnership would make them appreciated and even indispensable to the other—and it made no sense to them that they were, in the end, quite expendable indeed.

Noteworthy in these cases is how readily a hypergiver's need to be needed turns into a tendency to be overresponsible; the diligent effort expended on behalf of a social system—be it business, church, or family—reinforces a hypergiver's internal sense of security. But this role also means that one may be taken for granted, or even exploited by someone who is underresponsible; later on, a hypergiver may bitterly conclude that h/h dedication was masochistic. Applied to marriage, whatever the voluntary and gladly given contributions of a hypergiver, extra burdens are imposed when the countersymbiant is underresponsible in terms of preserving the relationship. Eventually, the hypergiver may leave because too gross an imbalance exists in the giving: receiving ratio of the relationship, but it takes a lot to drive a hypergiver away.

THE PYGMALION COMPLEX

Because hypergivers often base their emotional investment on some need or weakness of their partners, they tend to seek control by becoming engaged in a perpetual effort to sustain, mold, or reform their chosen objects. This attachment style brings to mind Laing's (1969) concept of "transpersonal defenses" in which "self attempts to regulate the inner life of the other in order to preserve his own" (p. 13). Laing suggested that such unconscious manipulation may be experienced as persecution by the object, who feels denied h/h individuation by the press to conform so that the caretaker can survive. Thus, a subtle self-serving dynamic can be involved even in what appears to be the most noble love.

The need of the hypergiver to reconfigure the partner shows that, like the countersymbiant, h/s tends to renounce the actuality of the partner in favor of an idealized image. However, whereas the countersymbiant's dread of engulfment may lead to breakup of a committed union so that h/s can set out on a quest to find a more exciting new object, the hypergiver tends to remain enmeshed, resisting the anxiety inherent in separation either by persistently devoting energy to reforming the partner or by denying or ignoring the partner's fallibility. Like Pygmalion of the Greek legend who carved a statue of his ideal woman so real that it came to life, the hypergiver is in love with a creation of h/h own imagination. But, as depicted in the legend, such a project must result in failure. Having carved the statue according to his inspiration and naming her "Galatea," Pygmalion could not resist Galatea's beauty. Yet his courtship soon proved to be in vain; once transformed into a living creature, Galatea took on her own personal ity, including a contrary will. Pygmalion's ardor was slated to be thwarted by a statue that ultimately craved life on autonomous terms, even if such terms were (in the eyes of the sculptor) those of a mere statue.

In object relations theory, whenever a real person is turned into an idealized object, the Pygmalion theme is repeated: "Through internalization, the other is stripped of his or her wholeness, subjectivity, and freedom and is transformed into a thinglike object. However, this thinglike object gets its revenge by having a life of its own and possessing, tormenting, and persecuting its possessor" (Seinfeld, 1996, p. 7). Thus, an ironic twist awaits any hypergiver trying to change the object in conformity with internal needs, shaping a partner who supposedly requires only a redemptive hand to smooth out particular lacks and reach h/h true potential. In the final analysis, this is a contingent, limited way of loving.

From the countersymbiant's standpoint, the caretaking of a hypergiver initially provides the safety and benefits of having an enmeshed mate. Moreover, should the mate become too controlling, distancing defenses are always available to keep the relationship in equilibrium. Nevertheless, although this format is psychologically viable for the hypergiver (who counts more on being needed than on being loved), it does not work as well over time for a reciprocal, who—in fact or fantasy—may outgrow the dependency so reassuring to the hypergiver. For the countersymbiant, the relationship as it stands at some point may appear to block self-actualization on h/h own terms; marital crisis then occurs when enough security and self-esteem is developed to burst free of the enveloping aura of the hypergiver. At this juncture in their history, the pairbond's interpersonal dynamics have put them on a collision course. If breakup ensues, the hypergiver will regard the now estranged partner with a sense that there is much to rue and much to resent for having so unstintingly invested in this ungrateful consort.

NARCISSISM IN THE MASOCHISTIC HYPERGIVER

Cooper (1989) has tried to synthesize the extensive literature on narcissism with the relatively sparse study of the phenomenon of masochism. He viewed these two personality variables as intertwined aspects of a single clinical entity: the narcissistic–masochistic character. In his formulation, "pathologic narcissistic tendencies are unconscious vehicles for attaining masochistic disappointment, [whereas] masochistic injuries are an affirmation of distorted narcissistic fantasies" (p. 551). He proposed four indicators to diagnose masochism: (1) setting up victimization and defeat so that another is seen as in control of key sectors of one's life and using the other's "control" to bring about a sense of humiliation, helplessness, and loss of opportunities; (2) a compliant acceptance of painful circumstances, or exaggeration of the pain experienced, as the affective component of masochism; (3) a readiness to succumb to guilt and depression as its superego component; and (4) a self-centered approach to life, including the conviction that no one else suffers as much as the subject does, as its narcissistic component.

Solomon (1989) similarly synthesized narcissism and masochism. In a section describing narcissistic defensive organization in love relationships, she concluded that "narcissistic needs may be overtly acted out in grandiose fantasies and expectations, or covertly expressed by filling such needs in others" (p. 57). The latter case obviously applies to our hypergiver. Solomon found that in transactions between troubled spouses, often "what was given was neither requested nor wanted" (p. 58) and was offered because of narcissistic vulnerability on the part of the provider, as well as fusion fantasies as if the other were an extension of the self.

If the syndromes of narcissism and masochism are two sides of the same coin, the narcissist must have a masochistic side (which we discuss in Chapter 19) and the masochist must have a narcissistic side. Masterson (1993) has written about the "closet narcissist"—the individual whose thematic defense in intimate relationships is "idealization or devaluation of the omnipotent object to regulate the grandiose sense of self" (p. 5). Such a "false defensive self" is maintained by seeking to mirror the object, often a manifest narcissist, which permits the closet narcissist to "feel special or unique in the glow of the . . . other" (p. 13). But if the object should defect, the idealization turns into devaluation as if one had been betrayed by an inferior, defective partner, so that again the grandiose sense of self is shown. The dynamics of the closet narcissist are consonant with those of our hypergiver; both terms describe a person combining devoted idealization with a fear of abandonment so that the object must be controlled or transformed in order to protect an image of self as worthy of love. Concerning a businessman who came for psychotherapy with a complaint of "codependency" after "having subordinated himself to his mother and then two wives" (p. 16), Masterson declared that this patient had internalized a need for involvement with dominating women and emotionally invested in external aggressors to reinforce it. The implication of this comment is that closet narcissists tend to choose partners who demand masochistic abdication of self during the relationship. However, if such partners leave, they are then devalued by the forsaken mate, making masochistic pursuit following breakup all the more self-demeaning.

All in all, the aforementioned theorists agree that the narcissism of a hypergiver lies primarily in the sense of being connected to an idealized object, and secondarily in the assumption that one is taking better care of the partner than anyone else would. Even if the caretaking is laudable, such investment in the partner is pathological because it occurs in the absence of receiving, or perhaps even wanting, anything close to an equivalent return. Although the hypergiver may need at least some symbolic response from the partner in order to maintain this type of involvement, the partner need not be greatly committed, or greatly available, since the barest contact or assurance can reinforce a hypergiver's illusory idea that there is a mutual love. If breakup or some other event occurs that is incompatible with maintenance of an internalized conception of the union, a sense of emptiness flows from loss of that aspect of self delegated to the introjected object; so much is invested in this setup that the hypergiver must immediately struggle to regain the partner in order to maintain the desired state of fusion with the introject.

To demonstrate the lengths to which some mates will go to retain the narcissistic–masochistic illusion of a mutually loving relationship, we consider the Amy Fisher case (Fisher & Weller, 1993), which has received much media attention.

> Amy, a high school student, shot the wife of her married lover, Joey Buttafuoco. The wife, Mary Jo, survived a head wound but was neurologically impaired. She vehemently defended her husband

against any taint of infidelity during Amy's trial for attempted murder and even during her husband's own later trial for statutory rape. Mary Jo's account was the basis of the script for a CBS-TV movie, *Casualties of Love*, according to which Amy only fantasized that she had an affair with Mary Jo's husband, as if Mary Jo could possibly know what had transpired between them (other than what Joey told her). She waited for her husband to be released from prison to resume what she saw as a good marriage, still regarding Joey and herself as victims of the nefarious Amy, and receiving much public support for her resolve to "stand by her man." However, when detectives sympathetic to Mary Jo as a crime victim showed her evidence that Joey had been intimate with Amy, they found her "past denial"—for example, when they produced a dozen motel receipts from Joey–Amy trysts, Mary Jo said, "Then a dozen times, I'll just say that *I* was in that motel room with him" (pp. 238–239). This inane defense of her husband amounted to *pseudologia fantastica*—Mary Jo had subordinated her own interests and reality testing to preserve an internalized image of Joey as innocent.

Mary Jo's extreme behavior encapsulates many trends relative to the narcissistic side of masochism and serves as a model (if not a caricature) of hypergiving attitudes. In the course of creating a self-soothing sense of being indispensable, a hypergiver tends to overestimate h/h value to the partner so that projection-based complacency and denial-based gullibility will be readily seen. But unconsciously, there is dread that one may not be needed after all—a dread activated into awareness only if a threat of loss emerges that cannot be evaded. When the partner is shown to be not only imperfect but (far worse) not fused with the self, the result is fragmentation, despair, and emptiness, to be defended against by massive denial leading to restoration of the object (Masterson, 1993). Thus, although the hypergiver's orientation to the committed union may appear largely altruistic, implying a dearth of narcissism, this is only a defense, because h/h self-esteem rests so greatly on the putative role assigned the partner ("putative" because the introject may have little relation to the actual partner). In effect, some narcissistic investment in self as part of good mental health is superseded by vicarious benefits anticipated from devotion to the introject representing the partner. Thus, the hypergiver is narcissistic in striving to be a perfect (and therefore secure) mate, although not necessarily claiming to be a perfect person.

SADOMASOCHISTIC DYNAMICS IN BREAKUP

Sadomasochistic phenomena have been seriously misunderstood in the clinical literature, so a cautionary word is necessary before delving into the subject of such relationships in divorce. Historically, the mental health field has defined both sadism and masochism as sexual perversions in which erotic arousal and orgastic release were contingent upon inflicting or receiving pain. Later, "masochism" was extended to describe a personality type, but a taint of paraphilia still adhered—that is, that submission to pain was associated with sexual pleasure. Thus, those deemed to exhibit masochistic traits were said to somehow enjoy their suffering at the hands of a love-partner, which then explained why they stayed in abusive relationships. However, this chapter should have made clear by now that *any drive for libidinal pleasure pales alongside the drive for attachment.* Sex after fighting may at times be more passionate, but in general eroticism has little to do with such a character style. As we see it, a sadomasochistic union expresses pathological forms of attachment on the part of both parties—this is the way a polarized couple deal with their closeness–distance issues. If they no longer can live together, to varying degrees each feels empty without the partner. But, at the same time, because it will be a long time before either spouse can tolerate loss of the other, there is an impressive stability to these interlocking self-destructive patterns during the separation process.

Accordingly, attachment theory may offer the most informative approach to understanding the paradoxical phenomenon whereby a forsaken symbiant—contrary to emotional balance and self-interest—courts a rejecting partner via protestations of eternal fealty, dramatic importunities, and ready forgiveness of past misdeeds. We have already noted that Hazan and Shaver (1994a) insisted such clinging derives from a cognitive model of anxious–ambivalent attachment, so that in intimate relationships "anxiety apparently intensifies the need to be near another person and makes that person's security-promoting potential more salient. [It] is a signal to get closer" (p. 10). We would add that for a symbiant, "closer" means becoming ever more hypergiving as h/h most immediate and hitherto reliable device to pull a countersymbiant back into h/h role as a relationship partner. But what the symbiant does not foresee is that in the situation of breakup, such overcompensation to recapture a disengaging partner now makes that partner feel even more ensnared, leading to more pronounced distancing, which in turn leads to further and ever more futile hypergiving, and so on in a vicious downward spiral as the couple's enmeshment unravels.

There are certain endemic features to these encounters. Let us first look at a typical program of a countersymbiant in breakup and then a symbiant's typical reactions. To avoid guilt, a countersymbiant often casts the other as the culprit responsible for the marital problems, regarding h/h severing of the conjugal ties as essentially reactive and self-protective. Accordingly, the disengaging partner is apt to manipulate the other's behavior until it coincides with h/h internal image of an intrusive, domineering spouse who always rides roughshod over the countersymbiant's wishes and needs. Instead of acknowledging a reciprocal influence, the countersymbiant may selectively isolate just those behaviors that prove that the mate is noxious and should therefore be rejected. Thus, behavior that provokes the symbiant is an integral part of a blaming defense needed by the countersymbiant, and retaliation by the symbiant will supply renewed motivation to struggle against any relenting in the militant determination to leave. Hence, a countersymbiant tends to incite just those traits that are most objectionable in the former mate. This is done by exploiting any vulnerability that arouses wrath, quickly turning the ex-mate into a hostile, reprehensible, and implacable foe—the very monster from whom the countersymbiant had to escape. By goading the symbiant into a retaliatory attack, the countersymbiant is now contending with a disturbed, perhaps dangerous individual whom any sane person would keep at a safe distance. Such instigation also allows the countersymbiant to confirm that h/s is being repulsed and disrespected at every approach to the former mate. Thus, even failure to reconcile can be blamed on the symbiant.

Meanwhile, the symbiant tends to take the bait. Rather than refuse to have anything more to do with an "agent provocateur," the symbiant at first often wants to placate the displeased partner and is highly distressed by the fighting to the point of being upset for days afterward, as if the relationship were now "lost." Excuses for the countersymbiant are made as the symbiant grovels, offering constant apologies for faults, intolerance, or misunderstanding. Where possible, other people are likely to be held responsible for the countersymbiant's current behavior, such as a lover, parent, or mentor. Later, as all these efforts fail and the provocations of the ex-partner escalate, the symbiant starts to impose retribution in ways that invite reprisal, and in short order a sadomasochistic battle is joined until the disengagement of letting go dims the passion or reconciliation (temporarily) resolves the problems. Consider the following three cases, involving couples comprised of a narcissistic countersymbiant and a hypergiving symbiant.

Ecstatic to be out of his marriage, a man still resisted his wife's pleas to get him to remove considerable remaining property from the apartment he had recently vacated. He refused to call before visiting the children, using his old keys to let himself in. He expected his wife to cook for him whenever he came by, tried to have sex with her, and on one occasion accused her of neglecting the children because she went out on a date—he insisted that, with him gone, "The kids need you more than ever." He refused to divulge his new address or phone number, delayed drawing up a financial agreement, and declared that he could not provide any funds right away because of the many bills he had incurred in moving. The couple fell into quarrel over each and every one of these actions on his part. He would then call her "bitchy" or "bossy" and march straight through the door to his residence where she could not reach him. *And how did the wife react to all this?* When the man exercised the prerogative to enter and exit his former home as he pleased, he initially found his wife fairly cooperative, because she had hope of talking with him about their situation, extracting money for child support, and possibly reconciling. She wept after every argument and begged him to be "considerate" and "to work out their problems." She told the children to be nice to their father and made excuses for him when they asked how they might get in touch with him. Nevertheless, she gradually became more hostile in her attitude: she finally changed the lock on her apartment door, took him to court for financial support despite his objections, and kept the children from him. He became livid at these reactions, complaining that she was now making it impossible for them to be together in any way. Taking him at what sounded like his word, she slept with him once again, but when these efforts proved abortive, she felt relieved to be apart from him.

A man came home for Thanksgiving dinner with a family he had left several weeks before. He met his ex-wife's digs and taunts with the comment that she always had a "big mouth" and had nagged him out of the marriage. He then warned her that if he should choose to reconcile, she must not throw in his face ever after that he had left her. In other words, he was saying it was her fault he had departed, but should he want to return, she must not criticize him lest she force him to walk out again. In this manner, the externalization of responsibility is carefully marked out: he would come and go only in relation to what she did. *Here again, what did the wife do in response to this crazy-making setup by which she was held accountable for the maintenance of the relationship out of which she had just been expelled?* She apologized for her "nagging" ways, entered therapy to "become a better wife," and accepted his terms for another try at marriage—only to be left again, and blamed again, because she could not contain her recriminations about the man's absences from the home and lack of concern for her feelings.

A forsaken man told his ex-wife that his suspicion that she had long been involved with a certain other man kept them from establishing a climate conducive to reunion. He offered to clear up matters once and for all by calling the person in question. She blanched and exclaimed, "You see what I mean? If you do that, I'll never speak to you again!" She accepted no responsibility for protecting a privacy that exacerbated his problems in trusting her; instead, her version of their cause–effect impasse pointed to his jealousy as the factor keeping them estranged. Thus, she was hinting that his lack of faith in her could conceivably drive her into the arms of the nonexistent rival. *And what did the husband do?* In the end, he never called the phantom "other man" and the couple reconciled, without any exploration on their part as to why she had left and why she had returned.

In the preceding cases, it is clear how a countersymbiant can take a pivotal position in stirring up a row, while exhibiting scant interest in h/h own contribution to the process. This attitude can insidiously impel an ex-mate either into collusion with h/h own humiliation or into intemperate actions that become material for the ex-partner's "grievance collecting" as well as calls for more "space." In either eventuality, a sadomasochistic bond ties the couple in an emotional knot, and this can go on long after breakup. Furthermore, in acting out an underlying need to punish the mate, the countersymbiant may consciously experience only that h/h tentative overtures for amicable relations in separation have been subverted by an archcritical and vindictive symbiant. All told, the countersymbiant's mode of dealing with attachment and guilt often requires just this volatile atmosphere, while the symbiant colludes by staying emotionally engaged, trying to find a way to overcome rejection in love, but eventually becoming angry enough to fully corroborate that h/s is (and always was) impossible to live with.

The behavior most damaging to a symbiant's ability to escape sadomasochistic interactions with the ex occurs when the rejecting partner appears as "Mr(s). Nice Guy." From a countersymbiant's point of view, the "provoking" strategy turns its object into an enemy toward whom h/s had to be cold, unforgiving, and harsh, but once separation is safely in hand, it may be possible to be more magnanimous. With this new attitude, the countersymbiant's self-image is not so negative; after shedding the mate, h/s often feels rid of the "bad" part of the former self. Thus, once breakup is assured, h/s may pointedly bear no grudges, try to be helpful, and ask that others recognize that separation was hard for h/h too. Once family members have adjusted, no one need be mad at anyone.

The symbiant is quite vulnerable to any displays of caring, concern, and helpfulness. Behavior along these lines appears to suggest potential reconciliation, or at least a softening of the disapproving attitude of the countersymbiant. At first, these are seized upon as opportunities for contact, either in a couple or family context. The symbiant will do everything possible to reward the countersymbiant for such overtures, so reminiscent of the "old" partner. But because the Mr(s). Nice Guy stance is episodic, taking place only when it suits the countersymbiant to be dealing with the forsaken symbiant, it cannot fix the symbiant in role for long.

The countersymbiant will be genuinely pained when the symbiant is no longer receptive to h/h benevolence, including willingness to let the couple and family unit sometimes be together as before. But the symbiant may have learned to assess this goodwill as shallow and contrived if the countersymbiant's caring breaks down as soon as consistency or commitment is sought. Usually, as these issues come up, the genial Mr(s). Nice Guy pose tends to give way to the agent provocateur, which is the other side of the mask. It is ironic that should the symbiant rebuff what seems like pseudoattempts at "niceness" between the ex-couple, the countersymbiant is apt to construe this as an inexplicable and unwarranted assault just at a time when a better relationship is at long last possible. However, for the symbiant, such rebuffing makes it possible to let go more quickly, without being confused by the double messages of the ex or by h/h own internal needs for the ex partner's love.

THE POWER—AND POWERLESSNESS—
OF THE "VICTIM"

When breakup occurs, a symbiant continues on as before by upholding the connectedness of the couple, although now miserable in the absence of that connection. In h/h estimation, the estranged partner has exploited the benefits of their relationship and leaves the stronger for it, whereas the forlorn symbiant is now helpless in the face of injustice. Thus, the symbiant interprets h/h plight as that of a victim, with its attendant pain, outrage, and wish for revenge. Although the victim role is a psychic consolation, it is also one of abject weakness that ultimately is inconsistent with personal dignity. As Vaughan (1986) remarked:

> Some partners forever wear the badge of rejection, [initially attracting] attention and support from family, friends, and perhaps even the initiator. . . . [As other interests] atrophy, these partners, by default, invest increased energy in the victim role, intensifying their focus on the relationship and their loss. They dwell on and recount the episodes of their perceived victimization. . . . [They] eventually alienate well-meaning others, who tire of the seemingly endless introspection, anger, and negativism. (pp. 163–164)

Nevertheless, for a long time it is hard to give up the sense of victimization. This is not just because of lasting resentment, for the victim role turns out to offer some surprising forms of empowerment. Despite initial shock, a symbiant finds that h/s is not helpless in the face of rejection: a unilateral breakup can be met by refusing to countenance the partner's deed as legitimate or permanent. Accordingly, symbiants tend to mobilize their resources to wage war on the perceived ambivalence and vulnerability of their estranged other; there will be no breakup without a sharp struggle. This mobilization provides some feeling of mastery in that the course of the separation will now be influenced not only by the choices of the countersymbiant, but also by the actions of the symbiant. Although much of the symbiant's efforts directed toward countering the separation prove futile, we must still take account of four types of pressure exerted to crack the will of the errant partner.

The Power of Courtship

Driven by fear of separation and the pain of mourning, a symbiant will try any means at h/h disposal to seduce the lover back into the relationship. At every opportunity, the symbiant wants to work on the problems of the couple. H/s seeks contact, earnestly discusses issues, tries to be accommodating and sensitive, and is filled with erotic longing. It may be hard for the countersymbiant to pass up these opportunities for sexual dalliances so that occasional successes may attend these efforts. But there are limitations to the power of courtship; seldom does carrying a torch ignite the passion of the partner. The symbiant's situation is akin to that of the compulsive gambler, throwing good money after bad. Such courting is largely wasted, because if a countersymbiant wants to escape the dominion of a symbiant, additional blandishments can only reinforce the need to flee. Yet ever believing that it is h/h behavior that is ultimately responsible for the fate of their union, a symbiant tends to hang on, desperately seeking the "right" approach that will prompt the partner to admit still being "in love" with the forsaken mate.

Goode (1956), a family sociologist, offered an explanation as to how spurned lovers preserve the relationship by projecting their feelings of love onto their partners, despite abundant evidence that there is no reciprocity. Thus, they carry their courtships quite far until finally forced to accept the rejection as genuine. However, psychoanalytic theories have long offered explanations of such projection as the basis for attempting to salvage an essential relationship. Going back to Freud's familiar premise that traumatic object loss recapitulates early separation anxiety, Masterson (1981) held that the child's bond with the mother establishes a condition whereby withdrawal of love will precipitate "abandonment depression," one aspect of which is that separation from the object is equivalent to loss of a vital part of the self and therefore tantamount to death. In order to ward off abandonment depression, defensive clinging and fusion mechanisms occur, because it is so painful to accept that the object is no longer available. If the separation–individuation process of childhood was impaired, such defensive operations persist into adulthood, still carrying the conviction that loss of the most significant other will annihilate the self. Thus, projection of love feelings to the disengaging partner is only one example of the primitive compensations used to deny the unacceptable reality of object loss; defensive operations will lead to manifold screen maneuvers that ward off abandonment depression.

In a successful treatment exemplifying this conceptual approach, a woman still ardently pursuing her estranged husband developed an obsessive concern that she had cancer and was going to die. Her therapist's formulation was that her morbid preoccupation constituted a symbolic equivalent of her unconscious belief that separation from her husband meant certain death. Moreover, the specific nature of her fear showed that she had taken her object inside her through identification but, in separation, the object had become a malignant foreign body that could only do her harm. Nevertheless, the woman had developed this hypochondriacal symptom to occupy the psychic space reserved for her ex-husband; her persistent preoccupation with cancer was a monument to their marriage. By holding onto this symptom, as she had once held onto him, she could avoid the final step of separation, which would entail recognition on her part that she could go on living without him.

Coercive Power

Frustration of courtship efforts is bound to lead to aggressive feelings that must somehow be expressed. A symbiant may thus develop strategies of punishment to alternate with strategies of courtship. But such punishment too may be designed to force the ex-partner back and can therefore be just as symbiotic as courtship, working in tandem with it. Hence, plans now tend to be initiated aimed at cutting a supply line that feeds the postseparation adjustment of the countersymbiant in order to ruin or nullify the other's "independence." The ruthless implementation of such aggression will be justified as "fighting fire with fire."

By a logistic assault on the necessities of the estranged partner's new life, the symbiant intends to coerce a return to a (comparatively better) old one or, at the very least, to leave the partner unhappy apart, penalized for the decision to leave. For example, a countersymbiant who has left minor children in the custody of the symbiant may find that visitation is now hindered, that children's attitudes have been negatively influenced, or that accusations of child abuse are being leveled. Other vengeful ploys may be intended to sabotage the economic viability of the countersymbiant—for instance, onerous claims in property settlement or for child support, attempts to damage the ex-partner's professional reputation, or the rampant running up of bills. Of course, there are many other opportunities for making trouble. Wherever privation or conflict can be fomented, a symbiant stirs the cauldron, hoping to conjure up the thought in the ex-partner's mind that in bringing about a breakup a terrible error was made, disastrous consequences impend, and reconciliation should be considered.

Nevertheless, to the consternation of most symbiants, even the best can't-miss schemes seem somehow to miss. In general, the more painful the punishment inflicted by a symbiant, the more resentment by a countersymbiant; for the latter, such intrigues soon become yet one more reason to resist reunion and keep safely away.

Moral Power

A forsaken symbiant cannot help but let the ex-partner know how much has been suffered—this grief is natural and cannot be concealed. It should not be dismissed as manipulation, because there is so much real loss to mourn and this distress is part of the protest and process. However, the symbiant often lays punitive "guilt trips," a behavior extending beyond normal mourning. Such behavior starts out as moral indignation at the defection of the partner but is soon carried to the point of intending humiliation through making the partner feel as culpable as possible for having left. Such attempts at guilt induction are common in unilateral breakups, in which one small way to extract vengeance is to attack the self-esteem of the countersymbiant. Thus, in meetings after separation, a symbiant may level accusations at the other's character or judgment, with caustic asides, quips, and diatribes inserted at opportune moments. Yet, beyond impugning the integrity of the other, there lurks in these attacks an underlying magical wish that the partner can be shamed, worried, or nagged back into the fold.

Moral considerations are not irrelevant in breakup. The countersymbiant may have curtly dismissed a devoted mate, been unfaithful and deceitful, impoverished the family because resources were diverted to private needs, treated the children poorly, and so on. If such behavior occurs, respect from an ex-spouse will certainly be diminished. But many of the reprimands do not address issues like this; rather, they are aimed at forcing a countersymbiant to behave as an ideal love object for the symbiant. In the latter's eyes, the real crime of the countersymbiant is that h/s does not love the symbiant. But an estranged partner cannot be criticized into reinstating the relationship, nor shamed into personality change, nor coerced into wanting to hear all this. If the partner were such a poor specimen of humanity, the symbiant would keep well clear and forbear to waste words. To the contrary, what the symbiant is eager to do is to inform the other that h/s is selfish, foolish, weak, spoiled, and so forth. This self-righteous bludgeoning has no pragmatic value, but it serves an intrapsychic purpose for the symbiant as a defense against h/h own guilt concerning the breakup. Through guilt games, the countersymbiant is cast as an unworthy partner, whereas the self did nothing wrong except to love unwisely.

Insofar as reunion is concerned, guilt games must prove to be futile, for moral power is no substitute for sexual–romantic power. Attempting to instill rectitude will not heal emotional alienation.

The Power of Desperation

A forsaken symbiant's desolation can be overwhelming. Yet there is no doubt that many symbiants behave in a fashion that exacerbates their plight, making a bad situation worse. In psychoanalytic theory, the wrecking of one's well-being in order to hurt a significant other is known as "masochistic aggression." It is cutting off your nose to spite h/h face. In marital breakups, a symbiant may want to ensure that the disengaged partner will not be afforded the relief of seeing the forsaken mate recover as if no serious harm were done. Instead, to compel the other's recognition of the tragic consequences of rejection, the symbiant may arrange to have the countersymbiant watch h/h fall apart, and perhaps even be caught up in the swath of destruction.

The bereft lover is already undergoing sorrow over loss of the beloved, but masochistic aggression inserts a wild card into the deck. Instead of maintaining h/h prior overresponsibility, the symbiant is now determined to impose on the countersymbiant h/h "fair share" of devastation. In taking the stance of a person crippled by rejection who has lost everything and no longer cares what happens, a symbiant awash in this brand of self-pity is prepared to sink down to rock bottom. Self-hatred attributed to rejection in love gives license for heretofore unthinkable actions imposed on self, the estranged partner, or those dear to the partner. Because there is nothing to lose, masochistic aggression may slide into pathological channels as diverse as alcoholism, suicide, crimes of passion, or use of children as pawns (as always, the choice of symptoms is determined by character and circumstances). The only substantial barrier to reckless desperation by a desperate symbiant are those remnants of self-esteem that forbid or contain certain impulses as too base to indulge. But self-esteem in a crisis of rejection in love may be frail. The symbiant is unloved and therefore acts out the part of the unlovable. It does not matter that in so doing, h/s is validating the lost partner's worst perceptions of who one is, making exit from this relationship appear wise in retrospect.

The "Power of the Victim" Summarized

A symbiant may make immense efforts to resuscitate a failing marriage, but such approaches as courting a rejector, coercive machinations, guilt games, and masochistic aggression tend to drive the ex-partner farther away in the long run. It has been said apropos this context that you can't beat a dead horse. The symbiant would retort that perhaps the horse isn't dead, only comatose—but then again, you can't usefully beat a horse in coma either! Our conclusion must be that a frantic symbiant can stir up some response from the countersymbiant and keep the relationship going in that sense, but reunion can rarely be accomplished by the methods just described. Nevertheless, beyond momentary satisfaction or hope, there is, after all, some psychological value even in these futile endeavors. This is protest behavior, needed as a way of looking back and checking one's location, before turning up the road to letting go.

WHITHER A MONOGAMIST WITHOUT A MATE?

Although a forsaken symbiant may be preoccupied for a long time with the dream that the partner will call to announce a change of heart, there is still the daily reality of functioning without the love object. In order to recover from rejection in love, a symbiant has to overcome the attachment still monogamously invested in the lost partner, each step along the way reflecting diminution of this investment. Once this problematic attachment is severed, there will be coping with existential loneliness before a new bond can be forged to another—and, one hopes, better—partner.

There is also reparative work to do in regard to self-concept. A symbiant tends to enter separation with a perception of self incorporated into h/h psyche through identification with the aggressor: I am an unworthy lover. Caught in the mirror of the other's rejection, the symbiant is apt to remain stuck on this note for a long time. So long as the disenchanted ex-partner's negative definition is introjected as to who h/s "is" as a mate, a symbiant will feel shorn of previous allure—desexualized and hence unable to attract or keep a fresh partner of suitable quality. Thus, a symbiant has to rebuild self-esteem after a crushing debacle, and this will take a series of experiences that are ego enhancing.

The course of the symbiant's recovery will likely find h/h swimming in many strange waters, but from a psychological point of view the most crucial are experiences that lead to questioning of hypergiving patterns. Indeed, sometimes the symbiant is thrust into the role of countersymbiant in new situations. In one such case, a woman still pining for an ex-husband finally began to date a serious new candidate for her affections, a man who relentlessly wooed her, promising that he would do anything to make her his. She was wary of the intensity of such ardor and cautious about being trapped by his pursuit. Nevertheless, she was impelled toward him: "It's the first time in my life," said this 41-year-old woman, "that I've allowed someone to pay attention to me. But I just don't know if I can love him." In so stating, she was now learning what the view is from the other side. This new perspective at last made her doubt that sheer devotion in love, useful and appealing as it is to its recipient, is what ultimately makes a committed relationship secure and enduring.

~ 5

Leaving

When the goal is separation, initiators cannot afford the luxury
of sentiment. . . . If they are affected . . . they dare not show it,
for the partner would take even the smallest signal as a possible
change of heart. [They] cultivate a stance toward the partner
that is sufficiently angry or benevolent or detached to allow
them to proceed to physical separation, insulating themselves
emotionally from the partner.

—VAUGHAN (1986, pp. 115–116)

THIS WAY OUT

"Leaving" is a project many countersymbiants have had under consideration for a long time. But no matter how each potential scenario is
rehearsed, the problem of doing it "right" still eludes solution. Many
aspects of the process seem laden with unavoidable anguish: imparting
the bad news to the symbiant mate, the impact on children, being
excoriated as the one who wrecked a family unit, finances, and so on.
A countersymbiant may be too compassionate or too fearful to go
through this ordeal—to be sure, many troubled marriages seem held
together by little more than a would-be rejector's inability to confront
the spouse with h/h wish to be out of the relationship (Kayser, 1993;
Lubetkin & Oumano, 1991).

To get out, a countersymbiant must pass a point of no return. It
is first of all necessary to develop a view of the symbiant as having
unbearable faults to justify the impending breakup, for as Vaughan
(1986) sarcastically noted, "it seems, we really cannot leave someone
we like" (p. 43). An assessment of the symbiant as an unworthy or

unsuitable mate now serves to override any feelings of compassion, so a callous or belligerent attitude is cultivated; Vaughan described cruelty on the part of many initiators getting ready to leave as they express their unhappiness by "irritability, drunkenness, rudeness, displays of temper, absences, silence, [and] withholding love" (p. 101). During the preparation phase, both decreased interaction with the symbiant and increased willingness to let negative feelings show have a dual purpose: to emotionally condition and toughen the countersymbiant to deliver the coup de grace, as well as to weaken the symbiant's resolve to fight for preservation of the union. The final step is to "go too far" in abusive or extrusive deeds so that a scene is set up in which the dread proclamation of breakup can be issued. At some point, at the initiative of either mate, planned or unplanned, some incident will trigger an encounter that sets the separation in motion. To succeed in getting free, the countersymbiant must be steeled—relentless in disregard for the mate's plight so as to get through confrontation and emerge from the grim scene with separation in hand. Whatever the stirring of sympathy, guilt, or dread, h/s must stand adamantly on the line announcing, "I don't love you anymore."

This is not the most felicitous of scripts. Indeed, telling a symbiant mate that the relationship is over is arguably one of the most searing endeavors to befall an ordinary person, and initiators can seldom fulfill this task without hurting. In the abstract, candor obviously has advantages, saying what has to be said and causing minimal confusion. But the mate's pain on being told of the breakup is increased by frank dialogue, for every statement that explains why the countersymbiant's commitment is being rescinded causes corresponding agony to the symbiant. No matter how resolved a countersymbiant may be to relate in explicit terms h/h discontent within the union, as well as current sexual–romantic aspirations, and no matter how much the symbiant asks to hear this information, the countersymbiant is prone to be overwhelmed by the symbiant's distress, prompting a glossing over of the most damning features of the narrative. Thus, to cushion the devastating blow, initiators tend to equivocate about their wish to escape the orbit of the partner by exaggerating reluctance to leave, affection felt for the mate, and intention to abide generously by financial and parental responsibilities. In the circumstances of enforcing a breakup, Mark Twain's aphorism comes to mind, that the truth is highly overrated.

Hence, many countersymbiants invoke a strategy that in some fashion aborts, curtails, or dilutes a wrenching separation scene, but not the separation itself. For example, despite affirmations that everything possible has been tried to make the spouse aware of a countersymbiant's unhappiness within the relationship, h/s may still depart with a startling lack of prior communication and scant warning. Accordingly, the leave-taking may be announced just prior to going through the door, or even afterward when "the incident that finally succeeds in getting the partner's attention may be the initiator's departure" (Vaughan, 1986, p. 104). Weiss (1975) made a similar observation about such surprise exits:

> It may seem unbelievable that the husband or wife . . . visited by these sudden announcements really could not have anticipated them. Yet individuals whose marriages ended in this way insist that they had no warning, received no hint or threat that they felt they should have taken seriously. And they appeared to be no less sensitive, no more given to denial, than others among the separated. Some of them knew their spouse to be . . . unhappy, although they did not suspect that [h/s] was contemplating departure, [whereas] others had thought their marriage was a good one—until they were told it was over. (p. 61)

As can be seen, one "out" for the countersymbiant is to make the barest announcement so that there is virtually no discussion that would delay or change things. In a very different "out," the notification may be sugarcoated to make it almost palatable when delivered. Thus, to contain or manipulate the symbiant's reactions, a countersymbiant wanting to leave on favorable terms may dissemble about motives and plans, project an image of being reasonable and considerate, and structure ongoing future dealings to offer some hope of reunion. Nevertheless, no amount of niceness, concern, or friendship can for very long totally neutralize a symbiant's perception that rejection by the countersymbiant is a hostile act.

Internally, a countersymbiant must deal with h/h own feelings in respect to crucial dimensions that determine just how the breakup is actually conducted. To begin with, the countersymbiant must set a comfortable *critical distance* that will ensure enough "space" to fulfill burgeoning new needs, while at the same time allowing whatever is desired of access to the safety, comfort, and supplies of the ex-mate. Further, *guilt* about abandoning family commitments will play a part. Where guilt is forthrightly faced, appropriate concern about the well-being of those left behind is shown, which requires more involvement. However, when guilt is not faced, there is a conviction that neither apology nor restitution for leaving is necessary, which translates into less concern and more entitlement. Finally, there is the issue of how to regulate *aggression*, which has complex sources and may reach irrepressible proportions. The sources of aggression start with the unforgiven problems that the mate ostensibly created in the marriage, setting a baseline level of anger at the symbiant as a "bad" partner. In addition, the countersymbiant's need for—and fear of—the discarded mate may be unconsciously responded to as if h/h own ego-dystonic dependency needs were the symbiant's fault, and at the extreme, even compliance with separate lives by the symbiant may be regarded as defection by a perceived parentified partner whose job it is to be there, no matter what. Thus, the real and projected faults of the symbiant combine to generate the countersymbiant's hostility, which is then made manifest after breakup in the actual punishment of the symbiant, perhaps going beyond studied indifference to the imposing of gratuitous humiliations and torments. In summary, all forms of disconnective anger are enacted to put more distance between the couple, which is needed by the countersymbiant to make the breakup workable. Yet at the same time, such distancing is often being used in the service of aggression because nothing hurts the symbiant more.

In the following review of various ways to break apart from a mate, these intrapsychic choices will be starkly evident in the program each countersymbiant forges for the kind of separation that will result. The course and outcome will reflect h/h need to vent hostility carried over from the marriage, to deal with guilt about leaving, and, most important, to set the critical distance boundary just so—certainly not too close and sometimes not too far.

THE CLEAN BREAK:
EXTRUSION

One often hears that the most humane way to leave a lover is for the parting member of the pairbond to refuse to have any more contact with the ex, except for necessary financial arrangements, legalities, and child visitation. The rationale for such a drastic mode of severing stresses that the ex-mate must not be permitted to have illusions about reversing the decision to separate; once the finality of breakup is understood, h/s will have no choice but to reorganize life on the assumption of a permanent split, with less suffering in the long run. Thus, it is counterproductive to keep in touch, show undue concern, or offer more than nominal friendship (at least in the early stages of a separation), lest these well-intentioned actions have the unwanted effect of increasing the longing of the ex-mate for restoration of the dissolved union.

Walder (1978), a psychoanalyst, has been a strong proponent of the "clean break," urging strict emotional disengagement in marital separation for the benefit of both parties. Walder depicted a sharp struggle around breakup in which the countersymbiant's caring and involvement tends to be elicited by the anguish of the symbiant; however much it hurt, the countersymbiant has to beat back the pleas and importunities of the symbiant and give priority to h/h own needs to end a bad relationship by refusing to take part in it any longer. Walder called for a militant attitude, stirring his target audience of the unhappily married with martial metaphors:

> There's no halfway measure. Either you break loose from your spouse or you don't! For this operation to be effective, you'll have to be prepared to see it through to the end! You may have to fight for every inch of ground. You may be in for a grueling battle. You'll have to mobilize all your resources. For a while, the outcome may be in doubt because you'll be tempted to retreat or to give up. But in the end you'll be victorious because you're fighting for a good cause—*freedom*! (p. 193)

In this war without mercy, the countersymbiant is counseled to react to h/h symbiant by "emotionally hanging up," interpreting all objections to breakup as the faintly disguised clinging of an ex-mate who fears autonomy. The misguided but wily symbiant can be expected to try to turn panic at the prospect of being left into interactions contrived to keep the countersymbiant enmeshed. Walder listed five categories of manipulation to this end, the first four of which are guilt, pity, physical illness, and threats. In order to avoid these snares, naturally solicitous feelings must be suppressed so that whenever the symbiant calls with problems or complaints, Walder recommended literally and figuratively "hanging up." But the fifth category, suicide, represents a more serious menace: "The survivor of a suicide may be plagued with guilt and remorse. The children of a suicide may feel responsible for driving their parent to it. The family of a suicide may be stigmatized by the community" (p. 190). Although Walder did not list the ex-mate's death as one unwelcome consequence of suicide, he thought this sort of entrapment had to be handled differently, for a countersymbiant could not practice emotional disregard toward a potential suicide without heightening the risk of its implementation. He therefore recommended that the countersymbiant assist the symbiant in developing a "lifeline"—a helping relationship with someone else, perhaps a therapist. By shifting responsibility for the ex-mate's well-being to another person, the countersymbiant could then safely get back to the usual pattern of "emotionally hanging up."

Although Walder claimed his tactics are ultimately useful to both parties, and he wished the symbiant mate well after divorce, he directed his support solely toward bolstering the ego of the countersymbiant. He reported that he advised his clinical patients to summarily quit an unhappy marriage and adopt an attitude of ruthlessness once out. He expected the compassion that might momentarily overtake these patients in the course of breakup, but he then immediately pointed out that divorce is a struggle in which no quarter can be given. In his estimation, the conflict's source could be traced to the noxious dependency of the symbiant and this person must be taught to be on h/h own. To impart this harsh but necessary lesson, the countersymbiant must resist being counted on in any way. Walder's rules of disengagement prohibited expressions of concern or tenderness during the separation, and "friendship" is not a word he cared to mention. He was always insistent that ending a committed union unilaterally is a bloody business—the squeamish need not apply. For example, in respect to property division within the divorce settlement, he worried lest the countersymbiant be "screwed by . . . guilt. [In this phase of battle, you must] know your enemy! Are you susceptible to feeling guilty? If you are, take your lawyer's advice!" (p. 217). In advocating confrontation over finances, Walder set up attorneys as agents who grant permission to countersymbiant clients to overrule any sentimental compunctions.

On therapeutic grounds, Walder sought to minimize the guilt and trepidation of countersymbiants struggling to achieve a marital separation. But, in so doing, he ignored significant psychodynamic issues in favor of fostering and condoning behavior that could aggravate already extant problems with commitment and empathy. Under the aegis of the "clean break," he elevated callousness to a matter of principle: ending a bad marriage was held to be akin to shooting a crippled horse—a decisive act to end unbearable agony. With this rationale, the countersymbiant could slough off criticism about being a cold, calculating person who stayed with a mate when beneficial, then cast that mate aside when expedient.

Despite disclaimers, Walder's disinterest in the symbiant's fate was never recognized by himself as provocative and hostile; he seemed unaware that the drastic disengagement he advised had anything to do with anger, emphasizing only that distancing is a technique to assert autonomy and to avoid enmeshment and misunderstanding. But this is disingenuous, for if "emotionally hanging up" is how one disengages, animosity is expressed and resentment from its recipient is inevitable. The symbiant will learn soon enough to "hang tough" so as to match the ex-partner in willful disregard. When this happens, as the ex-couple have occasion to deal with each other, a clean break transforms into a filthy brawl.

Further, although the clean break purports to guarantee decisive leave-taking, deliberate aloofness cannot achieve the dismantling of closeness–distance ties because the nexus of the couple continues in separation through what will soon be *mutual* provocations. Their getting apart may actually be prolonged by hostile machinations in which they somehow no longer "think" of the other when they are deliberately doing things to hurt the other. Moreover, this approach places such great mental strain on parting partners in their struggle to outdo each other in disconnective anger that it will never be a very popular prescription—it is just too bleak a demonstration of the brutality of divorce. Even when a clean break is intended, few among the population of those who disband their marriages sustain this policy. Drastic severing serves best the countersymbiant's mustering of concerted aggression to burst free of the centrifugal pull of the relationship, but once this aim has been attained, h/s is often willing to restore some contact. In addition, despite the advantages of a clean break, the majority of countersymbiants do not want to depart in an uncaring manner that leaks so much enmity beneath an outward detachment; most are sufficiently concerned about the well-being of their ex-mate that they do not just walk away and never look back. Still others desire the friendship of their ex and go to great lengths to bring about breakup in as prudent and considerate a manner as possible. There are also countersymbiants who want to keep open the option of a return to the marriage. All in all, countersymbiants rarely follow Walder's strategy. Even though, in a pragmatic sense, the clean break works (you do get out of your marriage), it can hardly be regarded as an ultimately humane way to leave your lover.

THE ESCAPIST APPROACH: UNANNOUNCED DEPARTURE

The most radical mode of breakup is abandonment of the marital ship, which immediately sinks. In frontier times, when divorce was hard to obtain, desertion was commonplace (Scanzoni, 1979). Yet in spite of the modern availability of divorce, departures still occur without notice, forwarding address, or financial arrangements; it is now just another way of leaving, conveying through acting out that the committed union has been unilaterally abrogated. With the sudden cutting of attachment ties, a countersymbiant "disappears" without having to bother with explanations and creating instant breakup as a *fait accompli*. An onlooker can only suspect that the abandonment is fear-induced: the countersymbiant must feel *terror* at the prospect of having to state in plain language an intention and a plan to leave. Indeed, anticipation of violent reprisal does motivate certain people to depart in clandestine fashion—the most obvious example is the woman who goes to a shelter so that her husband cannot beat or kill her for leaving. In such cases, an unannounced separation is warranted, though it would probably not have occurred in this way had another recourse been available. However, except for the common basis in fear, the "battered wife" situation usually does not fit into the pattern of marital desertion we are presently describing. In cases known to us, desertion seemed a counterphobic response to what was felt to be prior submissive behavior within the marriage; quietly slipping away was preferred to announced breakup because the symbiant appeared to be so overwhelming that confrontation was best deferred until one was safely out of range and could then call or write within the context of an existing separation. In her uncoupling research, Vaughan (1986) found that desertion did not alter the former mate's reaction to breakup, but geographical distance delayed an initiator's having to deal with that reaction and reduced susceptibility to any change of plan.

In terms of aggression, unannounced departures deliberately leave the symbiant paralyzed by doubt—wondering and worrying whether the missing partner is alive or dead, or whether the absence is voluntary or involuntary. This compounding of the inherent hurt of breakup speaks for itself, indicating not only a wish to get away from the symbiant but also a lack of respect for the other's needs or rights. This avoidant style of leaving is a kind of vengeance, for it humiliates the symbiant, showing, through acting out, the limits of the latter's control, as well as passive–aggressively punishing h/h for what is felt to have been a loss of autonomy in the marriage. At the same time, abandonment also presupposes the symbiant to be strong enough to manage alone. As for feelings of guilt, such concerns seem to play a negligible role in regulating the manner in which the countersymbiant conducts breakup.

Two case illustrations follow. First, a husband went to the bank, withdrew the balance of the couple's joint savings account, bought a motorcycle, and telephoned his wife several days later from 2,000 miles away to inform her that he had decided to terminate their marriage. This method of departure gave his wife no opportunity to dissuade him or to protect herself from his sense of entitlement to a better life at her financial expense. Second, a wife went off on a Caribbean vacation with her new lover, without telling her husband anything of her whereabouts, so that he, worried about possible foul play, reported her absence to the police as a missing person. A week later, she wrote and declared that she wanted a divorce, without any mention of the existence of her lover. The husband immediately replied that he was relieved to hear from her inasmuch as she was alive and well, but he was astonished at this turn of events because she had seemed so happy lately!

When a committed union is sundered by the vanishing of a partner, particularly if nothing is heard from this party for a very long time or ever, the leaving will ultimately be experienced by the deserted party as a selfish act perpetrated by a coward. It is certainly the utmost in lack of consideration: no arrangements have been made, spouse and children are thrown onto their own resources without preparation, and the family's emotional disengagement occurs in relation to a "ghost." In addition, the symbiant is left to speculate about what h/s might have done to drive the partner away or what should have been known about the partner's feelings. All told, the symbiant will not forgive the lack of caring or responsibility on the part of the absent partner, and this scornful attitude will be saved up until the couple meet again, by chance or necessity. For example, a man who had deserted his family some 5 years before turned up at their apartment after being tracked down and accompanied back by a teenage son. There was much curiosity about his activities in the interim, but he basically received a lukewarm reception from his erstwhile family. He appeared to be out of touch with the extent of the resentment awaiting him, saying that he had hoped they would be glad to see him and that it was always in his mind to come back someday and make amends. But the very confrontation with his wife avoided at the point of their breakup had merely been put on hold until this later encounter. She now insisted on talking to him about her many personal and financial grievances. He left abruptly and was not heard from again.

TRIAL SEPARATION: STALLING FOR TIME?

Living apart for a time, as a mode of separation, can be accused of inauthenticity. Consider Vaughan's (1986) description of initiators who state they temporarily "need some space," but say this in leaving merely to bring "the other person to accept the idea that the relationship is unsaveable, to force the partner to rely on outside resources, [and] to initiate the physical breach gently" (pp. 120–121). Yet in defense of trial separation, it may be the only formula that allows a particular couple to get apart without immediate trauma. The countersymbiant announces a decision to leave in a tentative or uncertain manner and asks for time to reconsider the relationship while h/s lives apart. The reason given for this request is that the countersymbiant needs to decide whether independence is what is really wanted; if not, h/s will return forthwith. In this situation, the symbiant may be all too eager to grasp at any ray of hope and thus acquiesces in this so-called experiment; the estranged countersymbiant is then able to pursue new relationships while simultaneously being waited for and courted by the symbiant. Because the countersymbiant can presumably go back whenever h/s wishes, the only gamble is that the symbiant will lose faith and become involved with someone else. Still, even this may suit the countersymbiant perfectly well, but if not, the risk of such an eventuality is remote because the least hint of eventual return goes a long way toward keeping the symbiant steadfast.

Trial separation preserves the cosmetic facade of a committed union, permitting each partner to cling to the vestiges of a past that once had substance and to envision a future as a reunited couple. But its present is something else again: the pair are far more separated than they are married. As Lubetkin and Oumano (1991) noted: "A trial separation is appropriate when you know you need space and . . . want to keep your options open. You're not absolutely convinced you want to bail out, but you are leaning strongly toward that decision. You need time and space to consolidate your choice" (p. 163). As can be seen, although a trial separation buys time for both parties inasmuch as each one has reasons to stall or to cling to an ambiguous status quo, the usual trend is toward divorce.

When a trial separation eventuates in breakup, there are ample grounds for retroactive suspicion that the countersymbiant has, at best, only let the spouse down lightly; at worst, it is sheer exploitation. If the countersymbiant never had plans to return, or reached that decision soon after separating, the symbiant feels duped and used. When the dire reality is finally exposed, reactions often occur because the symbiant may be unable to contain the long-stifled anger held in abeyance while there was yet hope of reconciliation. Woody Allen's film *Interiors* concerns a marriage in which the husband tells his wife that he is not quite sure whether he wants to be on his own, but can find answers only outside the home. He departs, soon meets another woman, and gets divorced. On the day of his second wedding, his ex-wife shows up at the ceremony and commits suicide on the premises. The man is then chastised by a daughter for stringing her mother along. She argues that throughout the trial separation, he knew he was never coming back.

As a means of dealing with breakup, a trial separation offers latitude to the countersymbiant to come to grips with ambivalence about the issue of leaving. This is true as far as it goes, but is usually quite misleading: *if the countersymbiant has real doubts about leaving, h/s does not.* Trial separation very often amounts to sleight-of-hand to ease a way out of the relationship without hurting the spouse too much (at least, not at first) or having to conduct a breakup as such. As the countersymbiant "provisionally" goes through the door, h/s may over-emphasize how hard it is to risk losing the spouse and that h/s may want to return once proper perspective is gained. The trial separation can thus be a useful artifice: the countersymbiant—looking confused and bereft—makes a perfect getaway by backing out.

In terms of distance regulation, trial separation offers as much contact with a symbiant mate as desired, but keeps the countersymbiant outside the centrifugal pull of the relationship so as not be drawn back against h/h will. Strong guilt feelings about hurting the symbiant may require a fitful type of leaving, with temporary reassurances if the symbiant becomes too distressed. But guilt notwithstanding, the aggression of the countersymbiant is marked: not only is the mate left, but placed in a tormented limbo for an indeterminate period. However hidden this hostility is by sporadic shows of caring, the symbiant is being cruelly *dangled,* pushed and pulled about with little control over h/h own life.

Are trial separations ever genuine? Theoretically, yes. If the partners make a covenant that the purpose of the separation is to test whether they miss each other, while giving attention to the ailments of their flagging union under less pressured conditions, the arrangement makes sense (Lubetkin & Oumano, 1991). Reunion is conceivable, though hardly assured. But if affairs are found to have secretly occurred during or, especially, prior to the agreement, a trial separation will quickly strike the symbiant as a sham, with definitive breakup as the most likely sequel. Consider the following illustration. A husband was rather suddenly left by wife and infant child; she explained that she had never lived on her own and needed this experience to "find herself." This she proposed to do by moving far away, taking a job, consulting her husband not a whit about these serious decisions, and leaving him to wait while charged with selling their old house. She conveyed to him her wish to resume the working marriage in about a year's time. He wrote her love letters, called frequently, and hastened to her side when she invited him for visits. He felt optimistic about the prospects for reunion, pointing out that his wife was facing financial and single-parent responsibilities that would make her a more mature partner. He observed a strict sexual fidelity, and his wife said she did too. The husband seemed virtually unaware of any resentment toward his wife for working out her "identity" by unilaterally forcing a trial separation; he lived for the future. On his third visit to what would eventually be their new family home, several incidents took place that raised suspicion that his wife had a lover. He even wondered whether this particular man had played a part in her decision to leave and to relocate where she did. He did not tarry to confirm his conjectures; instead, he met someone soon after and told his wife he wanted to divorce. His wife readily accepted his change of heart, and their marriage ended.

OPEN MARRIAGE: ENLIGHTENMENT OR HYPOCRISY?

It is possible for a couple to be emotionally divorced and still live under the same roof. In such cases, their estrangement may be covered by a fig leaf of "togetherness." Sometimes the couple has occasional sexual relations and view themselves as partners in a working marriage, but there may be much hypocrisy involved. This brings us to the concept of "open marriage" as set forth by Nena and George O'Neill (1972) in a best-seller by that name. The O'Neills burst into prominence when their book suggested that marriage is a flexible arrangement that can be altered by mutual consent of the partners to fit particular needs. It was widely assumed that they were advocating negotiation of marital fidelity; indeed, the term "open marriage" became synonymous with jointly condoned extramarital sex. It suggested that divorce could often be avoided if an open marriage format permitted both mates to be involved in outside affairs; partners would only have to state their respective sexual bents and then barter to reach mutual accommodations. The public ignored disclaimers from the O'Neills, and George went to his grave complaining that the book was never meant to legitimize adultery (*Time,* 1980).

Despite the popular interpretation of open marriage, there is a core to marriage that the parties cannot negotiate without compromising the meaning of marriage itself. For most people, this includes monogamous attachment, or at least the ideal of monogamous attachment. Couples tend to frown upon sexual affairs; seldom do they legitimize them by organizing a quid pro quo, because the elastic of marriage can be stretched only so far. The problems inherent in open marriage can be seen in Wolfe's (1975) study. She presented cases in which one marital partner is caught up in an affair, much to the distress of the other (pp. 199–215). Rather than give up the affair or go the divorce route, the adulterous partner puts pressure on the nonadulterous mate to find a lover of h/h own. This solution is one way for the partner who is unfaithful to deal with guilt, from which both will be exempted by mutual commission of the same marital "sin." And now, in this open marriage, a perverse outcome can ensue if an "accommodator," fearful to lose the partner, accepts the offer and so takes a lover too. This balancing often proves unsatisfying, because an affair is not what the accommodator really wanted. So the lover may be dropped, with the pretense afterward of going out with someone in order to maintain the illusion of reciprocity and thus keep the marriage functional. Wolfe notes that whereas in conventional marriage one hides an affair, in open marriage one may have to hide the absence of an affair! After a time, the perversity of the situation is revealed and divorce initiated by the accommodator follows.

What Wolfe pointed out is that open marriages are often not genuinely mutual: "negotiation" may be taking place for one mate at the point of a gun held by the other. In other words, a shocked and reluctant mate may be forced to accept this arrangement in order to keep the marriage. The aggression of this negotiation consists in making the mate complicit—perhaps the worst kind of humiliation.

The paradox of open marriage becomes evident in the renowned union between the French philosophers Jean-Paul Sartre and Simone de Beauvoir (de Beauvoir, 1984; Schwartzer, 1984). These lovers maintained an "open" relationship for 30 years; their disdain for the norms of bourgeois society was manifested by their agreement that neither was bound to the other. They made no vows of exclusive commitment, did not marry, had no children (although Sartre adopted one in later life), had numerous lovers, and were so protective of their independence that they hardly ever lived together (when in a hotel, they usually rented separate rooms). De Beauvoir insisted that the union with Sartre was her finest accomplishment. But their "beautiful" relationship was threatened as each became involved with a younger person. They ultimately renounced their paramours in order to preserve what was, for them, the more important value of their mutuality. But this is what monogamous ideals are all about!

In summary, open marriage very often turns out to be a euphemism for "closet divorce." The couple prefer not to live apart, although they may no longer sleep in the same bed, perhaps not even in the same bedroom, and sometimes do not come home at night. This arrangement can go on for years, perhaps indefinitely, as a substitute for separation or as a transition to separation. Until a breakup occurs, the shell of a marriage is maintained as they make no effort to hide their affairs and take pride in their lack of deceit and jealousy. But this is not to say that such emotions disappear—the partners cannot make emotional demands on each other for preeminent intimacy without risking the breakdown of the relationship. On a pragmatic basis, an open marriage works only if both partners are detached emotionally. Closeness–distance boundaries have to be set far apart, but then again, if there is too much space, the marriage itself is drained of meaning.

We can offer two examples of open marriage at this bleak level of alienation. The first involves a man who walked out on wife and children only to be run over by a bus. His wife, detecting divine intercession in his misfortune, took her husband home from the hospital to be lovingly nursed while broken bones (and marital disaffiliation) mended. However, the man insisted on staying in the basement, where he could recuperate without unduly disturbing the family unit. After his convalescence, he continued to live "at home" in the basement, going about his business as if he were a boarder. He did not hide the fact from his family that he had a lover whom he saw daily. He did not care what his wife did.

The second example comes from Spotnitz and Freeman (1964, p. 102). A man could not get his wife to agree to a divorce so that he could marry another woman. She had found out about his affair, but could not face the prospect of separation. The couple developed an accord whereby he spent late evenings with his lover and returned home to wife and children by 6:00 A.M. The marriage was retained in this fashion until his death 15 years later.

CLINGING/DISTANCING:
A BALANCING ACT

Although some couples contrive to be separated while appearing to live together, others seem to preserve their marriage while living apart. Weiss (1975) described how many couples in separation still have sexual intercourse several months after breakup, but we are concerned here with couples who do so far beyond any period of readjustment and even retain such relations exclusively with each other for years. Although they have dismantled the domicile they once shared, they still see each other frequently—often daily—to the confusion of the surrounding social network. The couple may even have divorced, but the relationship remains unchanged in its format before and after this technicality, as if the couple could not fit into any fixed definition of their marital status. Indeed, they are quasi-married, quasi-separated.

The pairbond has averted the problems of incompatibility they encountered while living under a common roof, now conducting their marriage from a more amenable distance. At this level of controlled proximity, they sustain enough intimacy to feel connected despite physical separation. However, this arrangement seldom comes about by mutual consent. Typically, a countersymbiant designs the format by leaving the marital abode, but not quite leaving the marriage. Meanwhile, a symbiant goes along with this program in hope of eventual full restoration of the marriage, but at the same time shows h/h own problems with intimacy by continuing to pursue a partner whose overall intent is to distance and thus, through collusion, demonstrates a fear of either being alone or finding a different kind of relationship where mutual closeness is possible. All told, as in trial separation, one partner is both married and single at the same time, while the other clings to whatever vestige of the marriage is available. Patterns vary enormously, but what all have in common in this type of semiseparation is that the couple have measured out the critical distance that allows the relationship to survive while they are living apart, but with a concomitant sense of still being married. As for logistics, whereas some countersymbiants go to a more or less distant town, others simply leave the conjoint marital residence to move back in with their family of origin, or take a nearby apartment.

In marriage across two households, the partners must often improvise to find time to be together. Sometimes the call of respective careers tends to take precedence over maintenance of a common abode, typically with one spouse choosing to accept a position in a distant locale while the other chooses to stay put. In regard to sex, monogamy may still be a norm in the relationship, with the couple going to a motel in some cases so as to protect their privacy from the scrutiny of disapproving parents or children, or, in contrast, they may pursue active affairs with outsiders and meet each other only sporadically or at prearranged vacation times. At certain points in time, the couple consider themselves "separated"; at other moments, they consider themselves as apart only by dint of more or less interim circumstances. The fact of breakup is an equivocal reality.

One young couple accepted respective jobs in two fairly remote regions. The wife was deeply unhappy with the marriage and had many affairs; she would have divorced if they had tried to coexist in a unitary home, but she did not find this necessary, because now the couple seldom saw each other. Another couple broke up and the wife moved a new man into her home, but the husband was ever hopeful of reconciliation. However, the original pairbond continued to see each other during his daily visits to the children, and they also were sexually intimate about once a month. Four years later, the wife put her new mate out and the former mate thought they would at last reunite. But she did not permit him to move in, and they went on as before, which as of this writing has been 3 years. Still another couple had severe problems getting along in a year together and so returned to live with their respective parents. They put their furniture in storage and "dated" on weekends. They went on in this vein for 4 years until the man left town without notice. The wife, working toward reunion, was furious and filed divorce papers. He reappeared after a year and wanted to resume where they had left off, but she now refused. A final example is a wife who asked her husband to leave but continued to see him every day during visitation of their child. They slept exclusively with each other and attended therapy. Three years later, they have sometimes talked about reconciliation and sometimes about definitive separation, but have actually settled for an indefinite truce until the wife has more resources to make a full break or until the husband regards his efforts to turn her around as a waste of his time.

As we have seen, a countersymbiant who wishes to leave a committed relationship has the prerogative to declare trump (the plan for the separation), and, for a time at least, the symbiant tends to follow suit. In this case, an ambivalent countersymbiant has fashioned an ambiguous separation that yields much of the freedom of living apart but still keeps the symbiant "dangled." Here it is the countersymbiant who appears to cling, not able to dispense altogether with the security represented by the mate or to cope with a wanted but frightening independence. Thus, the clinging countersymbiant *covertly* demonstrates much the same difficulties with dependency that are *overtly* problematic in the largely forsaken symbiant. In the end, such a couple hold onto each other for an extended period, carrying out a confusing compromise between marriage and divorce unless one of them ultimately calls a halt.

In a quasi-married, quasi-separated relationship, what seems like ambivalence in a partially distanced countersymbiant is very easily misread, and it usually takes a symbiant a long time to catch on. The countersymbiant may have many doubts about h/h ability to manage autonomously, but this is not the same as ambivalently wishing to reconcile. Clinging is not ambivalence—rather, it is making sure that one has a safety net. It has no bearing on reunion (other than in the symbiant's mind); instead, it represents the countersymbiant's need to hedge against failure, while at the same time obtaining succor in the course of what may be a protracted period of readjustment. Indeed, the countersymbiant may never be ready to dismiss the mate totally, but by the same token h/s is often even far less ready to reconvene the half-severed marriage. In this exploitation of the mate, aggression is expressed via an imposed separation and the lack of candor about actual intentions, and guilt feelings may be assuaged through shielding the mate (at least provisionally) from the rigors of full-fledged breakup.

THE ACCIDENTAL APPROACH:
AN AFFAIR TO DISCOVER

Not every discovery of a sexual indiscretion by a spouse is an "accident," for the unconscious often has a hand in these matters; as one initiator stated, "I didn't think so at the time, but now I wonder if I took my lover out publicly so my wife would catch me at it" (Vaughan, 1986, p. 102). However, Vaughan also noted that many initiators were far more deliberate in their intent to be found out. In being caught, the countersymbiant perhaps has little to lose (a marriage not valued very much) and much to gain (a way to leave by being thrown out). As they get more and more reckless in their pursuit of an extramarital affair, countersymbiants often express growing indifference as to whether they will be found out in their evasions, as if resigned to eventual discovery.

Note that on being apprehended as an adulterous partner, the countersymbiant who wants to be out of the marriage is not really on the defensive. The mate will be outraged by the affair, the deceit, the lack of character, and so forth; but the partner's profound alienation from the marriage, not the affair, would constitute the true discussion if the countersymbiant cared to offer a rejoinder. However, the latter may prefer to be silent on that subject, relying on the affair per se to stand as an unspoken comment on the quality of the marriage; while the mate scolds, the countersymbiant has made h/h case through the medium of acting out. As the couple explore the implications of the newly discovered outside liaison, they will be implicitly evaluating the merits of their marriage in comparison with what the countersymbiant has in the third-party involvement. Moreover, the countersymbiant whose conscious or unconscious intent is to be sent packing will not seem in the least contrite (although perhaps a little nonplussed), a reaction that infuriates the mate and may result in the countersymbiant's being expelled from a union h/s may not have known how to escape. Were it otherwise—if h/s did not want to be thrown out—the countersymbiant could express deep remorse and promise to quickly bring the affair to a close, or pretend to bring the affair to a close, or even propose that affair and marriage carry on as before since the mate has lived with the affair all along. In failing to make any of these moves, one can only infer that on some psychological level the countersymbiant wishes to be shown the door. All things considered, in situations such as this, the countersymbiant has a large measure of control, despite having to submit to being morally flayed as h/s goes.

The countersymbiant has permitted this method of breakup to come about because it offers a way to vent aggressive feelings toward the mate: dissatisfaction is implicitly conveyed, without having to relate wishes and plans to be out of the relationship. In addition, if the spouse opts to toss the countersymbiant out into the night, it is the mate who must take responsibility for the breakup, thus alleviating some of the countersymbiant's guilt. Also, by undergoing an embarrassing fall from marital grace, the countersymbiant throws a sop to the mate's wounded self-esteem by letting it appear that the countersymbiant is being well punished for h/h sins, further reducing the burden of guilt. As for boundary regulation between the now separated pairbond, the mate's jealousy can be exploited for episodic closeness and the third-party involvement is used to create more distance when needed.

A man came into psychotherapy because he was concerned about his going on sudden drinking binges for a week at a time, much to the detriment of his business and to the alarm of his family. When not drinking, he worked 7 days a week and was a model husband and father. The therapist suggested that the man *plan* his binges—work for a time and then go on a week's vacation—so as neither to upset his family by "disappearing" nor to leave his business to founder during an absence. The man explained that this was impossible—he had a girlfriend, and his wife would never let him go on vacation for a week without including herself! This reply was a turning point in treatment. The therapist pointed out that his discontent within the marriage could not come up as an issue because he and his wife agreed that his drinking was *the* problem, but there was a downside to this cozy collusion: the man could go on a spree with his girlfriend only at the price of being branded a "drunken bum" by his employees and family. The binges ceased after this interpretation. The man soon made a "stupid" oversight, and his ongoing affair was discovered by his wife. She threw him out, and he immediately moved in with his girlfriend. The new couple started a business together and, at last report several years later, he no longer had a drinking problem.

THE DIABOLICAL APPROACH: LET JANE DO IT

Vaughan (1986) discussed the relative powerlessness of women in marriage that allowed men to manipulate them into doing the work of breakup and bearing the responsibility for it. This chivalric factor that says "Let Jane do it" (p. 221) operates on the premise that women tend to want breakup less than men. When women walk away after a major rule violation by a partner, but still hoping for a reconciliation, they often find that their leaving is then used as an opportunity to dissolve the relationship altogether. However, Vaughan believed that women were just as apt to let men do the dirty work of breakup when the power differential favored them.

The "Machiavellian maneuver" is what we call a premeditated, cynical, and sadistic effort to manipulate the feelings of the mate until they coincide with a countersymbiant's hidden agenda—that is, inducing the unwanted mate to sever the union and assume the mantle and onus of "rejector." Tom Lehrer (1981) sang a ditty about how such a procedure looked to one very confused man: he became a little bit aloof when his girlfriend threw him off the roof, but then she swore they'd never part! ("The Masochism Tango," p. 55).

Machiavellian countersymbiants engineer and perpetuate an intolerable situation for the mate, confidently waiting until, in self-defense, the mate has no choice but to end the relationship. The oft-heard reply of such countersymbiants to any complaints by the mate is along this line: "This is how I am—if you don't like it, leave!" More privately, among their intimates, they boast they are deliberately following a policy specifically crafted to torture the partner into calling a halt to the union. Hostility toward the mate is disdainfully inflicted, but the countersymbiant will stick around so long as the mate takes what is dished out.

Paradoxically, here is a paradigm that tends to prolong any separation crisis ad infinitum, for the true rejector forfeits the role of rejector. If h/h mate is a masochistic hypergiver, as is not infrequently the case, the countersymbiant has a reciprocal who can absorb enormous abuse and still remain in the partnership. In terms of aggression, the ploy of daring the other into calling it quits allows the widest possible scope for the countersymbiant to weaken and humiliate the mate through treatment that is cruel, self-indulgent, and mendacious. This approach also enables the countersymbiant to achieve an apparent mastery over the stormy relationship that renders it safe and amusing to linger in it, no matter how heatedly the mate fusses and fumes. In such fashion, the countersymbiant has projected unwanted dependency needs onto the mate, selecting someone for this role whose abject attachment can be ridiculed and exploited, at the same time using counterdependent defenses to deny that h/s needs anyone and punishing the mate for having the hated trait of "dependence." The closeness–distance struggle between two such contrary partners is especially acute: the countersymbiant's strategy is basically one in which h/s behaves like someone unencumbered by a mate by coming and going at will, but at the same time demanding that the mate behave like an accountable married person. This guarantees strife characterized by threats to leave from each side, without anyone leaving now, or possibly ever. As for feelings of guilt, the countersymbiant refuses to take any responsibility either for maintenance or for termination of the relationship.

A man tried to drive his second wife away by heavy gambling, withholding money, and spending much time with his ex-wife, to whom he confided that her successor was receiving treatment much worse than he had meted out to her when he broke up *their* marriage! Another man contrived to have his wife spend much time alone with his best friend, with whose wife he himself was secretly having an affair. The naive wife and friend eventually fell in love, and the wife sheepishly asked for a divorce! A woman spent extravagantly, took a lover more or less openly, refused her husband sex, and had temper tantrums whenever he tried to talk with her about their problems; she argued that he could leave if he could not make her happy.

These cases portray sadomasochistic unions in which the countersymbiant will not alter abusive conditions and announces indifference to what the symbiant does about it. As long as the symbiant stays, the countersymbiant can make sport of the impotent, clinging reactions of the mate and still enjoy the more tender moments they share. Separation can occur only when the symbiant has had enough—and whatever that takes, a Machiavellian partner can probably be counted on to provide. If breakup ever comes, it tends to be tempestuous and even violent, for Machiavellian maneuvers offer fertile spawning grounds for lurid crimes of passion.

THE INSIDIOUS REJECTION: DESERTING THE PARTNER FROM INSIDE THE MARRIAGE

[Just as] the "I want to divorce" message may be the means to shape up . . . the other spouse, similarly, the "I don't want to divorce" message may conceal a wish to separate. . . . One partner here attempts to force the other to make the decision, [a strategy that allows that partner] to feel the victim, dissipate guilt, and/or act out angry feelings. (Rice & Rice, 1986, p. 148)

When a recalcitrant mate is pushed into becoming an involuntary rejector, the partner who has been left may consciously want the marriage to end (as in the Machiavellian maneuver), semiconsciously want to be thrown out (as in letting the mate find out about the affair), or unconsciously induce separation, as with the insidious provoker (the type we are concerned with in this section). Dissociated thinking is generally involved here: the gratification of a dark side of the countersymbiant brings about rejection by the symbiant, yet on the level of the countersymbiant's awareness any such rejection is vehemently protested and bitterly blocked. For this partner, *what is at issue in separation is h/h way of being*—a pattern of behavior that the mate now invokes to justify breakup, while the insidious provoker refuses to accept that such an adverse judgment is warranted (although largely acknowledging that h/h behavior is as described). In sum, while the insidious provoker resists breakup, h/h objectionable traits make the mate walk away with a sense of having been thrust out by an intransigent partner whose attitude seems to be that egregious faults or pathogenic patterns should be overlooked, forgiven, or just plain lived with. But this cannot be, since the life style of the insidious provoker is incompatible with the mate's maintenance of self-esteem and is therefore incompatible with the survival of the marriage itself. Although it is evident that giving up the pathogenic behavior is the sole way to prevent the mate's departure, an insidious provoker will not admit the necessity for change, or will pay only lip service to it, viewing breakup as an inexcusable injustice. Thus, a wife batterer will be remorseful afterward, but once forgiven resumes the behavior. Or a credit card addict will curtail spending after an event that ruins the financial position of the spouse, but finds surreptitious new resources for spending at the spouse's expense before the dust from the last argument settles.

An insidious provoker manifests somewhat different facets of narcissistic personality than an identity-seeking rejector. Unlike the latter, the insidious provoker's sexual–romantic needs are not to find a more exciting new mate elsewhere but to be loved and provided for by the present mate exactly on h/h own terms. For the insidious provoker, it is inconceivable that the mate could reach a degree of disapproval whereby there will no longer be compliance with the existing relationship as it has evolved over the course of the marriage. Given this outlook, rage occurs at any threat of breakup, because this implies that the insidious provoker is in some sense a defective partner; instead, the insidious provoker insists that the union as it stands is all-important, demanding that it be immediately reinstated if broken, and generally showing alarming signs of dire characterological disturbance after the loss of the mate.

Unlike the person who finds ways of making the spouse be the "bad guy" who brings about breakup (in which case the agent provocateur responds with little sense of loss and easily slides over into an equivalent relationship), an insidious provoker will actively try to prevent the mate from leaving or to coerce the mate back. Not only does the insidious provoker take on the role of the "rejected" in the marriage, but h/s does so as a fanatic convert to the Church of the Forsaken. Although it is undisputed that breakup provides a broad field for malicious and vengeful behavior on the part of all those who have lost their love objects, the insidious provoker is remarkable for irrational schemes of revenge; hence, the unleashing of raw aggression and the ensuing separation strife will be particularly vicious. A telltale characteristic of the insidious provoker in this struggle is that h/s will punish the ex-mate by intensifying precisely those behaviors that induced the walkout to begin with—as a means to compel or justify reunion! This behavior is more subtle and predictable than may appear at first glance, for while one hand reaches out to restore the relationship, the other hand continues to smite in the familiar, disconnective ways of yore.

A woman asked her husband to leave because he was spending all his time and money with friends away from home. His reaction was to break off all contact, including refusal to support her and their two children any longer—unless she came back to the marriage. A wife took her infant and left her apartment because her husband was conducting a flagrant affair. The husband was deeply upset by her departure and used every sort of pressure, including threats of violence, to bring about her return—but he also moved in with his girlfriend the day after his wife left. A middle-aged woman married for a second time, but then spent little time with her new husband because she was so emotionally and financially involved with her two grown sons and their families. She demanded that her new husband work extra jobs and give all his income to her so that she could buy a house into which she would also move her sons, their wives, and their children. When the new husband left her because they were virtually never alone and he felt that he was being "used," she urged reconciliation—the couple would go on a Caribbean vacation, of course taking along with them the grandchildren. A husband and wife went through years of marital discord, including several near separations, because of his virulent criticisms of her. Marital therapy was to no avail, and she finally took her child and left. He was indignant when she repeatedly refused demands for reunion, but meanwhile brought a custody suit against her as an "unfit mother."

The closeness–distance struggle pits a countersymbiant who is requiring unconditional acceptance against a desperate symbiant who cannot work out a relationship based on mutual concern. Although there are surely many ambiguous cases, in order to distinguish insidious provokers from other discarded spouses who may more legitimately be considered "rejected in love," we again point to the former's two most salient features: (1) if the insidious provoker underwent characterological change (or at least modified certain selfish or destructive behaviors), the loss of the mate would not happen, and (2) insidious rejectors typically seek reunion in counterproductive but characteristic ways that effectively preclude reunion.

THE FINAL COMMON PATHWAY

We have it on the authority of songwriter Paul Simon (1975) that many other ingenious ways to leave your lover exist. Our survey attempts to identify what seem to us the most common patterns. We realize that there must be other exiting techniques we overlooked, and that many individuals never fit snugly into any scheme of classification without overlap and mixed cases.

But all roads lead to Rome. The countersymbiant forges an exit, in whatever fashion. Because breakup is ordinarily a grim business, one cannot impose parting of the ways and then persevere through the ordeal of separation against the fierce opposition of a symbiant without the requisite personality structure. It takes a certain determined kind of person, with both the resourcefulness and the defenses needed to reach such a denouement, in present marital circumstances and at this particular point in developmental history.

❧ II

Jealousy

Introduction

> In 70% of the divorces included in one study, one spouse has been involved with another person during the final phase of the dying marriage. Such triangles obviously contribute to the decision to end the marriage. . . . As in the ancient rite of killing the messenger who bears the bad news, the extramarital lover can become the target of responsibility for breaking up a family and be blamed for the guilt and disillusionment that often follow.
>
> —FRANCKE (1983, p. 45)

South and Lloyd (1995) tried to estimate how often a third party (a "spousal alternative") was involved in divorce; they found that 40% of those in their sample knew their spouses had been unfaithful prior to breakup and another 20% were not sure. However, because only 15% of respondents said they themselves were unfaithful, South and Lloyd split the difference and came up with a figure of 31%. This is likely an underestimate, inasmuch as the rate could have been cumulative; they would then have arrived at the more usual estimate of about 65%.

On an emotional level, separating from a spouse in order to be with a lover produces a bitter breakup. Triangles beget jealousy—a vindictive and violent reaction to encounter in one's future ex-mate. If one must leave, a triangular exit may be expedient at first, but ultimately it is the most problematic way to depart.

As for the mate who is left, the power of jealousy and one's own susceptibility to it is typically underrated, especially if there is no prior history of such behavior. Despite a self-image of being "above" jealousy, this reaction to loss will almost certainly be experienced. Jealousy stems from attachment, yet it often takes the form of a destructive vendetta that injures both its object and its subject. No wonder there have always been social controls employed to prevent or reduce its malevolence and dangers. With our long experience as a species beset by sexual jealousy, can human nature really manage "civilized" reactions to triangular breakup?

Chapter 6 argues that our society has shifted its values so that any overt expression of jealousy is now condemned. Although jealousy is somewhat differently elicited from culture to culture and is to a degree amenable to changes in public attitude, it is currently suggested that jealousy never had to be viewed as an ineradicable part of the human psychosocial repertoire, rather, it should be interpreted as a sign of pathological insecurity, fueled by one mate's coercive efforts to "possess" the other and culminating in paranoid suspicion and schemes of revenge. Accordingly, as we start to probe jealousy in modern society, we enter into what many mental health authorities would characterize as an archaic world of madness. But perhaps jealous passion is a fine madness, upholding a vision of object constancy that stands in marked contrast to the "rational" view that humanity can transcend symbiotic attachments and remain largely unruffled no matter what breach of faith a partner commits.

Chapter 7 addresses the geometry of the eternal triangle, describing the respective roles of three principals who comprise an interactive system. Although one may get caught up in any of the three roles during the course of a lifetime, personality traits determine which role will tend to have the most "pull" for each individual over time. The common vicissitudes of love triangles are then explored, with the eventual outcome of each determined by the synergistic motives and character issues of the three protagonists.

Chapter 8 introduces the "defilement taboo": the jealous mate's refusal to deal with anyone or anything sullied by intimate and/or voluntary association with the rival. The rival is immediately seen as toxic, resulting in ostracism from the jealous mate's world. Moreover, because the rival supposedly defiles everything h/s touches, the jealous mate imposes a taboo on all significant others whereby they must not support or have friendly contact with the rival—on pain of becoming defiled themselves and therefore also ostracized. This ban applies to all those within the social network of the jealous mate, but a special exemption is made for a still loved unfaithful partner when seen alone or within a family context; however, if it turns out that the unfaithful partner is unwilling to give up the relationship with the "toxic" rival, h/s too will ultimately be ostracized by the jealous mate as "defiled." The taboo can become tragic when applied to the children of triangular divorce, for youngsters must usually relate to the unfaithful parent *and* h/h new mate. Thus they readily get caught in the middle of vicious and implacable separation strife as the jealous parent seeks to quarantine the "illicit" couple to the greatest extent possible, while the unfaithful ex-spouse and affair partner fight for the prerogative to be parents in their own right.

∿ 6

Infidelity versus Jealousy
Social History of a Dialectic

Anthropologist Lionel Tiger [states]: "If a relationship is good, it
is worth fighting for. Put it this oversimplified way: There will
never be a gene for sexual generosity. If jealousy had not served
an important purpose, it would have evolved out of the
species. . . . "

    In sharp contrast to Dr. Tiger, psychoanalyst Robert
Gould believes, "Jealousy has its roots in unhealthy patterns of
development. It is tied up with possessiveness and ownership.
As such, it is always pathological."

                                       —FRIDAY (1985, pp. 33–34)

Contemporary society, including its mental health arm, has increasingly
come to view jealousy as a malign condition calling for a "cure" (Friday,
1985, p. 15). In other words, jealousy has now become an emotion of
which one should be ashamed. Whereas 30 to 40 years ago the
unfaithful partner would have been regarded as manifesting a character
disorder, nowadays it is the jealous partner who is apt to be considered
emotionally disturbed and in need of therapy. Hence, a therapeutic
deconditioning of jealousy is being prescribed whereby the mental
health professional serves as the cutting edge of our culture's progressive disavowal of traditional standards of fidelity and commitment. The
passion of jealousy is being challenged at the cognitive level, pivoting
around the contention that lovers do not necessarily owe one another
exclusive and enduring attachment. In effect, jealous motivation now
tends to be attributed to neurotic possessiveness and lack of self-esteem
rather than to wounded love. The transformation in social attitudes
can be traced back to the Great Sexual Revolution of the 1960s.
Previously, jealousy had been taken for granted as an innate reaction
on the part of an actually or potentially wronged mate, serving to fend

off sexual rivals and at the same time upholding monogamous and reproductive rights. As such, jealousy preserved family stability by regulating marital interaction on behalf of what was pledged, established, and divinely ordained. As a guardian force in the maintenance of a firm domestic order, jealousy had its uses, although in crisis it tended to be expressed in grossly destructive and even violent ways.

The cultural upheaval of the 1960s brought about a revamping of values and mores. A new sexual ethos emerged that mandated such changes as "recreational sex," the legitimacy of "living together," "swinging," legalized abortion, no-fault divorce, serial marriage, gay rights, reconsideration of male/female sex roles, reduction of sexual guilt, and communes as an alternative family form (Comfort, 1974; Libby, 1978; Reiss, 1978; Smith & Smith, 1978). All these phenomena were consistent with Fritz Perls's (1969) unabashed call for everyone to "do your own thing." However, sooner or later the rising cult of unrestricted individualism had to collide with the existing institution of marriage. Whereas before this time jealousy had been a socially sanctioned, normative response based on the expectation that a mate should honor commitments, in contrast, the *absence* of jealousy soon became more adaptive to a changing culture wherein sexual–romantic unions were "open-ended" or "as long as love lasts." The generation of the 1960s learned to look askance at jealousy once it was reinterpreted as an illicit means of control, aiming to restrict a partner's autonomy as well as being a barrier to rational restructuring of family life. This new attitude vis-à-vis jealousy gradually gained ascendancy to the point where it appears that our society has tacitly agreed to relegating jealousy to the waste bin of history as "anachronistic," and in some respects "antisocial." Indeed, jealousy is now often regarded as a self-created problem. The jealous lover is likely to be told that it is foolish to resist adjustment to the fact that the partner has made another choice and has every right to be with someone else. As jealousy within our culture has steadily been stripped of intellectual and moral respectability without much public discussion, those so afflicted usually find scant sympathy and can project little personal dignity. This chapter proposes to show that jealousy has currently replaced homosexuality as "the love that dares not speak its name."

PSYCHODYNAMICS OF JEALOUSY

Jealousy is a passion that for a time dictates a way of life. Basically a mourning reaction, it simultaneously protests and seeks to undo a loss in love. By turning in rage on a partner perceived as unfaithful, the jealous person concretely demonstrates that such defection will be ruinous to both parties—and therefore cannot be or should not have been. Yet the very pitch of resentment and vengeance reveals the attachment still vested in the partner. Meanwhile, the jealous ego remains depleted so long as attention is fastened on the sexual activities of partner and rival, vicariously countering the sense of extrusion by planning ways to return hurt for hurt in order to enforce a crucial symbiotic point.

Jealousy asserts the prerogative to demand exclusivity and account-ability from the partner; it draws a boundary around the pairbond to ward off any intrusion into the sanctity of their union. When extrane-ous involvement occurs, ambivalent love and hate tend to be mani-fested toward the unfaithful partner: on love's side, heightened romantic interest because fear of loss tends to make the object more valued; on hate's side, suspicion, outrage, and reprisal, which are regarded as justified reactions to "cheating." Toward the intruder, however, unambivalent hate usually prevails, often marked by a refusal to have anything to do with this person, and sometimes extending to a need to drive off or destroy the rival, on the theory that *then* the beloved will return to the fold. But this expectation often proves to be patently incorrect.

Because jealousy avows that the partner's loss would cause unbear-able pain, it is commonly perceived as an indispensable and incontro-vertible evidence of love. As St. Augustine stated, "He that is not jealous is not in love" (Clanton & Smith, 1977, p. 9). Lovers often tease by initiating external flirtations to test the extent of jealous involvement, for without it the partner's interest may seem superficial. Moreover, jealousy makes a couple keenly aware of each other by generating excitement and ardor. It can even renew a stale marriage when a third party encroaches. Overall, "jealousy is a boundary-maintaining emo-tion" (Bernhard, 1986, p. 95) that affirms a relationship as too precious to lose.

On the downside, when jealousy rears up in earnest, the world of two mates suddenly turns ugly. System craziness ensues: the offending partner is considered guilty of crimes of betrayal, chicanery, and licentiousness, and the jealous mate may feel impelled to spy on, stalk, threaten, assault, or even kill the partner. Jealousy drives many actions by which an unpreferred lover expresses narcissistic urges to own, control, and monopolize the sexual–romantic attention of the partner. Forel (1933) traced such primitive human behavior back to barbaric times when males used brute force to hold females captive, noting, "It is ten times better to have an unfaithful husband than a jealous husband" (p. 117).

Indeed, once a third party invades across the boundaries of a couple, things tend to spin out of control for all three people. To start with, one marital partner has two ongoing love relationships; to keep this arrangement operative, h/s must juggle, assuage, and deceive. H/s may complain about demands, impositions, and claims for exclusive love emanating from the two suitors, which h/s may perceive to range anywhere from a passing inconvenience to an intolerable assault. In the face of these competing pressures, h/s may even be forced to make a choice and reject one. It will also be necessary to cope with guilt concerning the suffering imposed on others (the two rivals and possibly children) because of the existence—known or unknown—of a triangle. The end result is that an adulterous mate tends to espouse an anti-jealousy philosophy, trying to convince one or both rivals that jealous reactions are silly, pointless, counterproductive, spiteful, selfish, and so forth.

Meanwhile, the two adversaries in the triangle each seek to court their common love object and somehow dispose of the other. Either may become desperate and deliver an ultimatum to a dually involved partner to resolve the triangle, so that one of the rivals "wins" the competition for love. It is therefore the unselected suitor within the threesome who must pay for the ego satisfactions of the other two, and the price is a state of jealous anguish.

"NORMAL" AND "PATHOLOGICAL" JEALOUSY

Wittingly or not, mental health practitioners have now in effect shifted the stigma of "psychopathology" from an unfaithful, jealousy-fomenting partner onto the mate consumed by its torments. Yet before the current tendency to regard jealousy per se as a sign of emotional disorder, a distinction used to be drawn between "normal" and "pathological" reactions. Freud (1922/1957) based the normal form on the developmental grounds of the oedipal complex (the child's wish not to share the opposite-sexed parent with the other parent) and sibling rivalry (the child's wish to be preeminent among offspring). The child's grief at the recognition that others also have their claims on a parent will be compounded by that parent's preference at times to be with such competitors. In psychoanalytic doctrine, real or potential loss in adult life of an essential source of love reactivates the wounds of early childhood, and jealousy will be more or less severe according to how well this prodromal phase was mastered. However, because the oedipal complex and sibling rivalry are universal aspects of development, jealousy is so normal when there is real or threatened object loss to a third party that its absence implies failure to form deep attachments. In the Freudian view, "normal" does not mean that the jealous reaction is rational, just that it is spontaneous and natural, occurring in a situation of potential or actual alienation of the needed love object's caring.

However, Freud drew the obvious distinction between jealousy based on real loss and pathological forms of jealousy that often cause loss. He attributed the latter to ego-dystonic homosexual impulses projected onto a falsely accused mate constantly suspected of, and punished for, infidelity. The clinical trick here was to distinguish jealousy that occurred in an actual rather than an imaginary context, but the dichotomy at least gave therapists a conceptual hook on which to hang their hats. As a result, whereas pathological (i.e., delusional) jealousy was of clinical concern, normal jealousy (a reaction to loss of the love object to another) received sympathetic attention from psycho-analytic contributors to the professional literature into the 1960s. For example, Saul's (1967) endorsement of "normal" jealousy emphasized its biological, survival-of-the-species value. He noted that animals will tolerate other species in their demarcated areas, but fight off their own species of the same sex. "Jealousy signals a threat to one's mate and young and home, and to all the powerful needs for love and depend-ence" (p. 161); thus, a "jealous" animal will fight with more courage than any rival. But jealousy is also painful, and Saul regarded the infliction of jealousy by humans as an act of cruelty. According to his position, jealousy is a useful sociobiological emotion that should not be a serious concern for a well-adjusted couple, but when jealousy does occur, Saul insisted that it pointed to character disorder on the part of the adulterous partner.

Also citing phylogenetic evidence to advance the proposition that jealousy is instinctive, Ardrey (1961) held that what he called the "territorial imperative" is an innate predisposition with eugenic func-tions in social primates. He argued that human beings have these ancient strivings within them, harking back to a mammalian social order wherein an alpha male and an alpha female fend off less well-endowed rivals to their exclusive reproductive domain—an arrange-ment conducive to the survival of the species.

In the social sciences, the staunchest defense of "normal" jealousy came from sociologist Kingsley Davis (1936). He argued that jealousy cannot be considered an instinct—on the contrary, it is socially incul-cated to protect the "sexual distribution of property"; it is also not antisocial, because society needs it. Davis made a solid case for the social construction of a passion. He started by asserting that it is not adultery that provokes jealousy but rather *standards of monogamy*. When one enters the role of "mate," one brings to it socially prescribed notions of rights, duties, and status, including the privilege of unshared sexual access to the partner. A third party thus trespasses on sexual property. Jealousy deters, warning those who might stray of the fearful consequences in store for them and their lovers at the hands of a spouse–cuckold. Davis believed that society expects, demands, and condones jealous reactions as a means to sustain the institution of marriage. The jealous mate personifies society's indignation at the violation of its norms and values. People are socialized to feel jealous, they cannot help but feel jealous, and they then become society's instrument for the punishment of those who have transgressed against established community norms. Davis went on to show that jealousy can be regulated and modified by social stratification, as in the medieval custom of the lord of the manor taking all new brides as his own on the wedding night (*jus prima noctis*) or in cultures in which men can "lend" their wives to visitors, thus making clear that a wife is the husband's property to do with as he pleases. In short, societies require jealousy to uphold marital boundaries, though what constitutes infringement that can elicit jealousy varies across classes, cultures, and epochs.

The traditional view of jealousy as a normative response to object defection has not been ideologically refuted or abandoned. Instead, a competing philosophy depicting even normal jealousy as pathological has vied with the traditional view until, as with money in Gresham's law, the newly minted theory has more or less driven a more venerable one out of circulation. This process is first glimpsed in the work of Sokoloff (1947), a psychiatrist. He still regarded jealousy as "normal and universal," but Sokoloff restricted normal jealousy to a temporary state—an emergency response of the organism to the shock of object loss. Like fear and anger, it was instinctive behavior based on adrenal–sympathetic activation. Jealousy was thus a stress reaction uncontrollably experienced at the traumatic moment of loss. However, when a mate afterward became jealously obsessed, Sokoloff held that a morbid predisposition was revealed, triggered by the partner's infidelity. Prolonged cases of jealousy indicated an absence of love, in that it was a contradiction to wish harm on a "loved" partner and it was rank self-indulgence to behave vindictively. Thus, jealousy was a condition in which wounded pride led someone who cannot love to demand to be loved; La Rochefoucauld has said that jealousy springs more from love of self than love of another. All told, in Sokoloff's view enduring (but in other respects valid) jealous reactions were roughly equated with a temper tantrum toward getting one's way—or else!

Sokoloff's presentation of enduring jealousy as selfishness masquerading as love bespeaks a Platonic approach in which love is real only if it meets *abstract criteria*. Instead of starting with naturalistic observation of how human beings love according to their needs and drives (the apposite approach for psychiatry), Sokoloff exemplified a tendency in our culture to define love on an ideal basis, along the lines of "unconditional positive regard." By this standard, any behavior is excluded from love's purview that does not fit a model of altruistic involvement—hence, love worthy of the name is seen only as caring that carries forward no matter how the partner behaves. In consequence, possessive or vituperative traits associated with jealousy cause such emotional reactions to be denigrated as non-love, because this behavior does not jibe with preconceived notions of what love should be. We characterize such a perspective on love as an effort to make the real conform to the ideal, or philosophy imposing on psychology.

The psychodynamic view is quite different: love evolves in a setting in which disparate human beings create, identify with, and become subsumed under a conjoint "we." Its essence is symbiotic attachment to a needed object invested with special attributes and importance. Love can occur without the object's consent, but it deepens when its object has fostered expectations of mutual caring. Sexual–romantic involvement with a reciprocal now means that this person's actions become invested with enormous import—both positive and negative— for one's well-being, as two interdependent entities push and pull at one another to have the relationship each desires. The crucial connection to the partner is reinforced over time and will not dismantle easily, even if the partner dies or goes away.

Because there is so much personal implication inherent in what a beloved does, especially when the relationship itself is on the line, measures taken in jealousy are readily understood by both parties as affirmations of the significance of the union—indeed, the jealous mate makes this statement for both. Sokoloff has it backwards: jealousy for which there is a valid basis results from non-love in the object rather than in the subject! To stigmatize jealousy as "selfishness" is a truism that clarifies little, for every human action betrays egoism—jealousy and even love included. The jealous mate often has some awareness that h/s is overwrought, malicious, inconsistent, and driving the partner away. Yet h/s usually feels compelled to act in this way because deeds of jealousy, in their fashion, avow the sacrosanct nature of the couple's bonds. It seems contrary to what is known about human nature to expect that any person who claims to love another will thereby be converted into a selfless angel vis-à-vis h/h partner.

Our objections aside, Sokoloff proved to be a forerunner of the direction cultural developments were to take. During the social ferment of the 1960s, reference to jealousy all but ceased in the mental health literature. Of the work published on related topics, jealousy tended to be mentioned only in passing as a pathological reaction denoting a preexisting psychological problem, just as Sokoloff had argued. Thus, Socarides (1966), a psychoanalyst, traced the roots of revenge (covering jealousy under this rubric) to the deepest traumata of childhood. Whereas Freudians emphasize developmental factors in the genesis of current symptoms, Socarides virtually discounted the present situation altogether, viewing it as simply an eliciting occasion for preexisting disorder rather than as a causative occasion in its own right. Hence, in respect to jealousy, he did not consider the unfaithful partner's actions, the relationship's history, or the community's mores in reaching a diagnostic judgment. And, of course, he did not explore the social ramifications of a leading clinician like himself postulating that jealous behavior per se indicated early emotional disturbance and a consequent need for long-term treatment. In short, Socarides was unwittingly fostering the psychiatric shrinking of the passions, at least so far as jealousy was concerned. As harbinger of the new outlook, he was already serving notice that vindictive aspects of jealousy would no longer be therapeutically countenanced.

What was happening in the mental health field paralleled trends in other disciplines. In sociology, Bernard (1977) declared that the Clanton and Smith anthology, *Jealousy*, was the first significant volume on the topic since the classic exposition of Kingsley Davis in 1936. She believed that in the interim jealousy had lost much of its appeal as a theme to academics as well as to contemporary novelists and dramatists, ascribing its lack of topicality to alterations within the culture that influence what scholars, researchers, and artists address:

> Marriage has apparently changed so markedly with respect to sexual exclusivity that jealousy is no longer viewed as a necessary prop to enforce it, and hence it becomes of relatively little interest. Community support for the norm of sexual exclusivity which jealousy formerly buttressed has itself suffered serious attrition. (p. 141)

According to the editors of *Jealousy*, the same neglect of jealousy as a social issue could be observed in women's magazines:

> Toward the end of the 1960's, the trickle of articles on sexual jealousy was interrupted. The magazines were relatively silent on the subject from 1966 to 1973. It is as though writers, editors, and publishers sensed that jealousy was changing somehow, that jealousy was becoming problematic in a way which worked against a continued dispensing

of conventional wisdom. After this lull, articles ... typically took account of a new concern: they began to question the appropriateness of jealous feelings in marriage. It was no longer assumed that jealousy was evidence of love. For the first time *guilt* about jealousy became an issue for large numbers of people. (pp. 15–16)

Thus, as the mass media press shifted its presentation after 1973, under the new sexual ethos not only was jealousy no longer of public interest, but alternative conceptions appeared that were designed to repress or outlaw jealousy. The contrast can be seen in passages from two articles in Clanton and Smith (1977). In "Confessions of a Jealous Wife," Viorst wrote in the traditional vein: "A man who wasn't attractive to other women, a man who wasn't alive enough to enjoy other women, a man who was incapable of making me jealous, would never be the kind of man I'd love" (p. 24). Here, the pain of jealousy is worthwhile because it signifies that Viorst is still in love with her husband. But in "Taming the Green-Eyed Monster," Lobsenz urged examination of pangs of jealousy as clues to personal problems:

In all its manifestations, jealousy springs essentially from self-doubt, a lack of self-esteem, feelings of inadequacy—all the things psychotherapists lump under the heading of "low self-image." [To convert such jealousy] from a negative to a potentially positive reaction requires that we stop concentrating on what the other ... is doing [and] turning one's attention to one's self [to] ask: "Why is my self-esteem so low in the first place?" (p. 34)

In fine, whereas Viorst saw jealousy as part of the process of loving, Lobsenz wanted to psychotherapize people like her out of the neurotic "inadequacy" that underlies jealousy. He envisioned close relationships free of jealousy as a feasible social goal—irrespective of the partner's behavior. To make his position credible, Lobsenz trivialized jealousy; his examples in the main concerned flirtations that incite jealous reactions rather than more ominous situations in which one's partner leaves for another or is discovered in a surreptitious affair. Even though Lobsenz described only the kindergarten of jealousy, even such relatively innocuous practices as flirtatious teasing can be serious in the sense that they portend the pain that would be caused if more consequential breaches in fidelity and commitment were to occur.

Under a new sexual order in which serial love relationships are normative, jealousy must be pruned to fit a new landscape. As Toffler (1970) suggested, modern existences are speeded up so as to compress several lifetimes into one; "future shock" has to be handled with aplomb for one to remain adaptive to fluid conditions. In this vein,

Carl Rogers (1977) described the new requirements for the "emerging person" in the modern world:

> These persons are seeking new forms of community, of intimacy, of shared purpose. . . . There is recognition that personal life will be transient, mostly in temporary relationships, and that they must be able to establish closeness quickly. In this mobile world persons do not [stay in one area, nor] surrounded by family and relatives. They are part of the temporary society. There is a realization that if they are to live in a human context, there must be an ability to establish intimate, communicative, personal bonds with others in a very short space of time. They must be able to leave these close relationships behind, without excessive conflict or mourning. (pp. 270–271)

Rogers was lionizing the countercultural "flower children" of the late 1960s as role models for future generations. Note that in these "expedited lives" jealousy has no place—the conception of "closeness" derives from the instant intimacy of encounter groups as well as the transient, informal ties of communes. Mazur (1973) added the twist that jealousy is an attempt to force permanence on the natural flow of relationships, at the expense of intimacy:

> Jealousy can be just plain fear: fear of losing someone special, fear of being lonely, of being rejected. To the extent that one's own value depends on a partner's devotion, one will be vulnerable to the fear of desertion. If there is a classic form of jealousy, this probably is it. . . . The strongest and most joyful relationships are those in which partners are not afraid to let each other go; attempting to control the duration of a relationship because of insecurity sacrifices the magnificence of every *now*. . . . Let the future take care of itself. (p. 17)

A dissenting cry of warning, however, was sounded by Durbin (1977), who was virtually the sole countercultural voice to speak for the inviolability of committed unions, including the despised jealous feelings that she complained had become "the new Sin of the liberated generation." She depicted her compeers' attitude as follows: "To be jealous is to be a kind of capitalist pig of the heart: you're being possessive, treating your lover like a piece of property with 'No Trespassing' signs posted along the fence. You are, in other words, politically incorrect. Shame on you" (p. 38).

Durbin tried to accept the new ideology, but she always came up against her own deeply personal need for a binding union with a man, with old-fogyish jealousy as her response to any threat posed to that relationship by another woman. A confrontation around this issue occurred with a male friend who took offense when she said that, on feminist grounds, she could not think of having an affair with a married man because she would be hurting another female:

> He really blew up on that one. "That's none of your business," he said emphatically. "You're interfering with the relationship between that man and his wife when you start feeling guilty about her! That's . . . emotional imperialism." *Emotional Imperialism?* I left the conversation feeling guilty because I'd felt guilty. And trying to figure out why it's not interference when I sleep with someone's husband, but it is interference when I feel guilty about it. This new morality was obviously going to be even trickier than the old one. (p. 38)

But Durbin's was a voice in the wilderness. The cultural currents she resisted have swept in the consensual view, popular and professional, that jealousy is pathological behavior because it infringes on the autonomy of others. Moreover, the belief that "secure" people are jealousy-proof has almost taken enough hold to make us aspire to never being alarmed about losing a partner, or to a rapid recovery of emotional equilibrium even if we do.

The most radical anti-jealousy polemic has come from Cooper (1970), a British psychiatrist who espoused group marriage and the communal family. Jealousy was the bane of the radical communes of the 1960s, prompting numerous breakups of otherwise congenial comrades because of the "bourgeois" tendency to pair off, with resultant sexual competition. Cooper (pp. 43–64) described four cognitive approaches he used in his ideological and clinical interventions with commune members afflicted by jealousy:

Approach 1. Possessive love is a parasitic relationship. *A*'s love for *B* is really love for a representation of *B* in *A*'s mind. In the so-called happy marriage, persons *A* and *B* disappear into a composite personal entity *A–B*. When *C* comes along, fracturing the symbiotic *A–B* pseudounity, *A* is thrown back into a separate existence and becomes responsible for forming relationships on an equal basis. *A* does not own *B*, but wants to act as if this were so.

The pivotal statement here is the stigmatizing of jealousy as "parasitic"—such attachment is seen as engulfing and exploitative. *B* can be with *C* because no consonance is owed to *A*'s expectations, regardless of previous pledges and involvement. Cooper then moved to a moralistic precept—*A* has no right to expect different from *B*! Substituting philosophy for psychology, *A* "should" not be jealous, thus imposing on *B*'s rights. In legislating *A*'s feelings, Cooper assigned the prerogative of having rights to *B*.

Approach 2. Cooper believed we are victims of the illusion that love is quantifiable. We have been taught that we have only so much love to give, so that if *B* loves *C*, there is less (or none) for *A*. Cooper proclaimed this to be "naive algebra," for lovemaking would then represent depletion instead of enrichment. He argued that the more sexual relations are fulfilling (and this may require a variety of part-ners), the more one's ego is enhanced and the more love one has to distribute all around. Again, *A* "should" not be jealous that *B* has *C* because union *A–B* will benefit from *B*'s growth in capacity to love. Relationship *B–C* is not necessarily a threat to *A* and may make it possible for relationship *A–B* to survive, or even thrive, because of the infusion of joy into *B*'s life.

Despite his training, Cooper rejects the psychodynamic view that infidelity can express hostility against the mate, rather than love.

Approach 3. *A* fails to acknowledge a debt of gratitude to *B* for becoming involved with *C*:

> If one traces back the history of the relationship, the point of the partner having the affair that the other did not "know about" was often a point of liberation in sexual and relationship terms for the other (the "betrayed" one). But the divorce carries on, of course, because there is false resentment instead of real gratitude. But then the only evil of divorce is the prior evil of marriage. (p. 49)

Again, *A* "should" not be jealous, because *B* has emancipated *A* from monogamy, which *A* did not have the courage to appreciate. *B* has vicariously met *A*'s unconscious needs for sexual liberation, which could surface only in response to *B*'s infidelity. Jealousy is thus a cover-up for envy of *B*'s sexual freedom, and *A* can now likewise indulge with multiple sexual partners and—as a bonanza—project blame onto B!

Cooper depicts *B* as a scapegoat for the monogamous mate. He thinks *A*'s best way to deal with grief is to have an orgy as soon as possible—which is what h/s secretly desired all along.

Approach 4. *A* is repressing homosexual wishes toward *C*, and if they had an affair, *A* and *C* "could have a good or at least clearly seen relationship between themselves" (p. 46). Cooper arranged on several occasions for such liaisons and reported good therapeutic results. He thus advocated the bisexual triangle as the "cure" for jealousy and identified mental health as *A–C/B–C*.

In making this particular argument, Cooper has taken Freud's position concerning the unconscious dynamics of delusional jealousy and perversely applied the theory to *all* jealousy. In such merging of "normal" and "pathological" jealousy, gratification of an ego-dystonic homosexual wish is a prime focus of therapy.

In review of Cooper's four approaches and his influence on the mental health field, it is clear that hardly any clinicians then—or now—agree with most of his ideas; his work has received little serious attention. Nevertheless, his theoretical stance is extrapolated from prevalent trends equating jealousy with mental disturbance. His position thus incorporates currently acceptable but largely unformulated views on jealousy, although at the same time it is a *reductio ad absurdum* of those views. Hence, it seems that his stance is studiously ignored because his outlook, however extreme, is an embarrassing sign of the times. In the current social climate a jealous mate must now contend with a surrounding culture that seeks—in the name of "mental health"—to legislate feelings, reshuffle involvements, and inure to object loss. It is no longer sexual longings that must be repressed (as in Freud's day) but object constancy. As Durbin (1977) exclaimed, "Have we all gone . . . mad? What sort of liberation is it that leaves us apologizing for our passion?" (p. 40).

When Friday (1985) surveyed the literature and interviewed leading therapists, she reported her impression that jealousy is nowadays often regarded not so much as a passion but, instead, as a misguided idea. Nevertheless, Friday concluded that jealousy was still very much around. She was quite correct in this conclusion. In a poll of the readership of *Psychology Today*, Salovey and Rodin (1985) received 25,000 replies largely confirming the ubiquity of jealousy in relationships, with negligible differences for race, class, and gender. In addition, White and Mullen (1989) cited a nationwide survey of marriage counselors, according to which jealousy was a major focus of counseling for one-third of client couples, up from 15% in a similar 1970 survey—an increase that suggests that as committed unions have become less inviolate, the more jealousy becomes a clinical problem brought to therapists.

INFIDELITY: THE OBVERSE SIDE
OF THE JEALOUS COIN

The classic adaptation of the person restless or unhappy in h/h committed union is the affair. Affairs range from furtive one-night stands (intended to supplement the union) to an intense new romance that competes with (and may finally supplant) the union. According to Hunt (1969), boredom—sexual or otherwise—is the chief precipitant of an extramarital affair. He reported that some spouses contended their flings hurt no one or even improved their marriages. Others said they needed the affair to render their marriage bearable and to ward off divorce. In the vast majority of his cases, affairs were discreetly conducted and the extramarital lover was given up if perpetuation of the affair posed any threat to the marriage itself. Even when a third-party involvement actually became the occasion for breakup, only half the divorce initiators married the lover for whose sake the marriage was apparently ended.

Hunt concluded there are two types of marriage: the romantic–puritan based on monogamous ideals and the pagan–courtly in which there is no expectation of fidelity. In the former model, adultery has implications regarding the marriage's viability. In the latter model, adultery is expected and may be necessary to the marriage's survival. But Hunt did not deal with the rather common situation in which one partner is in one model, while the mate is in the other!

Traditional psychiatric opinion has disapproved extramarital affairs. Caprio (1953) stated, "Infidelity, like alcoholism or drug addiction, is an expression of a deep basic disorder of character" (p. 7). Saul (1967) said, "Infidelity is often a neurotic . . . pursuit of exactly the [person] one imagines one needs. It is primarily a return to behavior characteristic of adolescence or earlier" (p. 144). Spotnitz and Freeman (1964) maintained, "Infidelity may be *statistically normal* but it is also *psychologically unhealthy*" (p. 28). Strean (1980) granted that mankind is biologically polygamous, but "an extramarital affair is *never* a healthy or mature act" (p. 202). These clinicians made distinctions between types of marriages, but they still assumed that even an open-marriage covenant is already symptomatic of psychopathology. Their point of view is that engagement in infidelity is a sign of a troubled personality unable to handle intimacy. An unfaithful partner does not work with the mate on problems of mutual concern but instead secretly goes elsewhere for compensation and support, at the same time punishing the mate for felt sexual–romantic deprivation within the marriage. From this stern traditional perspective, an affair can never be considered a harmless, let alone helpful, addendum to a marriage.

But in the Great Sexual Revolution, adultery, like almost all other forms of sexuality, has become progressively purged of guilt. Prior to this period psychiatry replaced the religious injunction against adultery as a "sin" with an equivalent psychological taint by which adultery became "character disorder." Since the 1960s, however, American society has slowly relinquished any psychiatric onus. Of course, the traditional view is still around and those inclined toward adultery must deal with the culture's ethical conflicts and confusion about the psychic import of such behavior. But the overall trend is clearly toward relaxation of standards mandating lifelong monogamous commitment. The AIDS epidemic has complicated this situation by making sex with new partners suspect, but people are not necessarily faithful these days predominantly out of monogamous commitment, and they are also less apt to accept psychiatric stigmatization of adulterous behavior. It has now become strikingly unusual to read comments in the professional literature like that of Mullen (1991), who stated that in spite of the decline in monogamous practice within society, jealousy still retains interpersonal meaning and social relevance because it is a response to infidelity, which Mullen insisted has a *moral* aspect.

Whitehurst (1969), a sociologist, exemplifies the contemporary revision in thinking about infidelity, basically stripping away any moral connotation. He held that ethical strictures around sexuality must be broadened so that people are not too readily labeled as "deviant." He panned mental health workers who ascribed adultery to a wish to be "partly single and partly married," while discerning at its core "sick, immature, narcissistic, neurotic, hostile, and maladjusted motivation denoting evil." Whitehurst went on to complain that "this type of social definition is . . . moralistic—it purports to separate the good guys from the bad guys" (p. 130). He countered with the contention that adultery is a natural outcome of marriage, where time takes its toll in the importance of the relationship, and the mates eventually tend to go in somewhat different sexual directions—without either being the "bad" guy.

Whitehurst also derided the psychiatric interpretation that an unfaithful spouse may be reacting to a negligent partner. In this way, he argued, infidelity comes to be seen as a symptom of unmet personality needs—which is true as far as it goes. But, Whitehurst said, nearly all human behaviors are a result of unmet personality needs and therefore this slanted approach explains little.

Whitehurst wanted the stigma conveyed by the term "infidelity" removed, so he preferred the more neutral "extramarital sex." However, to place an affair beyond reach of moral judgment, he had to consider it out of interpersonal context so that the event is empirical data—something that just "happens." He disallowed any psychodynamic inquiry into motivation and limited his research to the purely statistical, normative, and descriptive. Yet despite his efforts at a detached objectivity, the position of Whitehurst contains an intrinsic value judgment: he intimates that any condemnation of extramarital sex is unjust because only the institution of marriage can be properly blamed for its existence.

Although Whitehurst lent a sort of legitimacy to extramarital sex by framing it as a normal response to marital entropy, it was but a short step to advocacy of infidelity as a mental health boon. In "The Positive Values of the Affair," English (1971) took this step:

> It is often the affair outside of marriage that prevents the neurotic marriage from being made and neurotically maintained, and doubtless at times has prevented mayhem or murder, divorce, or complete disillusionment or misery to the children of this despotically neurotic enslavement to social form called "marital fidelity." (pp. 191–192)

Despite its having been written by an eminent academic psychiatrist, this passage is so polemical that it is tempting to dismiss it. For example, the word "neurotic" is thrice used, implying that mental dysfunction is the inevitable outcome of conformity to monogamous social norms. The need to diatribe against constraints of fidelity is so powerful that English even commits a non sequitur in speaking of an "affair outside of marriage" before the marriage has been made, but what was intended here seems to be that the couple should be openly unfaithful before and during marriage to forestall any imposition of sexual monopoly by either mate. However, despite dogmatism, the anguish of guilt-ridden lust and forgone pleasure can easily be read between the lines of English's text. In reaction to the loss of opportunity and perhaps sexual deprivation imposed by a mate's demands for fidelity, that mate runs a great risk of being resented, if not hated. In the final analysis, English bears poignant witness to the possibility that marital fidelity can cause suffering for one mate as does jealousy for the other. The problem with English's position, from our vantage point, is that he treats jealousy as a manacle on the wrist of the would-be unfaithful partner and not as a sorrow for the mate.

The use of a mental health rationale to celebrate adultery reaches its apogee in Albert Ellis's *The Civilized Couple's Guide to Extramarital Adventure* (1972). This psychologist elevated pickups, casual affairs, and inveterate promiscuity to the status of refined accessories to the sophisticate's primary love relationship. In his view, guilt is superfluous and jealousy is "the partner's problem." Despite warnings to avoid extramarital sex to those who "can't handle it," Ellis still managed to convey that a spouse must be neurotically inhibited to pass up the benefits of a robust affair.

According to a survey by Tumin (cited by Bohannan, 1971, pp. 9–10), the work of sociologists after World War II showed that they, as a group, tended to become apologists for an anti–monogamy and pro-divorce ideology. Tumin chided members of his discipline for their "tacit applause" of divorce as an appropriate reaction to "the implied malfunctioning of society" and concluded that the bulk of recent publications assumed "divorce and adultery are simply evil-sounding terms for expressions of spirit that rise above ordinary limitations of unjustified normative restraints" (p. 10). In effect, Tumin applied sociological principles in evaluating current practices in sociology; what he found was a contumacious attitude in his colleagues toward the basic institutions they studied. As Bohannan remarked, "the shock value of Tumin's analysis should not distract us from its validity" (p. 10).

Just as positivist research in sociology reflected a new social orientation toward infidelity—and helped create that orientation—Lasch (1979), a cultural historian, arraigned the latest forms of psychotherapy for similar offenses. Lasch bitterly complained about the dilution of conjugal commitment through what amounts to therapeutic sleight-of-hand:

> Our society . . . has made deep and lasting friendships, love affairs, and marriages increasingly difficult to achieve. As social life becomes more and more warlike and barbaric, personal relations, which ostensibly provide relief from these conditions, take on the character of combat. Some of the new therapies . . . celebrate impermanent attachments under such formulas as "open marriage" and "open-ended commitments." Thus they intensify the disease they pretend to cure. (p. 30)

One way to illustrate Lasch's complaints about "new therapies" is to cite the famous Fritz Perls (1969) "prayer" often displayed on walls in offices and homes across America throughout the 1970s:

> I do my thing, and you do your thing.
> I am not in this world to live up to your expectations.
> And you are not in this world to live up to mine.
> You are you and I am I,
> And if by chance we find each other,
> It's beautiful.
> If not, it can't be helped. (p. 4)

In Perls's radical espousal of individualism, one takes no responsibility for the fate of significant others; in the name of a mental health ethic, he has written a prescription for mass callousness. According to Solomon (1989), this "prayer" is just "a recipe for narcissism, with its concomitant loneliness and emptiness" (p. 11). Even fellow Gestalt therapists were singularly critical of what Perls had done. His biographer, Shepard (1975), quoted Bill Schutz: "I'm disappointed that it's so influential. I think it's had a negative effect as well as positive—a kind of 'Fuck you' attitude" (p. 4). He also quoted Laura Perls (Fritz's ex-wife): "[I'm] rather unhappy about it. Particularly the last sentence, for it abdicates all responsibility to work on anything" (p. 4). Any psychotherapist trained to the outlook of the prayer will have no difficulty identifying with an unfaithful partner but will not be able to empathize with a jealous one.

Mullen (1981), a philosopher, thought an attack on the nuclear family was inherent in looking upon commitments as "nonbinding," as therapists were now doing. "Whereas marriage [used to represent] an either/or, the present age clamors for a both/and" (p. 91).

In sum, there are trends within the mental health field and the allied social sciences that promote the thesis that a committed union is an inherently stultifying arrangement to be supplemented, supplanted, or paradoxically sustained by guilt-free extramural sex. According to this viewpoint, the "healthy" individual cannot readily be contained within a monogamous union. Moreover, the old-fashioned psychoanalytic conviction that adultery proceeds from a disturbed psyche or a disturbed relationship is scorned, if paid any attention at all. In the end, old and new positions coexist today, clashing within an ambivalent culture that plays out on macroscale (in its literature and mores) what the individual has to struggle with on microscale (in personal conflicts and values).

WITHOUT JEALOUSY?

Because of the potential for violence whenever jealousy is aroused, every culture must find ways to limit its expression. But in the wake of the Great Sexual Revolution, can our society move to its summary extirpation? In a chapter called "Without Jealousy?", Carl Rogers (1977) described his correspondence with a young man who claimed to be free of jealousy, having encouraged his wife into an open marriage and regarding her current lover as his own best friend. His best female friend was an even choice between his wife and his girlfriend (with whom his wife was also friendly). The young man denied homosexual proclivities on the part of anyone within the overlapping triangles. Rogers was intrigued, for he immediately recognized the theoretical significance of finding an "emerging person" who was demonstrating that jealousy could be eliminated from what is considered "human nature." But, as a clinician, Rogers was wary. He agreed to meet the man and, afterward, his wife (each seen alone) so that he could assess the situation. The wife saw herself as a woman who had two primary relationships at the same time, now liking an unconventional arrangement that was unimaginable to her when she married. However, she revealed to Rogers that her husband had made a recent suicide attempt! Despite the couple's pride in full disclosure to each other of their sex lives, the husband had secretly plotted his own death, took an overdose of pills, and barely survived 8 days in coma. True to form, his suicide note to his wife, like his letters to Rogers, continued to avow lack of jealousy: "I . . . want you to know that this is something I'm doing totally on my own. It has nothing to do with our chosen life-style. You have always been the best mate/partner/ friend and you continue to be even at this moment. Don't let the stresses of society and friends or relatives who don't understand what great things we've achieved . . . wear you down. Hang in there" (p. 216). Rogers was moved by the couple's story, but he recognized that the husband did not share significant aspects of his emotional life with his spouse and that there were problems in this trio he had initially hailed as "too good to be true" (p. 206). Rogers thus remained somewhat reserved on the crucial point that the husband was, indeed, without jealousy, but he approved the courage of the couple in living an alternate life style and he saw no evidence that jealousy was an impediment to their relationship.

A very different clinical formulation can be gleaned from Rogers' narrative. Can it be that this modern-day couple could speak frankly to each other about affairs, but not about feelings? What strikes us is that, in setting up an open marriage, in his own friendship with his wife's lover, in his suicide note, and in his correspondence with Rogers, the young man was proclaiming over and over again his imperviousness to jealousy. Perhaps he doth protest too much. His denial amounted to an obsession, demonstrating the centrality of jealousy the same way a recovering alcoholic shows the ongoing importance of alcohol by attending AA meetings every evening and twice on Sunday. The young man's stance can be interpreted to be an exhibitionistic reaction formation to the idea that jealousy could ever be a green-eyed dragon able to slay *him*. His wife almost left him after his suicide attempt to "run" to her lover because of his psychiatric problem, which later turned out to be manic–depression.

On the universality of jealousy, Freud (1922/1957) warned, "If anyone appears to be without it, the inference is justified that it has undergone severe repression and consequently plays all the greater part in . . . unconscious mental life" (p. 221).

~ 7

The Geometry of the Eternal Triangle

> All Mary Jo Buttafuoco wants is what she can't have: to go back
> to life the way it was. . . . By now . . . everyone knows the story of
> how 17-year-old Amy Fisher shot Mary Jo because she had the
> man the "Lethal Lolita" coveted. The sexual soap opera seized
> our collective psyche with its themes of jealousy, rage, lust, and
> violence. But lost in all the lurid details is the story of the victim
> who miraculously survived, [although] considered by many to be
> a fool [because she refuses to believe that her husband, Joey,
> and Amy were lovers]. . . . "I got forgotten," she says [about the
> scandal]. "It's always been Joey and Mary Jo. When did it become
> Joey and Amy? . . . It scares me to think that there's no end to
> this, that . . . we are locked into some eternal triangle."
> —KANNER (1993, p. 56)

A mate must deal with a devastating plight when the partner becomes seriously involved with someone else: the threat of breakup is compounded by the narcissistic injury of jealousy (Weiss, 1975). Applying Bowen's (1978) concept of "triangulation," one spouse has sought equilibrium within the marriage by turning to a third party, in this case a lover. Like most family therapists, Moultrup (1990) regarded affairs as products of a disturbed conjugal system, noting that an affair may sometimes stabilize a problematic marriage but also can destroy it. For descriptive convenience, we continue to use Cooper's (1970) system of notation introduced in the preceding chapter. Thus, in geometric terms, the eternal triangle can be represented as comprising three points—a jealous mate (A) in a relationship with an unfaithful partner (B) who has a lover (C). To use a mnemonic device, A feels *abandoned*, B is *between* two mates, and C is a *catalyst* for crisis in union A–B. Leigh (1985) preferred a nomenclature describing the principals as "victim," "cheater," and "cheatee," whereas Pittman (1987) utilized "cuckold," "infidel," and "affairee," but such terminology strikes us as judgmental to all parties.

Wittingly or not, most adults have been involved in a love triangle, inasmuch as endemic rates of extramarital sex are now being reported. Vaughan (1989) reviewed various surveys of the extent of marital infidelity over the past 40 years: for men, the Kinsey report in 1948 estimated rates of 50% by age 40, the Hite report in 1980 gave a figure of 72% after two years of marriage, and Halper in 1988 found 82%; for women, the Kinsey report in 1953 gave rates of 26% by age 40, a *Cosmopolitan* survey in 1980 raised the figure to 50%, and the Hite report in 1987 estimated 70% after the first two years of marriage. Atwater (1982) noted that the trend toward increased incidence is much steeper for women, suggesting major shifts in social values during this period, especially as the rates were pushed up by chronologically younger wives.

In the most comprehensive survey to date, Blumstein and Schwartz (1983) interviewed 300 couples, of whom 72 were married, 48 were cohabiting heterosexuals, 90 were gay, and 90 were lesbian. They found that concerns about the partner's fidelity were in general quite justified: unfounded suspicion ran only about 10%, 22%, 2%, and 16% for the respective subgroups. The greatest deception about outside relationships was practiced within the married category, but these couples also most strongly upheld the ideal of monogamy. Active church membership had no bearing on rates of infidelity. Unfaithful women were more apt to have had affairs with but a single partner (43%, as compared with a male rate of 29%), whereas unfaithful men were more apt to have had six or more partners (29% to 17%). The partner most likely to engage in an affair was the one who "loved less," and rates of separation rose markedly when one partner was unfaithful within a year preceding the breakup.

In a similar study of married couples in Great Britain, Lawson (1988) reported comparable statistics. The surreptitious nature of infidelity was again a major finding. For instance, 61% of spouses learned about the affair only when the partner finally told them during the separation process, whereas of those who were aware prior to breakup, 7% were told of this situation by other sources and 25% discovered some kind of evidence. Further, even after separation, 10% still had no suspicion of infidelity and 6% were "not sure."

Based on an extensive family therapy practice, Pittman (1989) stated that although nonadulterous marriages rarely end in divorce, in 100 cases he treated in which adultery was an issue the couples did divorce more often than not. However, he found that only 10 couples were in a "sexually dead" marriage; the other 90 still had active conjugal relations. He believed that therapy helped salvage some of these marriages otherwise headed toward divorce, particularly when the infidelity occurred late in the marriage and consisted of a single affair. Pittman concluded that bad marriages sometimes lead to affairs, but that affairs can ruin a serviceable marriage.

Surveys have also been done relative to the outside party. Most published data concern the long-term female lovers of married men, but Blumstein and Schwartz found wives just as prone to become involved with a long-term male lover. Thus, in marriages of more than 10 years, the rates for ever having been in a serious affair ran about 11% for both husbands and wives. Demographic factors may play a significant role in the "married man–single woman" relationship— Richardson (1985) pointed out that unattached women over 25 are in the majority and so must compete for all available men, including married ones. Despite popular stereotyping of the woman involved with a married man as "predatory," Richardson insisted the population in her sample was psychologically normal. Another factor cited in some surveys points to changes in women's attitudes toward the sanctity of marriage. For instance, actress Shirley MacLaine stated, "Because I can't ultimately take marriage seriously, I am not concerned with the morality of going to bed with a married person" (Leigh, 1985, p. 136). Eskapa (1984) interviewed 150 "other women" and found that generalizations such as "cruel" or "clever" did not apply. She concluded from her study that the panicky reactions of some wives more often ruin a marriage than the affair itself. As she put it, an affair is not necessarily the end of a marriage, even though both women, for very different reasons, may think so.

The extent of current extramarital sex means that a great number of people are involved as lovers of unfaithful spouses. Some will themselves be married and thereby be a *B* within their own marriages but a *C* in someone else's marriage. Obviously, however, many single people take the role of outside party, although we know of no survey to date that tries to quantify the prevalence rate.

GENERAL CHARACTERISTICS OF THE ETERNAL TRIANGLE

The tension within a triangle is generated by a dialectic of opposing passions: the sexual–romantic affair *B–C* is pitted against a jealous *A* concerned with protecting marriage *A–B*. In effect, *B* and *C* have joined forces to find happiness at *A*'s expense. *Their involvement may even intensify proportionate to A's jealousy*, because A's reaction can have the effect of driving them together. C does not necessarily feel that h/s has broken up another person's home, but rather sees h/h role as a precipitating agent whose advent gave B an opportunity to do something about serious dissatisfaction with A. Moreover, C too has had vows of commitment and so can assert a claim to B, seen as only on loan to A who happened to meet B first. But C will also worry that what befell A could also one day befall C: B might supplant A with C but then return to A, especially if there are children of marriage A–B. Or it is possible that B might surreptitiously have sexual contact with A after their breakup, thereby reversing the original roles of A and C. If A and C have bought into the same trouble—B—the two rivals could conceivably coordinate their respective information to combat any duplicity on B's part, but for this they would have to talk, and A will have nothing to do with C (and up to a separation crisis may not even know of C's existence). All along, of course, C relates only to B, not A, in part because B has often enjoined C to stay away from A.

Once A learns about the triangle, B may take the stance that relationship B–C is an immutable reality—jealousy will not change things. Such a B will be "nice" so long as A does not thwart affair B–C by threatening C or interfering with B's access to C. But A seldom accepts B's right to consort freely with C, and so a B in this circumstance becomes correspondingly aggressive—more brazen and belligerent until breakup, subsequently provocative and callous enough to make A realize h/s no longer counts. As can be seen, when an affair is serious, A is a symbiant by role and tends to be by character, and the same can be said of B as a countersymbiant.

As a subplot, A may try to rekindle B's love by introducing yet a fourth party (D) of whom, it is hoped, B might be jealous. But Ds are pawns, to be sacrificed whenever B returns to A, or soon after B makes manifest that h/s is not bothered by A having a D. Bs are usually only transiently jealous (B can get A back anytime) and, ironically, A's pseudoaffair may also backfire by alleviating B's guilt in respect to A. Hence, D is ordinarily a peripheral player in a basically triangular drama.

In the final analysis, there are many possible ways to resolve a triangle. If A never finds out about C, the triangle can continue ad infinitum. A may also have to face a situation in which B leaves the marriage to stay with C. Or B can offer to stay with A, provided there is no obstruction of affair B–C; A will then be in a dilemma as to whether to preserve the marriage while suffering jealous anguish, or to expel B despite the realization that B will go straight into the waiting arms of C. In contrast, if the affair is just a passing incident and B then returns to the fold, A's marriage may not be harmed in the long run and might even benefit in some way. However, even when B returns, A can sometimes remain fixated on the infidelity, constantly dredging it up in sadomasochistic diatribes (Framo, 1982).

Resolution can possibly be effected by B; h/s can spare A jealousy by giving up C. If B loves A enough, this is what will happen. Often, however, "leaving" C is only a mirage because, from B's viewpoint, marriage A–B has a fatal flaw and B cannot stay in it without C for consolation. Thus, in promising to send C away for A's sake, B may simply contrive to tryst secretly with C once again so that marriage and affair coexist as before, the triangle having returned underground. By now it should be clear that an intense B–C affair, often carried on over years, has enormous resilience and it is hard for B to give C up, even when pledging to do so or swearing that it has been done.

A very different resolution of the triangle can be brought about by the action of C, when B will not leave A, and so C finally leaves B. This is a contingency that C often threatens, but it may never actually occur, and even if it does occur, it is apt to be a long time in coming. If an exasperated C at last opts out of such a situation, hoping that B will *now* leave A, B may miss C enough to make the necessary break with A. On the other hand, B may not tarry long in finding a replacement for C to keep marriage A–B viable.

All told, although all three parties may wish for change, they often collectively preserve a triangular status quo over time. For their own reasons, each has a stake in the ongoing "system." We must therefore take a closer look at their respective situations.

THE POSITION OF A

A's ordeal usually commences with the discovery of affair B–C. In general, A resists the registration of such information for as long as possible (Friday, 1985). Occasionally, some fortuitous event forces A to stumble upon the partner's secret, but far more often it is the partner's increasing flagrance that insists upon ultimate detection, creating clues that A cannot overlook. Another common mode of discovery entails the anonymous note or phone call from C—or a confederate—designed to break up marriage A–B. Of course, if and when it suits B's purpose, h/s can always sit A down and reveal the truth. All things considered, because A does not want to recognize that there is a C, it usually takes something very pointed to puncture A's faith in a working marriage with B.

Once *A* grasps the idea, jealousy rules. *A* does not even have to have much information, just enough to be suspicious that something is amiss in the marriage, or to begin to harbor doubts about what *B* says or does. *A* will then probably start to observe *B* closely, checking up on h/h whereabouts, verifying excuses for absences, and perhaps even inspecting of mail, calls, and bills, as well as the contents of wallet, office, or car. *B*'s patterns of behavior will be minutely scrutinized: h/h coming and going, manner of dress on leaving, scent of body on return, sudden sporting of strange jewelry, financial management, and so forth. Any sexual unavailability on *B*'s part will be correlated with prior absence from the home. Moreover, if the identity of *C* can be ascertained, discreet inquiries will be launched concerning this person and *B* or *C* may even be followed. This entire process is likely to be attended by fantasies in which *A* fears the worst about *B*'s sexual conduct when out of sight. Caught between love and distrust of *B*, *A* readily becomes distraught, affectively labile, and obsessed with the triangle. If seen by a therapist, h/h turmoil and "pathological jealousy" may be regarded by some clinicians as indicative of a paranoid or borderline disorder, although in most cases this diagnosis would already be incorrect by history.

Meanwhile, as *A* attempts to ferret out the truth, h/s is not sure just what would be the better outcome. On one hand, *A* fears that an unbearable confirmation of *B*'s betrayal will emerge. On the other hand, if in fact there is no such perfidy, *A* would have to acknowledge that h/s suffers from a delusional form of jealousy. Both possibilities have frightening implications for *A*, but worse yet is to be in between, uncertain as to the truth.

As much as verification that one's mate has been unfaithful will cause pain, it is often the tricks used to cover *B*'s tracks that inflict the most damage to *A*'s mental health. Indeed, to ward off detection, *B* may choose to make *A* feel crazy. Laing (1965) called this interpersonal maneuver "mystification"—a defense with the function of preserving the status quo by making a significant other doubt legitimate perceptions and memories; in this way, the object attributes h/h problems to faulty mental health rather than to noxious treatment. Searles (1959) maintained that the conscious or unconscious effort to drive the other person crazy comes from a murderous hostility; however, to keep the person around for h/h utility and as a receptacle for malevolent projections, "psychosis wishes" replace "death wishes." Three case examples follow.

A college professor learned his wife was involved with a junior member of his department. He considered leaving the marriage and consulted a psychiatrist. He loved his wife and, as it turned out, she too did not want the marriage to end. The two discussed their problems, spent more time together, moved into a new house, and the wife agreed to forgo all contact with her former lover. The man remained in therapy even after the marital crisis subsided, with the complaint of recurrent suspicion of his wife, despite an undeniable improvement in their marriage. He was now determined to hire a detective to follow her. His therapist argued that the man was delusional, still not having worked through prior feelings of jealousy. Nevertheless, the professor soon did hire a detective, who informed him that his wife had actually never stopped seeing her paramour. This bitter news was sweeter than the unhealthy conjecture with which he had lived for so long, leading both him and his psychiatrist to question his reality testing. The man felt vindicated in that he was sensitive enough not to be taken in by his wife's mendacity. Ultimately, in learning the real state of affairs, the professor preferred an immediate divorce to continuing to be made a fool of as a "sane" and "rational" husband.

A mother of two engaged in several intense affairs, with the ironic motto that, if her husband suspected her, she should "lie like hell" so that the crucial tissue of trust between them would not be broken! This woman regarded as "immature" a cousin who revealed an affair to her own husband, which led to their separation; she thought the cousin should have held onto her marriage without destructive disclosures out of guilt or overinvolvement with a lover. Meanwhile, the breakup of the cousin's marriage because of an admitted affair had the effect of alerting the woman's husband to the state of his own marriage. She now had to meet her husband's more watchful demands for closeness, communication, and affection—without missing a stroke so far as her current lover was concerned; she simply had to work harder and lie better to keep her double life intact. One day her husband asked why she seldom wore her wedding ring; she indignantly replied that he was "getting paranoid over a symbol!" In such style she repulsed all queries emanating from his heightened vigilance. Before long the man was less wary and resumed complacent conjugal functioning. The wife took pride in having weathered a storm—she had spared her "emotionally fragile" mate an insight he could not endure. Unlike the preceding case, this husband seemed to want his suspicions quickly allayed. His own psychological defenses worked in tandem with her accusations of paranoia to stop his curiosity from pushing too far.

In Jong's autobiographical novel, *How to Save Your Own Life* (1977), a wife suspected her husband had sex with a particular lady and for some years pressed insinuations and allegations about this relationship, which the husband vehemently rebuffed. He became so irked with her "obsession" as to insist that she see a therapist to deal with her lack of trust. She did, their marriage went on, and the woman had a series of affairs and chose to remain childless as she wrestled with her problem. One day she came upon an old love letter in her husband's desk, with specifics corroborating her suspicions. Her husband was presented with this data, and he now confessed she had been right all along. She shortly left him for someone else. What upset her most about her husband's behavior was not the affair, which, though it hurt at the time, was brief and long since over. The issue was how he had undermined her self-confidence, forcing her to dwell in a land of murky guesswork for years and making her doubt her mental balance. She could forgive the affair more readily than the denial, which she insisted was based on his hatred of her.

Once there is definite proof that affair B–C exists and is no figment of A's projections, it becomes a tangible problem that can be discussed with B without obfuscation. Now real difficulties in the relationship have to be addressed instead of diversionary mystification. At this juncture, A needs to take a fresh look at B in order to arrive at decisions on crucial questions. Can A still live with B, even with C out of the picture? Indeed, will C be out of the picture? What sort of person has the affair revealed B to be? And, as a devastating afterthought, what sort of person has the affair revealed A to be—did A contribute to the affair by h/h own inadequacies or by neglecting B's needs, thereby prompting affair B–C to exist? Some of these questions need B's input, yet A alone must figure out where h/s stands on each and every point.

In terms of strategies to cope with jealousy, A has four basic areas to deal with: ambivalent feelings toward B, rivalry toward C, potential sexual compensation with D, and whether or not to let jealousy show. We will consider these thematic concerns in turn.

Ambivalence toward B

Some mates regard their committed union as hopelessly compromised by a partner's infidelity and depart more or less immediately. In so doing, a climactic act of hostility is often carried out in the moment of turning away. One woman arranged to have her philandering husband come home to find her and her pet gone, but instead discovering a pile of dog feces on their conjugal bed. Another woman quietly used her charge plates to furnish an elegant new apartment; when she suddenly moved out, she bequeathed her husband enough indebtedness to recall her mistreatment. A man took a knife and shredded his wife's wardrobe. Another man knocked his wife down with a car on his way out. These examples are acted out statements about A's rage, wishes for revenge, and the search for a memorable last word on the subject of B's honor.

Other jealous mates go to the opposite extreme, emphasizing chances for trust once the truth comes out about the dissatisfaction on B's part that culminated in an affair. Hoping to preserve the marriage, A attempts to place greater value on B's talking frankly about the couple's problems than on the fact of infidelity. The dilemma in this approach is that the lifting of secrecy around the conduct of the double life has already raised doubts about B's integrity. Even if B now discloses the whole truth, can trust be restored by belated admissions extracted only at A's behest? In addition, the affair exposes B as a very different person than A had supposed—as someone who, however charming, can be antagonistic and exploitative. To please this newly recognized B, accommodations by A are apt to be required that may exceed what A is prepared or equipped to do. All told, B's lack of honesty is a problem in its own right, but honesty per se does not resolve all the other problems. A will sometimes be terribly mistaken in the idea that candor by B in itself lays a foundation for reconciliation.

Nevertheless, some exceptional As persevere in squeezing from B an account of what is special about C, turning such communication into a regenerative opportunity. For example, a woman caught in her lies about an affair finally found her husband asking about and listening to things she had never dared say. She could finally share her resentment at his inhibitions about sex. When asked to compare husband and lover as partners, she complained about such "voyeuristic curiosity" but then reluctantly gave details about the lover's responsiveness to all her sexual inclinations. Despite the pain engendered by inquiring about his wife's involvement with another man, the husband saved the marriage from imminent collapse by seeking clarifications that subsequently enabled the couple to work out a better sex life and a higher level of openness.

Competition with C

The factor of sexual rivalry preoccupies A, with frequent fantasies about a clash with C. Either by accident or design, such an encounter may actually occur, often constituting the most dramatic confrontation imaginable. Restraint is generally beyond the power of the protagonists: they taunt or threaten, at times come to blows, and compel one or the other to leave the field humiliated. Given what can happen, A and/or C will normally veto any such meeting when organized on a planned, voluntary basis.

Yet there are times when A and C do attempt an interchange to their mutual benefit. Only by exchanging information can they check the validity of their interpretations, protect themselves from B's manipulations, and find out what each lacks that B finds in the other. Violent reactions can be contained, provided they talk as allied victims rather than as irreconcilable adversaries. In one case, a wife accidentally discovered a bill for a Ms. X's abortion in her husband's possession. She tracked down the stranger and called her. Ms. X was stunned, but she was also sympathetic to the wife's need for explanation (besides, Ms. X too had her own issues with B over this abortion—he had opposed it, even though he ended up paying for it). The two women did not hang up as friends, but their conversation was mutually instructive. B later found himself furious first at one, and then at the other, for disclosing his private business and getting him in trouble.

However, A–C chats cannot resolve the ills of the triangle. Even when both people control their emotions, such dialogues are inherently painful. Each may leave such an encounter with profound misgivings. By meeting on an equal footing, A fears lending respectability to an immoral affair, whereas C often does not want to be a party to saving a defunct marriage. More to the point, both A and C have to contend with a rival who is a real human being rather than typecast as a "defective partner" for B.

When a face-to-face A–C meeting does occur, it tends to be initiated by A, sometimes confronting C in B's presence in order to pressure B to leave with A. We are familiar with two instances in which a discarded wife took her children in hand and went to fetch "Daddy" from the home he now shared with a woman who had been his lover during the marriage. In one of these situations, the man went back with his wife, leaving the lover in despair. However, although the B–C relationship in this case soon resumed as a clandestine affair, it no longer worked for C and she shortly became involved with another man. In the other case, the sequence of events took a quite different turn. To her surprise, when the wife finally saw her rival for the first time, she found herself disgusted by her husband's taste. The rival, far from being a femme fatale, was someone in relation to whom the wife did not feel inferior, sexually or otherwise. When the estranged husband elected to stay where he was, the wife readily left him there, her jealousy—and love—now greatly dissipated. The lesson here is that in meeting the competition, A gets to see B in a new light that illuminates the qualities B has bargained for in a fresh romance, for which h/s is willing to sack the old marriage. Hence, C's fallibilities become B's fallibilities. In A's eyes, C had better be worth it!

Some family therapists attempt to bring C into the treatment of an *A–B* couple. Pittman (1987) is a strong advocate of such an approach; he maintained that bringing the three parties together in a session facilitates resolution of the triangle. On the basis of his clinical practice, Pittman reported that an affair sometimes collapses after *C* comes to a therapy meeting, although, more likely, *C* will not agree to participate or *B* will not permit it. If *C* does not cooperate, Pittman urged *A* to contact *C* outside the treatment:

> Ideally, the husband's mistress or the wife's mister should be considered part of the family system and included in the therapy sessions. . . . The persistent request for such inclusion clarifies and dramatizes his or her centrality in the family. Quite often the affairee will protest that affairs are supposed to be exempt from therapy. . . . Whether the affairee comes in or not, the cuckold should feel free to contact the third person in the marriage bed. The cuckold does not have to operate within the infidel's rules, and the affairee has no right of immunity. (pp. 122–123)

Compensation with *D*

After learning of affair *B–C,* many *A*s turn to a lover, *D,* in order to regain self-esteem, create a buffer against *B*'s loss, and give *B* a taste of h/h own medicine. Selection is made with a view toward maximizing *B*'s discomfort, so that a *D* is apt to be someone of importance in *B*'s network or a person of higher status. *D*'s main function is to upset *B,* being a person whose name and qualities—if and when revealed—will be a shock to *B.* Thus, one woman became involved with her husband's business partner; in another case, a man started seeing his wife's sister. Sometimes *D*s are chosen as informers, conveying news to *A* of *B*'s private activities: for example, a woman went out with the lawyer handling her husband's side of the divorce! *A*s who forge an affair with an eminent *D* often gloat over the thought of *B*'s reaction should h/s find out, and even *A*s who do not have a *D* nevertheless hint to *B* that they do, or soon will.

The new partner can be starkly exploited, so that some *D*s depart as soon as they discern that *A* is still fixated on *B.* Indeed, in *A*'s fantasy, *D* is meant to be expendable: *D* has been made a lover to induce jealousy in *B,* thus presumably prompting *B* to return to marriage *A–B* by offering to give up *C* on condition that *D* is sent packing as well. Or so *A* dreams. As noted earlier, however, this castle-in-the-air approach swiftly crashes to earth when *B* learns of affair *A–D.* This affair will most likely assuage guilt about *B*'s own affair, as well as reducing *B*'s concern about *A*'s well-being. Counterjealousy ploys just do not work. But this is not to say that the relationship with *D* has no value for *A*. By finding a lover, *A* starts to feel once more like a valued sexual object. *D* will also let *A* vent hostility toward *B*, providing reassurance and solace. Finally, *A* needs the relationship with *D* to practice being single again if *B* elects to keep on with *C*.

Should *A* Express or Suppress Jealousy?

In rounding out this section on the position of *A* within the triangle, we note a vexing issue that concerns the extent to which jealous feelings can or should be admitted. An *A* often does not want to give *B* the satisfaction of seeing h/h suffering, which would show how important *B* continues to be. An *A* may also be mortified by the malice of jealous impulses and so may disown these feelings or feign transcendence. But why should *A* want to be disingenuous about the effect of *B*'s behavior on *A*, as if *B* did not already know? Despite society's tendency to regard jealousy as an outmoded emotion of which one should be ashamed (Durbin, 1977), it seems to us that the jealous mate has every right to make a jealous statement, verbally or otherwise, and this statement must be such as to be unpleasant for *B* to hear, just as it was unpleasant for *A* to hear about *C*. There are very compelling reasons to control destructive aspects of jealousy, but no overriding reason to deny, hide, or apologize for the feelings. Once jealousy is expressed, if *B* makes no move to heal the breach in the relationship, *A* can only commence the difficult but ultimately liberating task of letting go.

THE POSITION OF *B*

A person in the role of *B* cannot readily be stereotyped as a sexual opportunist, inasmuch as unfaithful spouses are so because of a variety of motivations (Hunt, 1969). These range from a pursuit of a modicum of narcissistic enhancement to shore up an ego already depleted in an emotionally barren marriage (English, 1971), all the way to blatant narcissistic pathology in which no mate suffices to satisfy insatiable sexual–romantic entitlement (Saul, 1950). But it should be remembered that although an affair always involves some form of narcissistic gratification, narcissism is not a dirty word and we all need our fair share of it. Indeed, love relationships are inherently narcissistic (Solomon, 1989). A good marriage offers nurture, promotes self-actualization, and raises self-esteem. When those psychological benefits are no longer available within a committed union, it will not be long before serious emotional alienation from the mate develops.

At the extreme range of narcissistic needs, a countersymbiant B will demand a great deal in terms of being loved and is often ruthless in getting the supplies h/s craves. In such cases mates may be supplemented, substituted, or discarded, yet always with a feeling of deprivation on B's part, combined with outrage at anyone who criticizes or complains. Such Bs believe that what is good for them is ultimately good for everyone else. This self-centered approach not only distorts the basic interpersonal situation but is also bound to create repercussions that will inundate B and h/h significant others in constant entanglements and disentanglements.

Yet not all Bs are cut from the same cloth. Affairs can also occur where Bs are in the lower to middle range of the narcissistic scale and may even be the symbiant mate in their marriages. These affairs are hardly intended as shopping expeditions for a more elegant partner or as quasi-permanent adjuncts to a marriage; on the contrary, they tend to be ambivalent, guilt-ridden, and limited experiences because there is no doubt that primary allegiance is due the existing marriage. Although curiosity and opportunism enter in as precipitating factors, this type of B usually undertakes any affair with a sense that involvement with a lover will no longer be viable as soon as it interferes with the marital relationship, even though that union has its own problems. The existence of a third party may even be revealed to the spouse in order to strengthen the marriage and reaffirm the commitment; in such cases the third party has been made use of for the dyad's own deep purposes (Dicks, 1967) so that once the couple addresses their problems, the affair quickly withers away. Even if the marriage does not improve, the affair (known or unknown to the spouse) is still apt to fall of its own weight inasmuch as Bs who are not extremely narcissistic usually have little stomach for the moral and logistic strains posed by a sustained affair. In short, this sort of B does not stay a B long. For this reason, the classic B in the eternal triangle tends to be someone struggling with excessive needs to be loved.

And what does this classic B really want? Does B want to have h/h cake and eat it too, retaining both A and C? Or, conversely, is h/s just awaiting the right moment to leave A and go to C? The answer is complicated. If A and B could work out their issues, there would be no C; if they cannot, C becomes instrumental. C is B's ticket out of marriage A–B. Then again, once having purchased this ticket, B can paradoxically remain a bit longer. In other words, despite the discomfort, Bs can get very attached to a format of marriage-plus-affair. In B's conduct of a double life, A's role is to provide a secure and stabilizing home, and C's role is to serve as the exotic, forbidden incarnation of B's erotic or romantic yearning. Thus, the two relationships can complement each other, gratifying diverse aspects of B's personality. Many Bs tend to hold fast to both partners, resisting loss of one or the other, even when pressed to the limit for exclusive commitment by an adamant A or C. In the end, such a B often contends that the ideal mate would be a combination of A and C, but in the absence of a partner who is a perfect "10," h/s can only settle for two "5s".

In object relations terms, Fairbairn (1952) has described B's two partners as a *libidinal object* (C in our notation) and an *anti-libidinal object* (our AS), both of whom are inadequate mates in different ways. According to Fairbairn, the anti-libidinal object provides a secure base. This person is central in upholding social identity, but is also experienced as enmeshing, moralistic, and controlling. Fairbairn held that fusing the roles of mate and parent within the perception of the anti-libidinal object disrupts the sexual dimension of the marriage because of too many oedipal associations, with the result that an external libidinal object is needed to fill a sexual void, but not necessarily by someone with whom marriage is either feasible or desirable. In sum, Fairbairn postulated that the anti-libidinal partner is a responsible but desexualized caretaker of B and A–B's children, while B's libidinal drives are satisfied by an outside consort in furtive fashion so as not to sully the marriage to the "parentified spouse." In the final analysis, B's double life solves immediate conflicts by object splitting, denoting a developmental failure in ego integration.

Beyond psychodynamics, there are legitimate practical reasons that B might procrastinate about leaving A, or even be determined never to do so: it may be financially unwise, children can be hurt, reputation within the social–religious community will be damaged, and so forth. In short, promised departure to C may be repeatedly postponed as long as the marriage still fulfills some pragmatic function. No matter how unhappy B is in the marriage, h/s may be able to deal with its stresses and reap its benefits so long as C represents an escape hatch. Besides, insofar as C is primarily a sex object, B will not always be eager to make C a complete mate anyway (though, naturally, this goes unmentioned to C).

Typically, in order to preserve the three-party system, B must go beyond mere discretion about an affair to keep A in the role of symbiant spouse. H/s must also insidiously mislead A as to the ascribed quality of their marriage. B often purposely leaves many problems in the conjugal relationship unmentioned and unaddressed, because if A were to be alerted to B's misgivings, A might become vigilant enough to see signs of infidelity. The simplest course for B is to lull A into complacency by following stable marital rituals, despite what may be considerable absence from the home on *B*'s part. This self-protective, conflict-avoiding stance within the marriage partially accounts for the fact that so many *A*s are caught by surprise about affair *B–C*, for not only are such *A*s reluctant to face up to their partner's unhappiness, but *B* may have been silent quite deliberately, letting the fact of the affair itself, known or unknown to *A*, eloquently speak for *B*'s discontent.

As for *B*'s moral issues, very few people can cheat within a committed partnership without some guilt, though when the stakes are sufficiently high, many *B*s can go pretty far on a tankful of bad conscience. Until discovery, jealousy on *A*'s part is only a hypothetical proposition. *B* can always prevent it by vowing that *A* need never know about *C*, thus ostensibly protecting *A* while *B* goes about h/h sexual business. In most cases, it appears that so long as a marital crisis is averted, so too is a crisis in conscience. Although some *B*s get so fed up with their hypocrisy that they dissolve the triangle, it is more usual for *B*s to labor to keep the triangle intact, often trying to do so even after *A* finds out about *C*.

Although relationship *B–C* can be hidden from *A*, it is scarcely possible to hide marriage *A–B* from *C*. Unless the affair is purely sexual, with no other commitment expected (and even then problems around *C*'s tacit expectations can occur), *B*'s devotion to *C* must be unequivocally and passionately reiterated so that *C* can feel special, having faith that *B* would be with *C* if not already married to *A*. Unfortunately, as *B* explains, h/s cannot let *A* learn of the existence of *C*, and so couple *B–C* must take precautions to make themselves invisible to *A*. *B* may also then add that leaving *A* is not yet possible—but, if and when h/s can, it will be to unite with *C*. It is not necessarily the case that *B* is insincere in these protestations, but such sentiments are not tantamount to plans.

To sum up *B*'s convoluted position when engaged in two serious relationships at the same time: either *B* must give up *A* or *C*, or else seek to maintain the two simultaneous unions through not allowing *A* to discern or to disrupt affair *B–C*, while at the same time keeping marriage *A–B* intact by not allowing *C* to disrupt or to depart because *B* has not left *A*.

THE POSITION OF C

Whether the existence of a lover is regarded as a threat to a committed union or a cause for jealousy will depend on the marital arrangement between particular spouses. But when a third party does become a threat to the viability of a valued relationship, jealousy is a virtual certainty. Consider the renowned "open" union between Simone de Beauvoir and Jean-Paul Sartre (de Beauvoir, 1964):

> There are many couples who conclude more or less the same pact as Sartre and myself: to maintain throughout all deviations from the main path a certain "fidelity." . . . Such an undertaking has its risks—it is always possible that one of the partners may prefer a new attachment to the old one, the other partner then considering himself or herself unjustly betrayed; in place of two free persons, a victim and a torturer confront one another. If the two allies allow themselves only passing sexual liaisons, there is no difficulty, but it also means that the freedom they allow themselves is not worthy of the name. Sartre and I have been more ambitious . . . but there is one question we have avoided: How would the third person feel about our arrangement? It often happened that the third person accommodated himself to it without difficulty; our union left . . . room for loving friendships and fleeting affairs. But if the protagonist wanted more, then conflicts would break out. (p. 64)

Just as Sartre and de Beauvoir had trouble envisioning how a third party—as an individual with h/h own needs—might react to their committed but open arrangement, family therapists too have trouble picturing the third party as a person of substance inasmuch as they rarely get to meet C and tend to view the triangle from a marital perspective. For example, Brown (1991) regarded the female "unmarried other" as a psychologically disturbed woman who was struggling with problems of dependency, boundary confusion, and pervasive oedipal conflicts: "The mistress expects to beat out her lover's wife, just as she beat out her own mother" (p. 193). A bias against the "unmarried other" is clear, for it is never shown just what data support Brown's assertions. Such stereotyping is rife both in society and in professional literature when it comes to the persona of C, as little scope has been afforded third parties to express their own perspective. But Sands's *The Mistress' Survival Manual* (1978) is a notable exception to this rule.

Sands (herself a former C) examines the plight of the kept or unkept woman who secretly sees a married man over a span of years, often hoping for his divorce so that she can become his wife:

> How often has a mistress wished with all her energy that his wife would find out about the affair? How many mistresses saw to it that his wife was informed in detail of her husband's liaison? . . . Hopefully for everyone involved in this triangle, it will reach a climax. He will reach a choice. [The wife] will throw him out. Someone will decide some-

thing. . . . It takes three willing participants to create a triangle. . . . If
any one of them opts for change, the triangle explodes. (pp. 240–241)

Sands disputed the myth that the mistress is a "home wrecker"—she
is just not that powerful. Sands also challenged the stereotype of a
"Faustian battle" between a mistress "dressed in that black negligee"
and a wife "frantically searching for that white peignoir left over from
her wedding night." To Sands, the mistress is an outsider who, at most,
serves as a catalyst. The marital problems predated the affair and would
have occurred without the affair. Although the married man is a very
willing partner in the illicit union, Sands insisted that he is often
uncomfortable in his double life; she argued that he gets indigestion
from having that infamous cake and eating it too. She was indignant
at the pious declamations of wives who are either too complacently
naive or afraid to lose their marriages if they dare confronting their
husbands about their suspicions. She even discounted the idea that a
married couple cannot work out their problems so long as an affair is
under way, declaring that discovery of an affair frequently opens up
lines of communication between husband and wife, leading to a
regeneration of the marriage. Because Sands espoused the cause of the
mistress, she was not pleased about such an outcome. She complained
that nobody is unduly concerned about the loneliness, the fidelity, and
the jealousy of the mistress to whom pledges of commitment may have
also been made. She contended that the mistress is condemned to years
of waiting on tenterhooks unless she pushes her partner to a timely
resolution of his dual involvement.

Sand's book is a striking exposition of the principle that a third
party cannot "cause" a marital breakup. In a sound marriage, either
there would be no extramarital relationship or it would not be allowed
to evolve to a point where it threatens the cohesion of the couple. The
betrayed spouse is apt to contend that if the rival had never appeared,
all would have been well. But this argument is untenable—it alleges that
marital problems arise from the seduction of an otherwise contented
spouse. As mentioned earlier, even when the unfaithful partner presumably gives up the paramour to work on saving the marriage, the
lover is quite likely to be called on again, or to be replaced, as soon as
the same old troubles reappear in the marriage. It is simplistic to
castigate the third party as the villain in the triangle. The third party
may do some unethical things, such as anonymously informing a naive
spouse of the affair, but the couple still have to look to their own
marriage for the causes of their emotional alienation and potential
breakup.

As already stated, *C* has options within the triangle. H/s can accept the situation for what it is—let B stay with A and make no outward demands that B do differently. Alternatively, C can mount an active campaign to persuade B to leave A, or instigate by hook or crook to have A throw B out. And, of course, C can refuse to participate further in a triangle. Sands urged the mistress who does not want to share her partner with A ad infinitum to issue an ultimatum, threatening to leave unless her married man gets a divorce. When the mistress actually puts the threat into effect, the married man must make one choice or another, in either case destroying the triangle. In so doing, a mistress takes a great risk, but Sands stated that it must be faced or else the three-party system drags on and on. She asked her readers to be aware that married men typically procrastinate for 7 to 11 years.

Sands concluded that the position of C has its own romantic rewards but is overall a frustrating experience. C will spend a lot of evenings and weekends in solitude, able to be with B only at the latter's convenience. Even allotted time will be subject to sudden cancellation or curtailment because of situations emanating from marriage A–B. C will feel a measure of jealousy toward A, who can enjoy B's companionship in many respects denied to C, such as in raising a family or appearing together in any public place. C has to struggle to preserve self-respect because of the illicit nature and subterfuge of the affair. Hardest of all, C might have had promises of commitment from B, which never seem to come to fruition. In her own personal experience as a mistress, Sands found that she could not continue on forever in this position and had to force her married man to make a dichotomous decision. As her either-or ultimatum turned out, he left his wife to be with her.

In *The Second Wife's Survival Manual* (1982), Sands examined the sequel to the eternal triangle, when the married man has at last left his wife to be with his erstwhile mistress. She reported that many ex-wives "end a career in marriage only to begin a new career in harassment. . . . These ex-wives want no cooperation; they want only confrontation over the past. . . . In these cases the second wives are truly victims of a new unacknowledged crime" (p. 235). Through A's enduring jealousy, the triangle carries on in a new direction, with C demanding respect from A for the second marriage that A feels was not accorded by C to the first marriage. For Sands, this added up to "a woman scorned victimizing another woman." She finished this book by refusing to concede that the ex-wife has any social or moral grounds to be vindictive:

> Ex-wives stripped of eternal sympathy will be forced to abandon spite and start concentrating on a new life. . . . The second wife will be the

voice of the future. It is she who will change the system, the government, and the people of America. . . . Perhaps we, as second wives, can raise society's consciousness. . . . Perhaps that higher plane will even embrace justice! (p. 237)

In this patriotic defense of the sanctity of second marriage, the new wife has picked up where the old wife has not quite left off.

Our discussion has so far focused only on the married man and his female lover. However, it does not appear that the dynamics of a triangle are significantly different when sexes are reversed (Framo, 1982). Men and women love with equivalent passion as well as folly. In one case a married woman was irked at her lover and flaunted yet another paramour. The lover retaliated by calling up her flabbergasted husband to complain: "Your wife is cheating on both of us!" This C's purpose was to get B into marital trouble for "infidelity," with A to do the punishing for both A and C.

In another "married woman–single man" situation a man was able to induce the married woman he had been seeing to divorce her husband and marry him instead. A year later, she divorced him in turn, returning to her first husband. Soon thereafter, she resumed her affair with her lover—a reinstatement of the status quo ante. This case exemplifies a pattern that should by now be familiar: neither marriage was as resilient as the triangle itself.

TRIANGLES DIE HARD

A collusive network is always necessary to keep the triangle eternal. Three lives are intertwined, and any one of these parties can destroy the system. Yet, for a long while, no one does. The enmeshment of the three is so powerful that sometimes even its demise continues to reflect the established triangular spirit. For example, a man walked out on his wife to be with another woman, with all the jealous repercussions ordinarily entailed. Several years later the new wife called up the former wife and said this man had proved to be impossible to stay with—would she please take her ex back? The former wife declined the honor. When the man learned of this conversation, he jested, "It looks like they're still fighting over me!" Though they were now fighting *not* to have him, the configuration of the triangle prevailed to the end.

～ 8

When Marriage Ends in a Love Triangle
The Defilement Taboo

If the father's new girlfriend is believed by the mother to have been responsible for the ending of the marriage, then the mother may feel that she has already lost a husband to the new woman and is unwilling to risk loss of her children as well. *Some women develop imageries of the other woman as unclean, and are in a panic lest their children be defiled by the other woman's touch* (italics ours).

—WEISS (1979a, p. 160–161)

THE DEFILEMENT TABOO

This chapter addresses one common resolution of the geometry of the eternal triangle (Pam & Pearson, 1994), only barely covered in the previous chapter, which occurs when *B* (an unfaithful spouse) leaves the marriage to be with *C* (h/h lover) and *A* (the jilted partner) must now deal with *B–C* as a couple. While the focus of this chapter is on *A*'s jealousy toward the new *B–C* pairbond, which tends to lead to unusually bitter separations, a collateral aspect of such strife involves the impact of triangular breakup on the children of marriage *A–B*, because *A* is obliged to deal with *B–C* after breakup in accord with visitation and custody terms. So far as children are concerned, if parent *B* ends a marriage to resolve a triangle, is breakup just another variation on the theme of divorce, presenting problems no different or worse than those of any other separation? Or are special dilemmas posed, generating hardships of a far more ominous order? We contend that the latter is more often the case. In our clinical experience, divorce in

167

triangular circumstances forces children into drastic loyalty conflicts between A and B–C.

The thesis we will now advance is that a person thrust into the role of A tends to regard C as a standing menace to everything held dear, bringing about the imposition of a "defilement taboo." By this term we mean the emotional demand imposed by a jealous ex-mate on all members of h/h social network to eschew any friendly or supportive contact with the rival in the triangle. Indeed, C is superstitiously perceived as exuding "toxic" influence, so that—for A—anyone who violates this taboo risks becoming toxic too. Except for B in delimited situations, the penalty to be levied on significant others who willingly let themselves be exposed to such ascribed defilement ranges from loss of trust to total ostracism. Even A's own children must take heed; they are not exempt just because B is also their parent. As Moultrup (1990) has observed, children too become triangulated into an existing parental triangle in a process he called "multiple interlocking triangles."

In short, our premise is that three-sided breakups are prone to be extraordinarily acrimonious; moreover, this acrimony will put children in a cross fire when parent B brings offspring around C so that such contact runs afoul of the defilement taboo imposed by parent A. The plan for exploring this premise is as follows: (1) empirical findings are reviewed from research on the children of divorce to see whether our hypothesis fits in with current data; (2) the anthropological concepts of defilement and taboo are examined in relation to modern psychological theory; (3) A's mechanisms of defense in jealousy are discussed; (4) the course of a defilement taboo is tracked by taking account of the commensurate experiences of B, C, and the children of marriage A–B; and (5) suggestions are offered to fellow clinicians who encounter this phenomenon.

EMPIRICAL RESEARCH ON THE CHILDREN OF DIVORCE

Wallerstein (1991) has complained that studies of children of divorce have thus far been too broad, ignoring patterns within the divorce population. Every breakup creates unique issues, occurring for many reasons and at different stages in the family cycle, whereas the roots of the postdivorce situation extend far back in time, encompassing the history of the two mates prior to marriage, the course of their relationship, and the nature of their parting. Assessment of the impact of divorce on family members is further complicated by cultural changes impinging on its incidence, social meaning, and research evaluation. Although Wallerstein held that what is most urgently needed is more longitudinal information, she was dismayed that for the most part the field is making do with research based on quantitative methods in large samples. In summary of the current state of knowledge, she stated that we now realize that divorce is not a brief crisis within a family transition—rather, it tends to weaken the family in its child-rearing and child-protective functions. Nevertheless, although acrimony and loyalty conflicts have been identified as noxious factors, she noted that investigators have yet to make much sense of the abundant data we already have.

Without investigation of specific factors, the impact of triangle-based breakup on children has not been addressed in research; thus, we can deal only with more generic studies. We will consider four studies reviewed by Wallerstein, plus an additional investigation, which have at least some peripheral bearing on our topic.

Block, Block, and Gjerde (1988)

During a 10 year child study, divorce occurred in 41 of 110 families so that serendipitous data permitted prospective comparisons. One salient finding was that fathers often disengaged from children long before leaving and that breakup coincided with mothers pressuring fathers to become more active. This study surprisingly suggested that marital unhappiness frequently took the form of conflict over child rearing, but it was unclear whether such strife is a primary cause of divorce or a displacement or consequence of other marital tensions. Without case histories, any patterns in these breakups cannot be discerned.

Wallerstein and Blakeslee (1989)

The sample consisted of 131 children from divorced families interviewed four times over 15 years. Wallerstein insisted her data was robust enough to show that divorce is enduringly harmful to at least a third of children, but her work has been criticized for lack of a control group (Robinson, 1994). It is ironic that Wallerstein herself has not yet used her own cases to draw inferences about families that might explain why some children in her sample fare well in divorce and others do not.

Johnston, Kline, and Tschann (1989)

One hundred children from families engaged in litigation around visitation or custody were seen 5 years after breakup and followed up

3 years after their parents first went to court. Contrary to Despert's (1953) dictum that children of divorce benefit from ready access to both parents, these children were not helped by such access. When applied to litigating couples, prior research was considered invalid because it was done with cooperating parents. In this sample, hostile ex-mates were often reckless about child welfare, but again no theory was developed from the cases to explain just why these particular families were different from other divorcing families.

Buchanan, Maccoby, and Dornbusch (1991)

To investigate the effect of loyalty conflicts on children in divorced families, 522 youngsters were interviewed 5 years after breakup. The expected correspondence between high levels of parental discord and a sense of being "caught in the middle" was confirmed. The feeling of being caught in the middle correlated with symptoms of depression, anxiety, and deviance. However, 40% of children whose parents had high discord levels were able to keep emotional distance from the fray, and a similar percentage whose parents had low discord levels nevertheless felt "caught in the middle." Here too, no explanation based on case histories attempted to account for these anomalies.

Ahrons (1994)

In the course of discussing the importance of "good divorce" for children, Ahrons reported data from a Michigan survey in which 55% of the children sample came from families in which an extramarital affair was a factor in parental breakup. Of these divorces, 75% were acrimonious over the long term, as contrasted with only 25% in the remaining sample after the first year. But Ahrons did not draw any inferences from these statistics.

The preceding studies tend to support—but are not focused enough to verify—our premise that triangular breakups lead to remarkably lasting and vicious fighting between separated coparents in which children are subject to being caught in the middle and thereby emotionally damaged. Moreover, just as Wallerstein pointed out, it is clear that an egregious theoretical gap exists in the divorce literature, for without qualitative case histories, quantitative research does not get at the "why" of the fact that some breakups are conducted more bitterly than others. None of the studies made a systematic effort to tease out the family circumstances of children of divorce who were having an especially difficult time. But this is asking too much of large-sample empirical research, because the value of the methodology lies in validating surmises from individual cases. To fill this theoretical gap, our hypothesis of the defilement taboo may offer future researchers some suggestions as to why some breakups are so acrimonious and lead to adjustment problems among the children of divorce.

FREUD: FROM ANTHROPOLOGY TO PSYCHOANALYSIS

Why anthropological language in a study of modern love relationships? We can reply by pointing to the quotation from Weiss at the beginning of this chapter; the passage shows that primitive thinking often characterizes the phenomenology of jealous mates in triangular breakups.

The *Dictionary of Anthropology* (Winnick, 1956) gives the following definition of defilement: "The state of being unclean, resulting from contact with death, disease, sacrilege, or similar associations" (pp. 160–161). The listing for taboo yields: "A prohibition which, if violated, leads to an automatic penalty inflicted by magic or religion. [It is a sign] of caution established to guard against basically dangerous things . . . with an incidental effect of maintaining society [and upholding] values" (pp. 522–523). In short, "defilement" refers to toxicity that emanates from a supposedly evil source, and "taboo" is the social injunction against any contact with the toxic source as a form of quarantine, so that a community protects itself from practices that bring shame upon it and threaten its core rituals, institutions, or beliefs.

In *Totem and Taboo* (1913/1955), Freud traced the sense of *taboo* from its ancient tribal meanings to its modern mental derivatives. Although the word is of Polynesian origin, anthropologists found a comparable concept in every culture studied; it was the oldest unwritten code of laws, predating even religion. A taboo operates in three phases—it designates the sacred character of things, prohibits sacrilege, and mandates sanctions. Its purposes are protection of important persons, sheltering the weak, warding off interference with the chief passages of life such as sexuality and marriage, avoidance of impure foods, securing hallowed property against pillage, and warding off the wrath of the spirit world.

In Freud's view the most significant aspect of taboo is that an act of defilement made the offender himself taboo. The entire community too is in jeopardy of being rendered "unclean" unless appropriate restitution is made through chastisement that befalls the offender:

> The punishment was [originally] left to an . . . automatic agency: the violated taboo itself took vengeance [so that offenders would fall sick or die]. At a later stage, when ideas of gods or spirits arose, with whom taboos became associated, the penalty was expected to follow from the divine power. . . . With further evolution of the concept, society . . . took over punishment of offenders, whose conduct had brought their fellow humans into danger. (p. 20)

Freud argued that taboos were the forerunners of what nowadays is called conscience; these early rules served as crude but clear guidelines showing how to avoid or constrain lurking evils:

> What we are concerned with . . . is a number of prohibitions [based on] a theory that they are necessary because certain persons and things are charged with a dangerous power that can be transferred through contact . . . almost like an infection. The *quantity* of this dangerous attribute also plays a part; some people or things have more of it than others. . . . Anyone who [transgresses] himself acquires the characteristic of being prohibited—as though the whole of the dangerous charges had been transferred over to him. . . . The word "taboo" denotes everything, whether a person or a place or a thing or a transitory condition, which is the . . . source of this mysterious attribute. (pp. 21–22)

Freud concluded that taboos are part of our unconscious mental endowment and are most apt to emerge in irrational obsessions. He went on to state that because modern morality has been built up from a substratum of taboos, people today are never so far removed from these atavistic experiences as we might like to suppose.

JEALOUSY AS A CRUSADE AGAINST TABOO VIOLATORS

In marital situations jealousy represents a frantic effort by a wronged mate to uphold moral–religious family norms against transgression. One's sexual prerogatives have been desecrated and righteous action may be seen as necessary to safeguard the social order. Although the issue is profanation of the intangible sanctity of the committed union by *B*, wrath tends to be directed mainly at a tangible third party, *C*, who is an interloper readily stereotyped as the incarnation of infidelity.

In contrast, anger at *B* is problematic in that it may lead to loss of a needed partner, not only in reality but also as a "good" introject. A decision as to whether the relationship to *B* should be saved or not requires working through a complex psychic process, but meanwhile jealousy often becomes a crusade against the breach of inviolate dyadic boundaries, either to repel the outsider and guide a suitably reformed prodigal back into the fold or, alternatively, to extrude an apostate spouse.

When the infidelity involves discovery of a long-term affair, or of a recent relationship threatening to supplant the established marriage, *A* can be expected to exude moral censure toward both *B* and *C*. This reaction tends to be along lines of recrimination and revenge, with the subjective stance vis-à-vis the illicit couple being "They can't be allowed to get away with this!" However, although the transgression of the affair couple has been conjointly committed, their respective offenses are seen as different: whereas a "perfidious" *B* has betrayed sacred pledges and responsibilities, the "predatory" *C* is stigmatized as an opportunist who despoiled a loving marriage. Overall, the stance of *A* is that of a guardian of the sanctity of hearth and home against a sinister consortium.

Such moralizing emanates from the psychological fact that *A* has suffered a grievous loss. The new pairbond have not only destroyed the marriage, but, in so doing, they have also undermined *A*'s self-esteem, especially where sexuality is concerned. Behind reproofs about *B*'s "cheating" and *C*'s "home wrecking" is a rage at the sexual self, incapable of defending its territory or affirming its own worth. This psychic wound is typically dealt with by the ego-restoring device of displacing anger outward for intolerable narcissistic insult; in such cases the wish to punish one or both affair partners becomes a vendetta. At a conscious level the jealous ex-mate is warding off what is perceived as violation of the integrity of the home, but unconsciously h/s desperately resorts to behavioral compensations to withstand a profound sense of loss, humiliation, and powerlessness (Clanton & Smith, 1977).

OBJECT SPLITTING IN JEALOUSY

Logically, fury at *B* (the real source of jealous pain) is more appropriate than fury at *C*. Psycho-logically, however, it is more likely *C* who is the recipient of fury, to be treated as a wicked being whose very existence precipitated a conjugal crisis and now has to be driven off. As Baumeister and Wotman (1992) noted, jilted lovers typically "stifle their negative emotions as long as they are only dealing with the person they love, but the accumulated anger and bitterness can all be directed toward the third person. One woman, for example, said the other woman to whom she lost her beloved was 'the only person I've ever really hated' " (p. 54). By displacing much of the rage that could destroy the marriage onto the accomplice in the partner's infidelity, the beloved can be comparatively absolved of blame and may thereby still be loved. *C* has come to represent the "bad" side of *B*; h/h adulterous traits have been projectively assigned to a third party as scapegoat. In this way, the jealous mind can portray even the partner as "victim" of the rival. *B*'s compliance with seduction can now be mitigated, viewed as weakness or confusion to the extent that *C* is seen as the cause of the triangle. Thus, a jealous ex-mate can readily hate the "bad" *C* and the "tainted" aspect of *B* which is drawn to *C*, but not *B*'s still untainted conjugal aspects. Dicks (1967) has observed that even in cases of "malignant adultery" in which the partner has flaunted the rival as sexually superior, the denigrated spouse often continues to rigidly idealize "the partner I married."

In sum, *B*'s unfaithful behavior may be incompatible with *A*'s internal image of *B* as a loving partner, yet *B*'s infidelity cannot be overlooked. When *A* is in this emotional state, it can be said that a good–bad "splitting" in *A*'s perception of *B* has occurred. Kernberg (1980) has defined splitting as a defense mechanism that "protects the ego from conflicts by means of dissociating or actively keeping apart contradictory experiences of the self and of significant others" (p. 6). An individual using this defense cannot bear seeing an object as having both good and bad traits but rather must see that object as either all good or all bad, almost as if the object were at different times two distinct people. In the circumstances of a jealous triangle, *A*'s object splitting allows preservation of an idealized view of *B* at certain moments, ignoring those facets of *B* that contradict the idealization; at other moments *B* is criticized and condemned, with this stance overriding all previous love feelings. Such shifts in ego state depend on context. Hence, insofar as *B* is associated with *C* in *A*'s mind, *B* is just as hated as *C* and may be attacked along with or even apart from *C*. Yet insofar as this very same *B* is subjectively associated with the marriage, *A* loves *B* as before, looking upon *B* as the person with whom wedding vows were exchanged, as coparent within the family unit, and as a lover who could someday reunite (minus *C*) with *A*.

What are the practical implications of *A*'s object splitting that makes *B* the recipient of both solicitous love and jealous hate? Situations determine which *B*—Dr. Jekyll or Mr. Hyde—will emerge at any given moment. Should *B* be encountered with *C*, wear jewelry or clothing from *C,* or speak well of *C, A* will react to *B* as if *B* and *C* were a fused entity. But when *B* relates to self (or extensions of self such as one's children) without any evident attachment to *C,* the attraction can be overwhelming, for it seems that jealousy has aphrodisiac properties—as Jong (1977) vulgarly but correctly noted in a novel, "The First Law of Jealousy [is that it] makes the prick grow harder . . . and the cunt wetter" (p. 61).

Fortunately, as Jong hastened to add, such perversely based passion does not last. In order for *A* to continue loving the "good" image of *B, A*'s possessive demands must be gratified, at least by *B*'s surface presentation to *A.* If *B* can keep *A* hopeful that *C* is out of the picture, *A*'s splitting defense remains viable and the Jekyll perception can predominate. But this defense soon crumbles if *B* is discovered to have kept on with *C*; then the fickle partner will be seen as "belonging" with *C* and thus deserving the same ostracism as meted out to *C.* When *B* has gone too far with *C, A* will at some point assign primary responsibility for the triangle to *B—where it properly belonged all along—* and the Hyde side of *B*'s personality thereafter becomes paramount in *A*'s eyes.

As the real situation clarifies, the jealous passions subside, gradually fermenting into disgust and, with the letting go process, finally into a pronounced distaste and disinterest, which are the last residues of what once was love. Surprisingly, however, this does not mean that *A*'s crusade against *B–C* is over. Although jealousy as an acute emotion mercifully diminishes over time, its derivative—the defilement taboo—is likely to take much longer to resolve and may even become a permanent legacy of the breakup. In this latter situation, *A* will now be compelled to acknowledge a capacity for grudge holding that may be quite at variance with previously more characteristic easygoing and tolerant ways.

THE DEFILEMENT TABOO IN OPERATION

As we have seen, *C* is regarded as an immoral intruder among the sacred objects of *A*'s world (mate, children, home, friends, etc.). Despite the affair, a marriage to *B* may still go on, or a reconciliation pursued, but the evil of the situation tends to be attributed to the contaminating touch of *C.* Accordingly, *A* is usually determined that there will be no mingling of the sacrosanct (the person and things *A* loves) with the profane (*C* and *B–C*). Thus, *A* may avoid a place that is the known site of a *B–C* tryst or may smash a souvenir of a rendezvous of theirs. As the most glaring example, should the rival have gained access to the conjugal bed, the bed itself—and perhaps the home—is regarded as polluted. A woman came home early from a trip and found her husband with his secretary in their bed; she put the man out but she could no longer use that furniture or stay in that apartment. A man learned that his estranged wife had let her lover stay overnight; he refused from then on to set foot in his old house, instead picking up his children at school. Another man demanded to sell his former house when he saw repairs made by his ex-wife's lover; to him, the building was irreparably marred by such "improvements."

Although the splitting defense allows A to partially exempt B from the defilement taboo, A's social network gets no such leeway: anyone who fraternizes with the anathema C or B–C, or condones the new union, cannot remain long in A's good graces. Such demands for loyalty from friends are strictly enforced. For example, the close acquaintance of a recently separated couple gave a dinner party to which he invited each of them. But because the host gave permission to B to bring along C, A now angrily declined to attend and brought friendship with the host to an abrupt halt. The invitation to B–C, not B alone, was regarded as treason within A's network.

Because B's family is likely to accept whatever current partner is in B's life, their relations with A, however strong in the past, will almost surely fall afoul of the defilement taboo. Willison (1980) told of receiving a letter from her brother-in-law urging her not to speak poorly of her ex-husband's family so that, for her children's sake, there would be no rift. Willison was offended: "It was hard to see his family forget about my loneliness as they went to have dinner at my husband's girlfriend's house and smilingly welcomed the presence of my replacement in their newly reorganized family circle" (p. 114). Although she still invited the paternal grandparents to her children's birthday parties, Willison began to question even this last courtesy. Her former in-laws should not have dined at the girlfriend's house and at the same time expected to get along with her. She had this thought whenever she met any of them or even heard their names mentioned.

The defilement taboo may even disrupt ties to A's family of origin. A forlorn man's mother visited his ex-wife daily so that she could be involved with her grandchildren as before, a practice she kept up even when the ex-wife's lover moved into the home. The man refused to talk to his mother as long as she "broke bread with the enemy": he insisted that she see the children only at her own place. He also became estranged from his sister when she defended what their mother was doing. He shortly moved to a distant city because, beyond his pain over breakup, he could not stand his mother's being polite to the other man instead of caring about him.

It is one thing to sacrifice a friendship because that friend treated *C* with civility, but it is far more serious when adjustment of children who must deal with *C* is involved. The defilement taboo causes virtually intractable problems in the restructuring of many divorced families, frequently wrecking otherwise viable visitation or custody arrangements. Weiss (1975) illustrated how parent *A* warns children against contact with *C,* despite granting the child permission for contact with parent *B* who is now living with *C*:

> I said to my thirteen-year-old, "Alice, I . . . feel that your relationship to your father is one thing, but if I am to maintain my sanity and run this home and work, I . . . have to be considered and I don't want that woman's hands on you, I don't want you to be around her." I just feel like I'm going to lose my kids to her too. And this is the first time I've ever been violent on any subject. (pp. 200–201)

No words are spared here as to how Alice is to treat *C.* Parent *A* is grimly prepared to thwart any possibility that *C,* toxic as ever after having lured away *B,* could now expropriate *A*'s children as well. Out of "consideration," youngsters are now admonished to keep *C* at a distance in order to preserve the remaining sanctity of *A*'s world. However, the same splitting we noted in *A*'s dealings with *B* (*B* alone is good and *C* is the bad part of *B*) is now applied to children. They can love the other parent, but must not love the rival, nor parent and rival together. This mandate co-opts youngsters, delegating them to ostracize parent *A*'s adversaries—or else cause a breakdown in *A*'s functioning, which will cost the children dearly, including the possibility of effective loss of parent *A*.

When a defilement taboo has been imposed, it is inevitable that lines will form up for an implacable war of attrition. On one side of the trenches, parent *A* forbids youngsters to be near or nice to *C,* demands they report back any problems they encounter, and implicitly supports their acting out around *C*. In the opposing trenches, parent *B* will try to induct children into h/h new family, hoping they will meet, accept, and like *C*. The children usually want to accommodate parent *B*'s wishes; after all, h/s remains their parent and being with this parent is often contingent upon being with *C* too. In addition, *C* may also want a good relationship with *B*'s children, partly out of affection but also to uphold union *B–C* by striving for approval as a caring adult whose only crime toward the children is loving parent *B* as the children themselves do.

The worst acrimony occurs when the new *B–C* couple want joint or full custody of the children, or at least entertain wishes or fantasies along these lines. They can expect fierce resistance from *A*, as seen in the following vignette.

> *B* visited his three teenagers regularly, but called *A* one day to say that it was time the kids met *C*, who after all was "a reality they all had to accept." He proposed next Sunday as a suitable day. On hearing the suggested date, *A* became livid, because that was Mother's Day. She immediately responded, "Over my dead body!" and hung up. Her best friend agreed with her that by making this insensitive request *B–C* were wittingly or unwittingly inserting *C* into the role of mother. However, the friend also counseled her that *B–C* had seriously overreached. If *A* could somehow stand to let her children go, such hurtful intent would surely backfire. *A* was persuaded to call *B* back to say that she had changed her mind. The next Sunday, the three youngsters arrived on schedule, remained half an hour, refused to eat a morsel of a sumptuously prepared meal, and announced they had to return home to be with their own mother on this occasion. The point here is that only the conviction that *B–C* would rue their behavior moved *A* to cooperate; otherwise, she would have forbidden the visit.

Some *A*s are so uncomfortable with the destructive situation the defilement taboo imposes on youngsters that they try to rise above jealousy, curbing any impulses to prevent or poison contact between children and *B–C*. They have seemingly come to terms with *B*'s loss, *B*'s involvement with *C*, and, hence, *B–C*'s involvement with *A*'s children. Some believe they even owe it to their offspring to celebrate a child's special occasions jointly with *B–C*, comporting themselves in ultracivilized fashion. But even acceptance of the ex-mate's new relationship may sometimes disguise a hostile wish to gain revenge. We get a glimpse of this in Weiss' (1979a) account of divorced mothers he considered enlightened because "they don't really wish their ex-husbands ill, and if their ex-husbands are happy, it may in marginal ways be better for the children at home" (pp. 161–162). Weiss offered several cases of such enlightenment, yet in our reading we detect in each of them an ex-wife fomenting trouble. For example, a woman invited ex and lover over to talk about why the kids can't visit there without arguments about "Daddy's" attention, and another woman advised her ex to have the kids meet his new partner in spite of the latter's reluctance.

Despite displays of tolerance for the ex-mate's new union, which nominally suspends the defilement taboo against *C* and *B–C*, cases like these may instead show how clever *A*s catch more flies with honey than with vinegar. Even if *A* is an admirable adult who can rise above jealousy to parental altruism, it will probably take time to reach the requisite level of emotional security. Short of this attainment, it can be anticipated that parent *A* is usually prone to set children on a collision course with *C* and *B–C,* using them to get *B* and *C* to fight with each other over their care, or even insidiously urging kids to refuse to relate to *C, B–C,* and in some instances *B.* All in all, marriages that collapse under the weight of a triangle will not readily overcome jealous resentments that parent *A* overtly or covertly transmits to h/h offspring. When antipathy exists, such feelings cannot be hidden or denied so that children do not pick it up. Indeed, they are seldom allowed *not* to pick it up, because parent *A* often fumes at their dealings with *B–C,* saying that *B–C* is hardly a wholesome couple for them to be around.

THE POSITION OF THE CHILDREN
OF MARRIAGE *A–B*

In triangular breakups, emotional damage to children is caused to some degree by the divorce precipitated through the actions of parent *B,* and to some degree by the defilement taboo instituted by parent *A.* The ensuing problems of the children are seldom sufficient to make parents change—say, by *A* being less judgmental or by *B* not bringing the children around *C.* As already noted, parent *B* usually resists parent *A*'s mandate that youngsters keep their distance from *C* and *B–C,* even insisting that *C* is a fact of life that the children must accept. But such facts of life may not be accepted, for youngsters can refuse to see, obey, or respect *C.* Thus, one boy hid in the closet when his mother invited her new boyfriend over, and another proclaimed he would do anything to prevent either parent from remarrying. Even without support from parent *A,* a child cannot be forced to validate parent *B*'s new relationship.

However, because children normally do not wish to offend either parent, they often compromise by meeting with *B–C* but upsetting their applecart in sundry ways, or by providing *A* with negative accounts of experiences in their home, or by purveying confidential information about *B–C.* The polarization of the two camps makes the psychic life of the child precarious, leading to delicate maneuvers to keep each parent assured of loyalty. But this does not mean that the child can be diplomatically adept forever or is without sympathies and opinions; sooner or later h/h own feelings prevail, at times leading to loss of trust by one or the other adult. At one extreme, when the child treats *C* as *persona non grata,* parent *B* will be offended. An 8-year-old girl refused to use, or even touch, a new hairbrush left for her by her father's lover. The girl did not like this woman, resented her presence during visits to her father's place, and saw her as the reason her family was no longer intact. Such an attitude sat well with her mother but exasperated her father, who felt she did not give his girlfriend a chance. Forced to choose between daughter and girlfriend, the man saw less and less of his daughter.

The other extreme offends parent A: the child idealizes parent B, defends h/h decision to leave the marriage, and gets along well with C. A 17-year-old girl, always her father's favorite child, enjoyed wearing the necklace he gave her on her birthday just after he had left home to be with his affair partner. Her mother became angry. She believed C had shopped for and selected the necklace, because B had never done this kind of task or shown this sort of taste. If the daughter persisted in wearing the accursed item, the mother advised her that the price of such "insensitivity" would be to leave and move in with her father. In saying this, the mother was aware that B–C would prefer that the girl not reside with them, so her statement was a way to drive a wedge between father and daughter or between father and girlfriend. But the daughter stayed, and war continued to rage over the symbolism of the necklace: for parent A, the defiling touch of the "other woman"; for daughter, parent B's love for her, which parent A wished to thwart. The girl felt her mother was driving her crazy and was glad to go away to college. As long as she was seen to be on B–C's side, she was hounded, threatened, and almost extruded from her home for manifesting a loyalty to father that was interpreted as disloyalty to mother.

WORST-CASE SCENARIOS FOR CHILDREN: THE MEDEA COMPLEX

An adolescent can often handle a problem with belligerent parents by leaving home, either going to live with the noncustodial parent or making some other arrangement. But younger children whose parents fight over their care cannot do so—a custody disposition determines where they will be. A dreadful situation will now be discussed in which parent A's defilement taboo has been so starkly framed that parent B's involvement with the children is circumvented. In this pattern, A's defense mechanism of splitting the counterpart into a "good B" (a coparent welcome to relate to the children) and a "bad B" (harmful to the children when in C's proximity) is no longer in operation. Instead, an unforgivably tarnished B has been merged with C into a joint "bad B–C" percept that applies to both of them, now constituting ostracism of a totally defiled former partner even when apart from the rival. Sometimes even a degree of hatred may be subtly manifested toward the children whom *B* has procreated with *A*.

Jacobs (1988) has coined the term "Medea complex" from the 5th-century B.C. drama by Euripides. In the Greek play, Medea is cast aside by Jason, who wishes to marry Creusa, the daughter of the king of Corinth. Medea poisons Creusa and Creusa's father, then stabs her two sons to death. According to Jacobs, Jason no longer cared about Medea, so suicide was not a viable vengeance; Medea killed the boys because Jason would keenly suffer from *this* loss. Jacobs then traced the same dynamic in contemporary marriage, providing the case of a wife who put her husband out and cut off his access to the children after she found him in their bed with another woman. Jacobs's Medea complex thus refers to an ancient form, whereby *A* literally deprives *B* of h/h children by killing them (a scenario that unfortunately still occurs), and a modern form, whereby *A* deprives *B* of access, in effect taking them away from *B*. In both versions, boundary loss is experienced in which abandonment of *A* by *B* is merged with the *A*-imposed "abandonment" of children by *B*.

Jacobs applied the Medea complex only to women. Although Pittman (1987) agreed that the legend is psychologically accurate, he pointed out that in modern divorce men sometimes abandon their children to hurt the ex-wife. White and Mullen (1989) also view the tale as having modern parallels, but made no gender distinctions in citing an American study in which 6 of 138 pathologically jealous felons attacked their offspring, as well as a British series in which 9 of 71 jealous murderers killed one or more of their children.

Let us consider two examples of a modern Medea complex. The first case concerns a 16-year-old girl who said in therapy:

> I'll never forgive my mother for keeping me from my father. She did everything she could to turn us against him. She said he didn't love us and never called but never told us she'd changed our number to unlisted and never gave us the letters he wrote or the packages he sent. He finally gave up trying after we moved three times. How could she do that to me? I spent eight years without a father, thinking he didn't love me, all because she hated him for leaving with another woman. (Everett & Everett, 1994, p. 114)

The second example is found in Tolstoy's *Anna Karenina* (1878/1965), which concerns an errant wife who is punished by denial of access to her children. Anna becomes involved with a lover, but her husband preserves the semblance of marriage on social–religious grounds, stipulating that Anna must exercise discretion and that her lover must never visit their home. However, Anna is pregnant by her lover, and during a serious illness she sends for him. He visits but is seen by the husband on his way out. After accusing Anna of bringing the man into their home for an assignation, the husband states that he is leaving to live elsewhere and sending their son to his sister's estate. To Anna's pleas, he replies, "I have lost even affection for my son, because he is associated with the repulsion I feel for you. But still I shall take him!" (p. 385). Mother and son are soon separated, the boy being told that Anna is dead. Anna later commits suicide. Throughout the novel, it is plain that Tolstoy had more sympathy for the sinning wife than for the sanctimonious husband.

Chesler (1986) discussed nonfictional cases in which women have lost custody because they had affairs. She noted that punitive custody suits are hardly rare, especially when the husband has a history of "macho" or potency problems (in a sample of 10 cases, Chesler found that 3 men were sexually inadequate and 7 were abusive or adulterous). She concluded that custody litigation by irate ex-husbands may at times have little to do with concern for their children's welfare or a desire for greater involvement in their lives; instead, the legal system is used to vent the sexist rage of "castrated" males. Such men cavalierly trundle youngsters off to be raised elsewhere, while placing the woman outside the pale of respectable society as too morally impure to be in the company of her own brood. Although Chesler's data are limited in that they come from only the female side, she showed that children can easily be caught in custody strife when their parents part over sexual issues. This point is confirmed in a larger series of cases studied by Hodges (1986), who concluded that men whose wives had left them for a lover were more likely than others to seek custody.

C'S RELATIONSHIP TO THE CHILDREN

McGoldrick and Carter (1989) cited evidence that in 70% of divorces one of the spouses was involved in an affair, although only 15% of them later married the affair partner. Still, even without a second marriage, more than 15% must have stayed involved with the outside lover for some extended time after breakup of the first marriage. This brings us to the subject of stepfamilies, legal or common-law. Children may have problems in adjusting to a new stepparent, but these problems are hardly insuperable as research has shown that remarriage tends to be beneficial to youngsters (Hetherington, 1989). Further, many stepfamilies have been successfully treated for conflict between ex-spouse and new spouse over the care of children (McGoldrick & Carter, 1989). However, despite the usually positive aspects of remarriage for children, it seems to us that the literature on stepfamilies by and large does not take accurate measure of the situation posed for youngsters by one parent's divorce and remarriage within the context of a love triangle. Scattered clinical and case history data exist on this eventuality, and they are not favorable.

As a nationally known advocate for women in the third-party role and thus a strong defender of stepfamilies in general, Sands (1982) stated that *C* typically feels like a surrogate mother to her married man's children long before breakup of marriage *A–B*:

> When you . . . and he are planning your life together at last, does the picture include step-parenting expectations? . . . Chances are you already have maternal feelings. . . . After all, during your affair his children have been discussed. You've heard about their childhood diseases, their ups and downs, and . . . conflicts your married man felt. You knew . . . who was having what problem, and you probably even gave advice. And so you . . . got to know his children and care for them, even . . . without ever spending time with them. (p. 168)

Sands stated that this attitude tends to disappear once *C* has become a second wife, dealing with the children from marriage *A–B*. She cited a letter from Betsy, married herself but childless when she became involved with her best friend's husband, who now graphically described disillusionment as a stepparent in her second marriage:

> I found what I was looking for in a man . . . but I also found misery with Stan's daughters. His ex couldn't accept any of the blame for their marriage ending, so I got all the blame from everyone. [The girls] are spending the summer with us and their hostility is everywhere. It's not the endless chores . . . it's that I get no appreciation. No one talks to me unless I ask a question. Stan's youngest loathes me. I can't even touch her. If I do by mistake—say we rub shoulders in the car or I fix her collar—she touches her shoulder or collar and smells her fingers. It's as if I'm diseased to a point that I have a foul odor that she's sniffing for. (pp. 175–176)

Betsy concluded that Stan's girls were "spoiled, ungrateful little tarts." She hated them and decided she was glad not to have any children of her own if this is what it is like!

Sands noted that two-thirds of second marriages fail, mainly because of the stress of dealing with stepchildren, which is even worse in "former mistress/married man unions." She quoted from letters she had received (pp. 180–182): "Before getting married to my married man I had presentiments—they were *his* kids and I liked them. After getting married I had post-sentiments—suddenly they were *her* kids full of her faults and I couldn't stand them"; "As a mistress I used to scream at him about how I didn't want to be a martyr for his kids while he stayed married. Now as a second wife I am a real martyr for his kids"; and "He keeps on telling me to hold on every weekend we spend with his kids. He says that they're getting older all the time. I have one comment for him, we're getting older too." Only one correspondent eventually surmounted resentment from and toward the children: "His kids made me feel like a dirty object. I had no name. I was referred to as 'her.' After nine months they began calling me Sandy. After two years they actually liked talking to me. And now . . . I really look forward to their visits! I thought it would never happen."

Wallerstein and Blakeslee (1989) scoffed at the validity of the expectation that children will learn to love the father's new wife—only 10% of subjects in their sample ever grew closer to their stepmothers. One stepmother, a *C,* said, "If I had known then what I know now about how difficult it would be for me and his kids to get along, I might not have married him" (p. 254). They commented that many stepmothers were angry about their husband's paying child support to the first wife and let this frustration spill onto the youngsters, and others resented the intrusion of children into their space. Hetherington (1989) reported that many stepfathers had similar reservations, tending to remain aloof and saying, "I married her, not the kids". Some men even omitted mention of the spouse's children when asked to identify members of their families.

In summary, successful integration of children from a first marriage into a second marriage is problematic enough, even in the absence of an acrimonious triangular breakup. But whereas in general stepfamilies can work through conflicts over the care of children from previous marriages, it appears that the professional literature is far too sanguine about prospects for reorganization where triangle-based divorce and remarriage are concerned.

THE DEFILEMENT TABOO ASSESSED: ITS COST VERSUS ITS SOCIAL VALUE

Parent *A*'s defilement taboo forces dichotomous choices: you are either good or bad, you are either with me or against me. Whereas jealous passion eventually passes, a defilement taboo tends to endure as a cognitive set stemming not only from object splitting in jealousy but also from needs to restore a sense of control. Though undeniably creating hardships for children, the defilement taboo is in many ways adaptive for parent A. Psychic survival is seen to depend on warding off any further encroachment by B–C (Brown, 1991). It is not necessarily "overwrought" for A to think of B–C as a threat to everything h/s cherishes; in A's eyes, not only has there been actual loss of a marriage but also, from the viewpoint of morality, making peace with the new couple would only acquiesce in—as well as ratify—an intolerable status quo.

In respect to the latter point, in an age when jealousy is frowned upon and divorce is "the new freedom" (Fisher, 1974), social conflict is widespread because the same society also views exclusive sexual access as a marital prerogative. A's outrage proceeds from the traditional view that union B–C constitutes an assault upon the sanctity of h/h marriage and the social order in general. Because B–C's subversion of A's marriage is now acceptable behavior socially and legally, the only way for A to express indignation is to ensure personally that the "illicit" couple do not escape unpenalized and unstigmatized. Without someone to flag them, their violation of conjugal sanctity becomes another type of "defining deviancy down" (Moynihan, 1992). Persons in the position of A may become even more vengeful when they discover, to their dismay, how little community support actually exists for their stance. Nordheimer (1987) reported increasing violence in family courts dealing with divorce, alimony, and custody cases. After repeated incidents in which judges, lawyers, and ex-spouses were slain in open court by an aggrieved litigant, he came to the conclusion that violence in family court now exceeds that in criminal court. He attributed this aggression mainly to the acrimony of divorce, but Nordheimer did not consider whether the violent spouses viewed court personnel as officially condoning an infamous situation. When A sees that B–C are in fact receiving the protection of the law for their union, h/s may resort to extremely nihilistic measures such as a crime of passion (even extending to court officers), a vindictive custody suit, child abduction, or hysterical accusations of sexual abuse.

Whatever the psychological value of the defilement taboo for parent A, we still cannot ignore its destructiveness. In many cases it is pushed to an extreme where it becomes gravely deleterious to the emotional balance of a child, especially when parent A defames, ruins, or drives away parent B. Taken to such lengths, it is not good parenting. But when primordial feelings of "defilement" strike, the impact is so overwhelming that self-discipline "for the children's sake" prevails only through sheer determination and then only after a long period of working through antecedent anguish and resentment. Although the consequences can be devastating for children, parent A's performance in triangular circumstances cannot be exempt from human limitations— a jilted mate can rarely cope with jealous loss without the taboo as a defense. In addition, A can also point out that in all fairness B was hardly an altruistic parent when h/s exposed their children to the trauma of family breakup.

Professional advice is meant to be helpful but is sometimes not practicable; moreover, the literature is often vague about how to attain recommended goals because therapists do not have special techniques to make a parent A work well with an unfaithful partner and lover. Thus, Ahrons and Miller (1993) viewed father involvement as crucial when mothers retain custody, urging treatment during the first year if there are conflicts that drive fathers away. But this assumes that triangle-based conflicts are manageable by rapid intervention and that mothers must make accommodations no matter what the conduct of fathers. Consider the case of the husband who became involved with another woman during his wife's pregnancy. He declared that he would leave when the baby was born, but that he and his lover wanted regular contact with the child thereafter because he wished "to be a good father." After delivery, he left home as promised, but the wife refused to deal with him or give him access to the infant—an outcome no therapist could hope to change within the first year. If a clinician aims at getting parent A to cooperate with B–C's wish to be involved in the upbringing of children, such treatment stands a very good chance of being received by parent A as grossly unempathic and amoral. On the contrary, no matter what a therapist's agenda regarding involvement of both parents in care of their young, the first priority might better be to understand parent A's attitude toward B–C and to work with parent B not to take for granted that it is h/h immediate right to bring offspring around C (although this may be possible later on). If the therapist follows the lead of Ahrons and Miller, intervention will only exacerbate the already raging divorce strife; after all, there can be no therapeutic success with either parent A or B over mutual care of their children without rapport with *both* adults in the treatment (Isaacs, Montalvo, & Abelsohn, 1986). A's defilement taboo is not the last word on the subject of B's involvement, but neither can it be ignored or obviated without serious consequences.

Unfortunately, much of the clinical literature on the subject of divorce lacks a tragic perspective. As therapists, it is natural that we want to reduce suffering of family members, especially where children are concerned. But not every problem can be fixed. When a relationship breaks up in a love triangle and a defilement taboo ensues, these issues may sometimes be ultimately worked out in a way protective of children, but it is at times beyond our therapeutic capacity because the human and moral issues are complex and both parties are locked into such different views of mutual entitlement and obligation. In short, therapists have to be realistic enough to acknowledge that we are dealing with a situation brought on by the passions, provocations, and limitations of both parents. However, although a triangular breakup and a resultant defilement taboo can polarize the family unit, perhaps the one benefit of this painful situation is that it clarifies for the children the deep characterological, philosophic, and spiritual gulf between two parents grappling in divorce war.

∾ III

Catastrophic and Other Severe Reactions to Rejection in Love

Introduction

A study of eight cases . . . revealed a consistent pattern. The
murderer was a severely disturbed man who killed himself
immediately after murdering his mistress or wife. The crime was
. . . a reaction to separation in a relationship marked by
prolonged turmoil. [My hypothesis] is that the threat of
separation brought about an ego regression in which rage was
directed at both . . . subjects and that the murder–suicide was an
acting-out of fantasies of reunion.

—DORPAT (1976, p 197)

Separation is a severe test of a forsaken mate's qualities as a human
being. Caring about the lost partner, ability to tolerate the other's
autonomy, and control of one's own destructive impulses will be
challenged to the limit. Needless to say, not everyone handles loss of
a partner with restraint. Some even go to desperate extremes, so that
embarrassed symbiants may later declare that at this time their actions
were sadly "out of character" (Baumeister & Wotman, 1992). Hetherington, Law, and O'Connor (1993) reported that "previously rational,
self-controlled individuals report such things as smearing dog feces on
their ex-spouse's face, following them and peering into their bedroom
windows, defacing their property . . . [and saying] 'I can't believe I did
that' or 'That wasn't really me.' " (p. 216) Such vile behaviors are a
rejoinder to any hopes the countersymbiant may have for a "friendly"
divorce and "civilized" comportment; vindictive behaviors are protests
that cannot or dare not be ignored. Whereas the countersymbiant does
not expect the symbiant to like the fact of separation, h/s nevertheless
wants the forsaken mate to come to terms with it and make no trouble.
The symbiant, however, precisely because of a desire for impact and/or

contact, is likely to make trouble, or to be in trouble, in just those areas in which the countersymbiant is most vulnerable.

In acrimonious breakups, a rejector in the relationship is forced to acknowledge that spiteful countermeasures are to be expected, although it may be unpredictable just what or how drastic these will be. As we have seen in examining various ways to leave your lover, one factor in the choice of a method concerns self-protection: a countersymbiant may try to alleviate the threat of possible loss of control by an ex-mate via timely displays of caring or, conversely, through instant disengagement. Ostensible caring aims at forestalling a crisis by deceptively raising hopes for reunion. This approach bargains for time in order to make the final break less crushing, but may only make matters worse when ambivalence about leaving is exposed as duplicity. As for the opposite pole, disengagement (the clean break) conveys disregard for the ex-mate's survival and can thereby trigger a devastating reaction because the symbiant must go to drastic lengths to avoid being dismissed as insignificant. Thus, both these options are perilous for the countersymbiant, as either can incite implacable resolve on the part of the reciprocal in which, regardless of cost, revenge now becomes the sole purpose in living.

In this section we will deal with forsaken symbiants who go to lengths that are harmful—perhaps fatal—to themselves or their partners. Society sets limits as to how far an unrequited lover may go in revenge. Aside from criminal penalties, social precepts have long condemned harming others, using children as pawns, or even being vindictive in general. Such limits are necessary in order to maintain a humane and orderly society; there can be no question about the wisdom inherent in having moral and legal standards to govern reactions in situations of rejection in love. Nevertheless, the standards are *ideals,* which are unfortunately not always realizable during a paramount romantic crisis when a distraught suitor may defiantly declare, "All is fair in love and war!" In these tragic cases behavior occurs in which the ordinary rules of social, legal, and religious practice are thrown to the winds. Thus, catastrophic reactions include placing one's health or mental health in jeopardy, but at the extreme will involve the literal sacrifice of either party.

Although most people rejected in love react in ways that are hostile, intrusive, or self-destructive to the point of causing temporary guilt, worry, or mayhem for the ex-partner, some forsaken mates act out unbearable tension by irrevocable sadomasochistic aggression. When this occurs, the underlying dynamic is the symbiant's attempt to bind the countersymbiant to the relationship, in reality or in "reunion fantasy". In cases in which there is violent interference with the partner's plan for a separation, the symbiant is sending a message that the pair are still in relationship, despite the pretensions of the partner that they are not. Up against this mindset, anything a countersymbiant does to demonstrate independence risks escalation of the separation strife to a disastrous level, because the forsaken mate may be grimly resolved to uphold a claim of *eternal connection and intertwined destinies* that can be more important than the forfeit of either life.

In regard to the use of deadly force, Chapter 9 deals with revenge suicide and Chapter 10 considers crimes of passion. With resort to either mode, the forsaken mate irrefutably shows that one partner cannot exist without the other. This primitive psychic fusion merges two separate principals into a composite unity, the unconscious meaning of which is to magically undo earthly separation by plunging either self, partner, or both into a symbiotic love–death. The couple's commitment vows can end only "when death do us part," and even then the subjective presumption is that the union abides beyond the grave.

The life-threatening catastrophic reactions can be classified as follows: suicide, crimes of passion, and stress-induced medical illness (the topic of Chapter 11). A forsaken mate may manifest all three reactions at various times and in varying degrees, indicating that these phenotypically diverse outcomes share a common genotypic base. In fact, as the catastrophic reactions are reviewed, it will soon be apparent that existing psychological formulations describe each in quite similar dynamic terms. They are interchangeable ways to fall apart in the absence of the needed object—expressions of the common psychic theme asserting that the two people are still emotionally bonded. All three have dynamics that include (1) symptoms that primarily express grief directly or indirectly for the lost relationship, (2) the fastening of guilt on the partner for what turns out to be the consequences of rejection, and (3) sadomasochistic indifference to the ending or ruination of the two lives if this outcome serves the overriding cause of symbiosis.

In Chapter 12, we add a fourth type of adverse response, but one neither violent nor lethal: reactive sexual dysfunction. Mates who are forsaken are almost uniformly subject to sexual disorders and/or inability to tolerate closeness. This lasts from several weeks to several years after breakup and may even prove to be more or less permanent. The multiple determinants of the sexual symptoms encompass (1) preservation of the bond to the countersymbiant through impaired or limited contact with subsequent lovers, (2) punishment of self for unworthiness in love, and (3) displacement of rage at the disengaging partner for damage to one's sexual ego by treating new suitors as if they were dangerous reincarnations of the rejector. Parallels to the psychodynamics of the lethal catastrophic reactions can readily be drawn, specifically in regard to symbiosis, mourning, vengeance, and self-hatred, all tracing back to an etiology of traumatic object loss.

In whatever form, the desperate symptoms of a forsaken mate represent a psychodynamically fueled protest against what the disengaging partner has done. Just which variation on a morbid theme a given symbiant elects will depend on characterological makeup, as well as on the special circumstances of the separation, including the key factor of the countersymbiant's conduct of the breakup. A forsaken mate who cannot stand the pain must do *something*—a something that can in some cases transform the grave misfortune of rejection in love into an irremediable tragedy.

~ 9

Suicide
In the Shadow of the Object

> Sociologists and psychologists who talk of [suicide] as a disease
> puzzle me now as much as the Catholics and Muslims who call it
> the most deadly of mortal sins. It seems to me be as much
> beyond social or psychic prophylaxis as it is beyond morality, a
> terrible but . . . natural reaction to the strained . . . unnatural
> necessities we sometimes create for ourselves.
> —ALVAREZ (1972, pp. 283–284)

SUICIDOLOGY

Some people commit suicide after rejection in love, many more attempt it but survive, and most probably have fleeting fantasies or impulses along these lines. But before addressing suicidality in the context of rejection in love, we review the generic findings.

The French sociologist Durkheim (1897) analyzed demographic data to identify the social variables most conducive to suicide. He found consistently higher European rates for men than women, the elderly in contrast to the young, the single, widowed, and divorced as opposed to the married, and Protestants as compared with Catholics. Durkheim believed social marginality accounted for such statistical patterns: men tend to be less embedded in family life than women, the elderly are more apt to feel superfluous than the young, the single person is more isolated than the married, and Protestants have a more individualistic religion than Catholics. As the requisite prodromal setting for most cases of suicide, he then posited a psychic state of *anomie* (without norms), defined as the at-risk person's sense of not being integrated into society. In a primary prevention application (Lester, 1992), divorce rates have been cited as one index of a suicidogenic culture (Stengel, 1965).

But clarification of the concept of anomie is still needed. Besnard (1988) called for distinguishing between an acute crisis in social identity and chronic social alienation. Alvarez (1972) also criticized Durkheim's method, which "in the very process of treating suicide as a topic for serious research, manages to deny it all serious meaning by reducing despair to the boniest statistics" (p. xv), and Hendin (1995) complained that Durkheim put people in social categories without any considera-tion of culture per se, which is the only way to determine the psychic meaning to that person of being in that category. This "meaning for the individual" gap was bridged by the case study method of Freud, so that Durkheim and Freud are regarded as the two seminal figures in suicidology.

Subsequent research has found marked demographic differences between those who actually die of suicide and those who survive an attempt. Whereas the former tend to fit the pattern of alienation outlined by Durkheim, the latter are predominantly younger females engaged in a social matrix. This indicates that "parasuicide" or a "suicidal gesture" has a distinctive motif, which is not necessarily to die. Although those attempting to kill themselves sometimes survive by accident and those not wanting to die at times overdo a gesture, by and large those who perish by suicide intended to die and those who survive an attempt are manipulating a significant other.

As to the relation of psychiatric diagnosis to suicide, Robins, Murphy, Wilkinson, Gassner, and Kayes (1959) concluded that mental illness is usually the primary etiological factor (in their sample, 94% manifested preceding psychiatric disturbance and 4% severe medical illness). This generalization is still accepted today. However, such post hoc findings reflect bias. Unless a psychiatric history is already on record, a retroactive diagnosis tends to seek foregoing signs of depres-sion that then "explain" the suicide. Further, although a preceding depression is indeed found in most cases of suicide, situation-appropri-ate reactions (as in cases of chronic pain or terminal illness) do not constitute mental illness. Even when it is shown that depression varies with neurotransmitter levels (Kramer, 1993), such levels are simply somatic correlates of emotion. Drug therapy is often beneficial to treat depression, but this does not mean that etiology has been discovered (Pam, 1990).

Unlike modern clinicians who make depression the primary cause of suicide, Durkheim never regarded suicide as a homogeneous phe-nomenon. He differentiated between altruistic and egoistic types of suicide. The former involved self-sacrifice for the sake of others (not to be attributed to anomie), whereas the latter concerned loss of status and self-esteem (to be attributed to anomie). This distinction is not well received nowadays, because boundaries are not always clear and clinicians tend to be wary of justifications for suicide—for example, witness the current debate over assisted suicide. Roman (1980) held that if functional ability is compromised, suicide is a "rational" act, and Szasz (1973) stated that "suicide" is a term used only by those who oppose it as a right, whereas "death control" is the appropriate term for those who favor that right. In rebuttal, Hendin (1995) has pointed out that mental disorder can distort judgment in exercising such control.

We mention this controversy to counter the tendency within the mental health field to pathologize suicide in a way that seems to explain it away as a mental aberration. Such a view may preclude empathic understanding, whereas it is the thrust of this chapter to consider suicidal behavior as the product of a *tragic situation.*

THE PSYCHOLOGY OF DEPRESSION LEADING TO SUICIDE

There are many models of depression that clinicians now draw on to treat this condition. Among the most influential has been Seligman's (1989) paradigm of "learned helplessness." He found that animals exposed to unpredictable, uncontrollable stress eventually give up problem-solving behavior. He proposed a cognitive theory of depression: inability to cope with a major stressor leads to loss of hope as well as resignation to one's fate, and the antidote is some sense of empowerment. This thesis was strongly supported by Beck, Steer, Kovacs, and Garrison (1985), who followed 207 hospitalized suicidal patients of whom 89 were assessed as high on a measure of hopelessness—13 of 14 subsequent suicides in their sample came from this subgroup.

Hendin (1995) noted that *despair* is the word clinicians tend to use to distinguish suicidal from nonsuicidal depressed patients, but he thinks this is imprecise. Despair arises from an inability to envision significant human connections; many such patients are simply resigned to their situation—they are miserable but do not attempt suicide. But patients who commit suicide show an antecedent state of *desperation*—they are not only "hopeless about change but also [believe] life is impossible without such change" (p. 20).

Paykel (1980) studied the relation of suicide to preceding stressful events. He found that dire life events peaked within the month before a suicidal attempt and that marital problems were the single most commonly reported precipitant—in particular, the exit of a spouse. In a sample of alcoholics one-third of suicides took place in the year following loss of a close relationship, usually within 6 weeks (Murphy & Robins, 1967). Strife in an ongoing marriage is also a frequent precipitant of suicide. Lester (1992) reviewed research suggesting that marriages in which a spouse becomes suicidal are unusually problematic in terms of communication and agreement; he noted that after a suicide attempt, 40% of couples separated and a further 25% experienced a worsened relationship. Thus, suicide can be the result of marital distress, but an attempt that fails can either foster eventual breakup or cause further estrangement by the partner living under this threat.

Freud (1917/1955) emphasized the close association between mourning and melancholia, attributing depression to real or symbolic loss that brings about a state of bereavement. Regression to a mental state of relative incapacitation occurs, whereby "the basic relationship with the world is that of a hungry infant dependent on [an object] for its vital supplies" (Monroe, 1955, pp. 288–289). Only magical restoration of the symbiotic dyad promises relief from the trauma of object loss. When this is not possible, the afflicted individual anticipates virtually inexorable annihilation. At the same time, libidinal energy withdrawn from a lost love object is relocated in the ego and used to recreate the loved one as an aspect of the self; it is as if "the shadow of the object falls upon the ego" (Freud, 1917/1957) and the shadow is now treated as if it were the object, although a demarcation still exists between self and this introject (Litman, 1970b). In other words, the lost object has been turned into an introject with whom one is in constant dialogue about the relationship, so that the missed–fused person is "still there."

In a well-known maxim, Freud also pointed out that depression is anger turned inward. According to this formulation, depression shields the abandoning object as still worthy of love by deflecting anger toward the self. Excessive guilt and masochistic behavior are thus characteristic features of depression, displacing anger at the object. In suicide this dynamic is intensified so that "guilt over hatred of an incorporated lost love object [underlies] the need for self-punishment. In destroying [the self] *and* the [internalized] object, the individual accomplish[es] atonement as well as revenge" (Hendin, 1995, p. 23). Recovery occurs only when one gets in touch with largely repressed hostility and can express such feelings directly, appropriately, and without apology. Even if the object has died of natural causes, anger at loss is still presumed to occur. In short, psychoanalytic doctrine holds that human beings are selfish enough to rage at loved ones who have gone away for any reason, as well as needy enough to try to love them anyway.

All in all, the intrapsychic primary gain of symptoms of depression is cathartic grieving for the lost object, which ensures that the object remains at the epicenter of awareness and is not subjectively "lost." This dynamic as well protects the needed object from one's own rage. In addition, an interpersonal secondary gain extracts a measure of solicitude and punishes the significant other through guilt. But whatever the secondary gain, depression is not a manipulative ploy. Its symptoms are involuntary, its dynamics are mainly unconscious, and it can be expected to manifest itself in some dysphoric form following object loss.

MAGICAL THINKING IN SUICIDE

Suicide is an action driven by thoughts about the continued viability of one's life, the nature of death, the effect of suicide on significant others, and the message implicitly sent by this deed. Shneidman (1970a) analyzed thousands of notes to understand the logic of suicidal persons and concluded that their thinking reveals a split in self-perception. On the one hand, there is I_s who is the self experienced by the person, e.g., "I_s am glad [my death] is going to trouble you"). On the other hand, I_o is the self in "the shadow of the object" (e.g., "I_o will get attention; that is, certain other people will cry, sing hymns, relive memories, and the like"). This split is not a fallacy in reasoning but rather a fallacious identification. It occurs in all people when we think about our own death, but is especially vivid in imminent suicides:

> There is a form of satisfaction to I_s in the following sense: although it is true that I_s ceases to exist after death and thus could not [benefit from] remorse felt toward I_o at that time, I_s can experience a satisfaction through the anticipation of the remorse felt toward I_o. This anticipation . . . takes place before death, when I_s still exists. It is a fallacy because in order to achieve the anticipation . . . he cannot experience it, except that anticipation of pleasure can itself be a pleasure. It is this psychic reward which may be one of the prime motivating aspects of suicide. (pp. 65–66)

Litman (1970a) listed unconscious fantasies that contribute to suicide: "*a tired wish* for surcease, escape, sleep, death; *a guilty wish* for punishment [or] sacrifice to make restitution; *a hostile wish* for revenge, power, control, murder; *an erotic wish* for passionate surrender, the greatest ecstasy, reunion with the loved dead; and *a hopeful wish* for life, for rescue, rebirth, a new start" (p. 298, italics ours). Litman (1970b) especially stressed the intimate connection between death and sexuality in which sadomasochistic eroticism is considered the cause of most suicides.

Gernsbacher (1985) saw suicide as the outcome of a grandiose self-concept, suggesting that those who die by their own hand are frequently far too sanguine in their expectations as to how their self-destructive behavior will affect others and for how long.

Turning now to irrational fantasies specific to suicide in situations of unrequited love, we come back to the psychoanalytic premise that regressive childhood fears are recapitulated in the adult experience of loss so that survival is at first felt to depend on getting the love object back. In desperation, various ideas will now be entertained in which the fate of the self is used to mold the partner's reactions: "What can happen to me that will force h/h to care, or to regret what h/s has perpetrated?" Although not physically attacking the other, the implicit meaning of such symbiotic ruminations is *masochistic revenge*. Suffering in one form or another now seems oddly appealing, provided it makes the partner reconsider or repent the imposed breakup. However, when there seems to be no way to make the partner return, the "charm" of a suicidal solution is that it is a perverse way to implement compliance with the partner's wish for separation, but, by taking that wish too literally and too far, promises to make the partner rue what was done! Moreover, suicide is seen as a transcendent fusion: the immolation of self appears like a triumphant enactment of the vow that love ends only "when death us do part." Thus, upholding love is given preeminence over upholding life, and this is the eroticism that makes such acts of suicide a love–death.

MASOCHISTIC REVENGE UNLEASHED

The conscious and unconscious motivations that lead to suicide are extensions of the thematic issues Freud outlined for reactive depression. Menninger (1938) identified three distinct motifs that combine to make up suicidal impulsion. First, rage at a significant other is so great that *someone* has to be murdered. Second, suicide expresses self-hatred; the self is unlovable and deserves to die. Third, suicide secures relief in one of two ways: whereas some rush toward death without letting anyone intercede because their plight is unbearable (the wish to perish), others select methods that leave space for an opportune reprieve by a significant other (a cry for help). Thus, in tandem with the demographic data, the clinical literature identifies two populations of those who commit suicide, people who acutely want to die and people who make a suicidal gesture, fatalistically placing themselves in danger by their own hand as a desperate device. Litman (1970a) noted that therapists who deal with less lethally inclined suicidal patients tend to be impressed by their manipulation, dramatics, and hostility, whereas the more ominous cases tend to come across as persons who are hopeless, overwhelmed, and resigned.

Menninger's analysis rearranged the formulation for depression when applied to suicide in some details, but the cardinal idea of displacement—anger turned inward—still holds. As Hendin (1995) stated, "Suicide can be a form of control of violent impulses by those who feel torn apart by them" (p. 114). The self is destroyed in lieu of the abandoning object, but a posthumous revenge is obtained via the imposition of a haunting guilt, hence, the self paradoxically lives on as an accusatory memory. Sullivan (1953) pointed to the enormity of needs to punish when he regarded suicide as "hatefully conceived and executed" and "calculated to have a prolonged evil effect in some other people" (p. 25). Further, the next chapter will show that about half of lethal crimes of passion are either preceded or succeeded by suicidal behavior and that murder followed by suicide has dynamic characteristics more akin to suicide than to homicide. Thus, aggression against the lost object and aggression against the self can be two sides of the same coin. Indeed, whether in revenge suicide or in a crime of passion, *boundaries between self and object are so blurred that to punish one is as if to punish the other.* We can tell from what happens when rage is unleashed in a crime of passion just how very powerful are the angry feelings toward the beloved that the depressed person seeks to keep bottled up in depression or to enact only against h/h own self in suicide.

Meerloo (1968) took the interchangeability of suicide and murder to its conceptual limits, contending that many suicides could more accurately be called "psychic homicide" inasmuch as victims were impelled to self-destruction through hostility and murderous wishes emanating from a very significant other. The person who commits suicide intuitively detects messages that h/s is "in the way," "no good," "a burden," and so on, and fulfills the emotional demands of the other to be gotten rid of by imposing h/h own death. In so doing, the person kills *in effigy* the significant other h/s is gratifying, illustrating once again the confusion of self–object ego boundaries. Meerloo gave this case as an example:

A doctor having an affair with his secretary denied his wife treatment by a colleague for her reactive depression. Finally, he took a vacation with his secretary and his little daughter (his only child), leaving his wife at home. After two days, she committed suicide in accord with his unconscious demand. The man remained unaware of his psychic homicide. (p. 94)

Meerloo was attempting to force out into the open the most uncomfortable judgments about the suicidogenic environment, in effect saying that the psychological autopsy of many suicides will implicate an intimate of the victim as h/h wishful "murderer." However, these death wishes are usually unconsciously conveyed and the significant other is not going to acknowledge them as such, almost no matter what their intensity or their consequences. For these significant others, the truth about their feelings and intentions are too grim to be faced. As Shneidman (1970b) noted, Meerloo had his own experience with the darker side of life as a concentration camp survivor and realized that human beings cannot admit certain things without jeopardizing their self-esteem.

Meerloo's approach to suicide is especially applicable to the plight of an unwanted symbiant. To be sure, the vast majority of disengaging partners do not hope for their spouse's death. Their foremost need is to get out of the committed union, and there are many ways to accomplish this without fomenting suicide. However, sometimes a symbiant poses such intractable problems in separation that the countersymbiant is bound to have occasional wishes that the vexatious spouse would conveniently just "disappear." These are the incipient death wishes—fleeting, inchoate, and ambiguous at first, but perhaps growing to provocative proportions.

> A husband hovered on the brink of suicide after his wife left him for another man. After breakup, she justified harsh measures to make him leave her alone by citing to him the hypothetical case of a dog in the path of a speeding car—it being too dangerous to swerve or brake, she said that "you simply had to run over the damn dog!" In response, he commented that it did not seem to matter to her whether he lived or died so long as he stayed out of her way. She reassured him that she did not want any harm to befall him and that she would not be better off with him dead. But a few weeks later she asked him about the status of his life insurance coverage. He was piqued and retorted that he did not want her to be the beneficiary and therefore would let the policy lapse. A row ensued: she was highly insulted by his reply, which assumed that she had a stake in his demise; he too was insulted by her asking about life insurance when she knew he was suicidal owing to her actions.

Gillis (1986, pp. 66–68) described how her marriage started to unravel at her birthday dinner at a chic French restaurant. Her husband told her there that he had decided not to give her any gift because it didn't "mean anything." She immediately became nauseous, went to the bathroom to throw up, could not eat but sat through the expensive dinner while he ate, and when they finally went home she took three pills for pain relief. The next morning he accused her of trying to kill herself. In addition, a few days later he took out an insurance policy on her life, stating that it was just in case she committed suicide so that he would not be left penniless. Gillis was not aware of giving any sign of being suicidal, nor was her husband the least bit sympathetic or supportive. At first puzzled, she saw this event in a more ominous light when her husband shortly announced he was leaving; his fear that she might commit suicide now appeared to her to be more in the nature of a projected wish.

It is too much to expect the party who wishes to terminate a committed relationship to be in touch with any unconscious demands (if such there be) urging an encumbering spouse to self-destruct. Even when under heavy duress from the symbiant, admitting such reactive wishes or needs to drive the mate to suicide would entail recognition of conscious malevolence and selfishness. Whether disingenuous or not, the expressed attitude of most people exiting a committed relationship is one of wanting only happiness after breakup for the forsaken mate or, at worst, a lack of concern.

IS THE "DEATH WISH"
OVERWROUGHT HYPERBOLE?

Meerloo's indictment of the significant other for "psychic homicide" is too serious to be left standing without very critical examination. Such an accusation is questionable, because no direct measure of the "unconscious" exists and a clinician can never be sure of the validity of inferences based only on observed behavior, especially when there are disavowals by the principal. Further, in a situation of breakup, does a death wish really emanate from the disengaging partner, as Meerloo suggested? Or are we dealing with a projected accusation coming from the suicidal person's own wish to vicariously kill the significant other, as Menninger suggested?

From the perspective of the symbiant, abrogation of concern by the countersymbiant in breakup is readily perceived as an insidious form of hatred of the mate for being "in the way" and can be construed as a message to commit suicide in order to set the partner free. This interpretation interfaces with the sense of the symbiant that h/h existence is more or less over anyway after loss of the partner's love.

In this light, Meerloo's proposition about psychic homicide will appear valid—it adopts the frame of reference already held by the unrequited lover. The symbiant feels suicide is merely a self-inflicted coup de grace administered after being mutilated by the disengaging partner's firing squad.

But this is a one-sided exposition of the cause for a suicidal tendency. It is too pat to ascribe responsibility solely to the countersymbiant, as if a suicidal symbiant were merely an innocent victim without murderous pent-up ire of h/h own. Moreover, it is the symbiant's reading of the rejection that converts it into a death sentence, in effect branding the significant other a "psychic murderer" by choosing the expedient of suicide. Alvarez (1972) pointed out that the self-empowerment inherent in suicide is often manifested as a somewhat romantic and theatrical statement, a sort of grand finale rung in to highlight one's view of life. Thus, in marital breakups suicide may demonstrate an unrequited lover's willingness to forfeit existence in an unforgettable way, but such dramatizing can only indirectly be blamed on the partner.

From the perspective of the countersymbiant, suicide seems like an act caused by the symbiant's psychopathology, for which the countersymbiant is not personally responsible. The countersymbiant seeks at great cost to live an independent life, which indeed causes unfortunate consequences for the symbiant; but does this amount to malevolence, as if the reason for breakup was to hurt the symbiant? Is it malevolence if the countersymbiant declines to be blackmailed by possible suicide into staying with, or coming back to, an unwanted mate? Insofar as a countersymbiant can admit any desire for the symbiant to disappear or die, such fantasies occur only because there seems to be no escape from the forsaken mate's incessant interferences. Moreover, the countersymbiant is likely to add that fantasies that come from being fed up with a situation hardly constitute an infernal plot to precipitate a suicide.

Yet this too is a one-sided exposition. The countersymbiant has usually made it painfully clear that the symbiant should "be nice and go away"—just how or where is left to the discretion of the latter. Furthermore, the countersymbiant largely creates the context within which the symbiant operates; tact in breaking bad news, the pace of change, and the extent of contact after breakup are factors under the countersymbiant's control. Given such leverage, the countersymbiant has either not paid attention to, or grossly underestimated, or recklessly dared this particular denouement. It is always speculative to aver that the countersymbiant enjoined a death wish upon a suicidal symbiant, but we will be on firm ground if we note that the countersymbiant was more concerned with promoting h/h own purposes than with any catastrophe that might overtake the ex. It is this refusal to be "thy spouse's keeper" that constitutes the felt hostility in psychic homicide, for where there is a symbiotic relationship, experiencing such indifference kills.

Each protagonist's interpretation of the meaning of separation leads to blaming the reciprocal as the cause of a suicide. As we see it, the value of Meerloo's contribution is his insistence on a "systems" approach: he underscored the psychological connections between the person who commits suicide and h/h most significant other. In the circumstances of breakup, when suicide is threatened, attempted, or accomplished, the emotional violence is such on both sides that death wishes can often be said to be "in the air." It may at times appear that the countersymbiant's wishes were served all too well by having the mate take h/h own life; yet despite incitement, assessment of responsibility remains complex inasmuch as the ulterior motives of either party cannot be minimized and suicide is a collusive outcome of their pathological relationship. Meerloo has drawn attention to a crucial precipitant—a significant other's cold disinterest or even callous instigation—but, in the process, this only highlights a dyad's sadomasochistic enmeshment.

A LAST WORD ON SUICIDE AS THE LAST WORD

In the circumstances of breakup, suicidality is behavior that emphatically declares that rejection in love has so devastated and disorganized the subject that only this desperate act can restore meaning and coherence to one's life. As the French poet Artaud (1965) promised: "If I commit suicide, it will not be to destroy myself but to put myself back together again" (p. 56). But despite the personal holocaust of unrequited love, a symbiant cannot stake survival on restoration of the relationship—this gives too much power to the partner. Nor can the countersymbiant be forced into the role of "evil genius" intent on fostering suicide, thereby giving h/h too much responsibility. In the final analysis, it is up to the symbiant to find a reason to live, if only to spite the countersymbiant.

A mother of four was suddenly left by her husband, who stayed away for 2 weeks and then returned, explaining only that he had been "drinking." Unbeknownst to him, she learned he had been with her best friend, the bridesmaid at her wedding. The wife quietly kept up her friendship with this woman, revealing nothing about what she now knew in order to observe the situation. Her husband soon walked out again, but this time she called her "friend," asking her not to see him so the marriage could be saved. The woman replied that he had promised her he would not come to her unless his marriage was completely over. The wife was skeptical; she retorted, "But he made *me* other promises at the altar—and you were there!" Several days later the man came home to "reconcile," but the wife ascertained through her sources that he continued his affair with the other woman. The wife could not bear to confront him—she wanted to keep a father in the house for her children and saw no way to support the family without his income. In due course she became suicidal, complaining to herself that she was unfortunately too healthy to die of tuberculosis or cancer; besides, everybody would feel sorry for *him*. As her husband was a subway motorman, she decided on death by throwing herself under a train. She rode the subway, selecting a suitable station for her leap, and made what should have been a farewell phone call to her home. To her astonishment, the call was answered not by her husband, as planned, but by the other woman. She went into a fury, concluding that her husband and rival were prematurely celebrating her death and taking over her family. She hurried back to serve tea as the hostess in her own home. When her youngest child finished high school, she put her husband out.

Although it appears that cues were being sent demanding the suicide that almost occurred, this wife did have a choice. In the end, she did not accommodate her husband's death wish for oppositional reasons—it would have made things too easy for him. Moreover, the validity of the formulation "anger turned inward" is confirmed by how this woman ultimately survived. The anger at loss of her husband was owned and directed outward simply by returning to her home, rather than by being indirectly, symbolically, and masochistically turned against herself through suicide.

~ **10**

Crimes of Passion

It is . . . clear that homicide "out of the blue" is exceptionally
rare. Almost invariably there are words or actions which
provoke the killer into the use of force. . . . That reactions and
counterreactions exist is a [fact] which ought not be ignored
when "innocence" or "guilt" are under . . . scrutiny. As George
Meredith wrote:

> I see no sin;
> The wrong is mixed.
> In tragic life, God wot,
> No villain need be! Passions spin the plot:
> We are betrayed by what is false within.
> —MORRIS AND BLOM-COOPER (1976, p. 71)

A MORE COMPREHENSIVE DEFINITION
OF CRIMES OF PASSION

Originally a French police term, *le crime passionel* refers to a lethal
assault of a lover or mate for reasons of romantic rage. Technically, an
out-of-love partner can commit such an act, but the passion is not
between killer and victim—rather, it is typically between killer and a
paramour, with the victim standing in their way and therefore subject
to elimination as an impediment (Godwin, 1978). However, in an age
of readily accessible divorce, the vast majority of crimes of passion now
tend to involve the murder of a love object perceived to be unfaithful,
abandoning, or both. The felt sexual inadequacy of an unrequited lover
can impel measures whereby the beloved is slaughtered, nominally to
punish for desecration of the committed union, but essentially to
restore to the ego some sense of control. Bromberg (1961) referred to
such behavior in men as the "cuckolding reaction," echoing
Guttmacher (1960), who described castration fears in "gynocide."

However, in similar situations women too can commit lethal crimes of passion (e.g., Spencer, 1981). In these cases, a countersymbiant victim meets calamity at the hands of a symbiant who "carries a torch" for this relationship to the point of igniting a conflagration. Yarvis (1991) has noted that a common characteristic of such homicides is that the perpetrator has recently felt disenfranchised from the community, and this loss too is blamed on the victim, adding fuel to the flames.

Although not every case fits into a set pattern, this chapter focuses on the most prevalent type—aggression committed by an "in love" mate upon a partner perceived to be unfaithful to the terms of the relationship. However, we have modified and elaborated the traditional conception of such crimes of passion in three ways.

First, we have extended the definition to encompass not only homicide, but also the use of any illicit means to ruin the new life of the disengaging partner, amounting to symbolic murder. Given this broader application, crimes of passion will be criminal but not necessarily violent, or violent but not necessarily fatal, or murderous toward someone dear to the partner but not necessarily toward that person per se. As examples, physical assault resulting in maiming or disfiguring the partner, the abduction of a child, and killing a partner's lover would all now fall under the rubric of our classification. All such deeds have in common *criminal behavior in a context of terrorizing–punishing.* We have to exclude from this definition actions that remain within the limits of the law but may be just as malevolent as an illegal act. For instance, bringing a custody suit may sometimes be as malevolent as child kidnapping, but it is not criminal. In summary, the typical crime of passion concerns an injurious, felonious deed put into effect to make estrangement as grave a misfortune for the countersymbiant as it already is for the symbiant. Havoc is wreaked with disregard for the human cost to partner, children, collaterals, and self, or, rather, this cost is vindictively used to show the partner's depravity for letting the relationship come to such a pass. Accordingly, a symbiant will often justify h/h reprisal as a valid response to the "real" crime committed when the disengaging partner wrecked the committed union.

Second, the phrase "crime of passion" connotes the abnormal behavior of a perpetrator so overwrought with rage as to indicate an "emotional disturbance." But we are uncomfortable with such labeling applied to diverse reactions and corresponding to no existing diagnosis. A crime of passion is indeed an infraction of the criminal code, but at the same time it is well to remember that it is only a drastic extension of the ordinary warfare practiced in acrimonious breakup. Beyond the ubiquity of violent fantasies and impulses in the minds of parting partners, physical aggression commonly occurs in separation (e.g., smashing things, slapping, pushing, etc.), even though such actions may not be deemed serious enough to call the police, or if called, dismissed as a simple "domestic dispute." Further, still within the realm of ordinary warfare, people rejected in love often express their resentment in nonviolent ways that involve breaking the law (e.g., slander, trespass, refusal to obey court orders). In short, a crime of passion differs from "normal" acrimony only in that it goes to an alarming extreme. It is not the rage that produces it that is abnormal, and we can all empathize: "Hell hath no fury like a woman (or man) scorned!" We are *not* contending that crimes of passion are psychologically normal, only that the rage that produces them is normal. Thus, we identify psychopathology in the person who commits a crime of passion not by rage but by *nihilistic loss of control.* This criterion is met if vengeful, destructive impulses can no longer be contained so that an illicit measure not only is taken beyond the bounds of what can be socially tolerated, but is also counterproductive because the perpetrator has lost any rational sense of "future." The criminal act is more notably self-defeating than self-serving. In terms of diagnosis, such behavior usually bespeaks a severe adjustment disorder that has been triggered by traumatic rejection in love, although often complicated by premorbid personality pathology. Because the character of a symbiant determines how h/s will deal with separation distress in general and control of aggressive impulses in particular, the more tenuous the ego strength, the more likely nihilistic loss of control will occur. Spouses with a marked propensity for fighting, drinking, or jealousy are the most apt to resort to gross violence in a lover's quarrel (Chimbos, 1978).

Third, although nihilistic loss of control stamps the symbiant who takes aggression too far as "disturbed," family systems theory teaches us that it may be simplistic to impute sole responsibility to the psychopathology of a perpetrator. Instead, the locus of the problem often lies in the *interactive patterns of the dyad, for which both are responsible.* In other words, the countersymbiant may be provocative enough to push the symbiant past the limits of what the latter can endure. When this happens, the countersymbiant has set up conditions conducive to loss of control, and the symbiant strikes the blow. Thus, a crime of passion tends to be a collusive transaction: both parties jointly (though not necessarily equally) participate in a process that results in tragedy.

The core idea in our formulation is that crimes of passion indicate powerful centrifugal–centripetal forces operating within a troubled symbiotic relationship. The enmeshment inherent in a crime of passion is often not only within the perpetrator's mind, but may also be a mutual dynamic impelling the two principals in an unfolding drama. As such, it is an enactment of "love gone wrong" in which a couple cannot bear to stay together or come apart.

COMPARISON OF SUICIDE
AND CRIMES OF PASSION

The psychic wellspring of both a crime of passion and suicide is the credo that life without the beloved is not worth living. Psychoanalysis has always stressed that they share a common denominator—in the unconscious, suicide is murder and murder is suicide:

> Freud pointed out the very close relationship of suicide to murder. It was his thesis that many suicides are disguised murder, though the act of self-murder only symbolically kills some hated individual. . . . The reverse is also true—there are murders that are symbolic suicides. . . . It appears that the individual is attempting to destroy . . . that part of himself that he has projected onto the victim he wishes to destroy. (Guttmacher, 1960, p. 68)

In the *depressive* catastrophic reactions, we saw the razor's edge that barely delineated between destructive behavior deployed against the self and violence deployed against the significant other in cases of suicide in which aggression was masochistically discharged—anger turned inward. When we turn attention to the *hostile* catastrophic reactions, we see the same close affinity between self-hate and object hate, but this time the balance tips the other way, with rage externally released while depression is held in temporary abeyance—despair turned outward. We summarize the difference between these two drastic resolutions as follows.

In depressive–suicidal reactions anger is vented directly at the self, and indirectly at the significant other by the imposing of guilt for the tragic fate of the self, but aggression is deflected masochistically to protect the significant other from overt attack. In crimes of passion anger is vented directly at the significant other, and indirectly at the self through assumption of guilt for harm inflicted on the significant other, but there is masochistic refusal to protect either other or self from the unleashed aggression.

In the preceding chapter, Meerloo's concept of "psychic homicide" was introduced—suicide was interpreted as the result of a death wish from a significant other. The equivalent concept in the field of criminology is Wolfgang's (1959, 1976) "victim-precipitated homicide." He studied a series of Philadelphia murders and found that in 26% of cases the victim had struck the first blow. Wolfgang was impressed by two findings: victim-precipitated homicide was even more prevalent when the parties were spouses, and the victim was more apt to have a prior record of assaultive or criminal behavior than the perpetrator. He concluded that in many cases there was a psychological provocation that could have triggered a lethal assault—the victim participated in the genesis of h/h own murder. Wolfgang thus established an interpersonal context for certain perpetrator–victim dyads in homicide comparable to that set forth by Meerloo in certain dyads in which suicide occurs. In each relationship, one party's behavior has an underside that fosters violence by the reciprocal, ultimately inducing the latter to perform a decisive deed to relieve unbearable tension between them. In either taking one's own life or a murderous crime of passion, one of the two must die, and the survivor is nailed to a cross of guilt.

Many other studies have confirmed Wolfgang's findings. For example, 32% of a series of murders in Baltimore were victim-precipitated—an even higher rate than Wolfgang found (McDonald, 1968). Goldenberg and Goldenberg (1982) reported that one-third of all murders in the United States are within the family; 53% of these are between spouses, a far higher rate than for any other related pair. They concluded that domestic murders were best understood from a systems viewpoint: "The locus of pathology is not the individual but rather the individual in context" (p. 199) and "a particular family climate must exist for homicide to occur" (p. 201). Daly and Wilson (1988) described a "spousal homicide syndrome" in which the victim was engaged in an affair, with breakup and reconciliation of the marriage preceding the killing. They cited one study of spousal murders in which 85% of the perpetrators blamed unspecified "sexual matters" as the cause of their crime, as well as a Detroit study in which 29% of spousal murders were over "jealous conflicts."

Forensic research has shown that persons committing "domestic" murders show characteristics more closely resembling the clinical picture found in suicide than in most murders—that is, they were more likely to be depressed than predatory. In both suicide and crimes of passion, the motive appears to be symbiotic union across the boundaries of life and death. Indeed, the killing of an intimate is frequently preceded or succeeded by powerful suicidal urges. In a survey of British crime statistics, Mowat (1966) demonstrated that some 35% of those who killed a significant other died of suicide after the murder and another 10% made attempts before the crime. West (1965) estimated that half of domestic-type murders are followed by an actual or seriously attempted suicide. He compared 148 random murderers brought to the bar of British justice and 148 cases of murder followed by suicide, finding that the crimes of the second group were associated with family quarrels more than with pecuniary motives, and that more persons were killed per murderer, sometimes extending to whole families, collaterals, or bystanders. This conclusion confirmed results earlier reported by Wolfgang (1958) in a parallel U.S. study. The murder–suicide group had far fewer psychopathic types, deviated less from community norms in terms of prior psychiatric or criminal history, but committed more violent crimes, involving multiple shootings or stabbings.

Given the similarity between crimes of passion and suicide, the two phenomena can be construed to stand as alternative aspects of the same malignant process. Dorpat (1976) offered clinical data illustrating their virtual interchangeability, especially when a couple are in conflict about separation. For example, a woman ran out of her house in an agitated state, waving a knife about, undecided whether to kill herself or her husband. A parallel case occurred when Jean Harris shot to death her longtime lover, Dr. Herman Tarnower, after he took up with a younger woman (Spencer, 1981). Harris had come to his house with a pistol, intending to kill herself on his property. According to her trial testimony, when Dr. Tarnower tried to stop her, she accidentally shot him as they struggled for the gun (this claim did not prove a viable defense—she could not explain why he had four bullets in his body). She then added that after shooting him, the pistol jammed when she turned it against herself (this point was credible because examination of the weapon showed that the bolt was bent). Harris lamented that she had not been able to join her lover in death; she thought of her life as over anyway, stating that his loss was more punishment for her than any sentence the court could impose. She was found guilty and sent to prison for life. Even this outcome can be seen as unconsciously contrived to be self-destructive. Had Harris allowed her attorney to plead extreme emotional disturbance as a defense instead of accidental homicide, she might have received a more lenient sentence.

Only nuances apart, every feature of the dynamics of suicide has its mirror image in crimes of passion. As noted in the previous chapter, Freud saw killing the self as psychologically equivalent to killing the object—here it is vice versa. We also reviewed Menninger's three motivational components in suicide: the symbolic murder of a significant other, punishment of an unworthy self, and escape from suffering. The analogues in crimes of passion for the first two components have already been discussed. In regard to the third component, the equivalent of the "wish to perish" or the less lethal "cry for help" occurs when extrication from suffering is sought by removing the partner—instead of the self—from the relationship, either through murder (in lieu of a consummated suicide) or through terrorism as a warning (tantamount to a cry for help in parasuicide). In the latter situation, a menacing eruption by a symbiant amounts to telling the partner to get out of reach immediately because control has been lost—only thus can murder be averted. Consider the case of Martin (Tennov, 1979):

Sarah was stringing me along ... she didn't care for me the way I needed her to and I began to look elsewhere. But Sarah couldn't leave well enough alone, so she'd come around on a flimsy excuse, roll her eyes at me and hint that she [wanted me to take her out] ... a temptation I never could resist. After an evening in which I paid the bills and she flirted with every man she saw, I was left high and dry again. I was an emotional slave. Finally, I couldn't take it anymore. I took a sledge hammer ... and stormed outside. ... I began hammering the first object I came to, which [was] a neighbor's car. I smashed the roof in. Then I smashed the window [of a shop] and broke about 30 more store windows before they stopped me, and the funny thing is, I don't think I was crazy. I knew what I was doing. I was trying to stop the pain and I succeeded. I spent six weeks in jail, paid $10,000 in fines, and had to face all those guys whose property I had damaged. [But] I never saw Sarah again. (pp. 152–153)

Martin's rampage was a cry for help; by smashing Sarah in effigy, he showed that she had gone too far in trifling with his sexuality and could no longer come around him without precipitating violence toward her. In this "macho" manner he counteracted any feelings of castration. Too vulnerable to leave on his own, he chose to drive her out of the relationship. Emotional letting go was not yet available—Martin first needed Sarah to keep away.

THE PERPETRATOR–VICTIM DUET

We have already postulated that inasmuch as the symbiant is only half of a two-party network, the source of violence may lie in the interactive pattern of the couple rather than in the aberrant personality of one. McDonald (1961) captured the spirit of a systems approach to murder when he quoted from a Franz Werfel novel in which a boy who slew his father exclaimed, "I, the assassin, and he, the victim, are both guilty ... but he is a little more guilty than I!" (pp. 65–66).

All students of homicide have been struck by the victim's contribution. Von Hentig (1948) stated that "there are cases in which [victim and offender] are reversed and in the long line of causative forces the victim assumes the role of a determinant" so that "in a sense, the victim shapes and molds the criminal" (pp. 383–385). Abrahamsen (1973) called for a new discipline he named "comprehensive victimology," which would stand as a departure from the traditional practice of criminal law: "This is not to say that the murderer is not guilty, or that the victim is not dead; it means only that the emotional interaction leads to an act of murder" (pp.

43–44). McDonald (1968) held that "some persons seem drawn to death by violence, not merely by an injudicious word or gesture at an inopportune moment, but rather through a persisting pattern of sado-masochistic behavior. They may be homicide-prone as others are accident-prone" (pp. 45–46). Morris and Blom-Cooper (1976) questioned just how applicable the term "victim" is when a murder occurs between principals well known to each other. Lester and Lester (1975) went so far as to speculate whether anyone ever provokes h/h own murder as a means to commit suicide, at the same time ensuring that the dyadic partner gets punished by the law.

In a crime of passion, the countersymbiant guides the process of separation, but h/h role is more or less confined to setting a stage for disaster, goading the symbiant to bring about a finale that provides resolution for the enmeshed couple. When the partner incites by uncaring behavior an extreme reaction from a symbiant, unverbalized (and later to be denied) death wishes may have been conveyed, which now boomerang on the countersymbiant. Even more than in suicide, in crimes of passion acting out goes to lengths that the countersymbiant will soon regret, in that the symbiant carries out with a vengeance the reciprocal's largely unconscious demand that the other must do something to sever their bonds. If irrevocable acting out were to be avoided, the countersymbiant would have striven to manage the separation so as to give the symbiant time and means to adjust. In brief, whenever a symbiant struggles with inclinations toward some sort of catastrophic reaction, the countersymbiant may be, on the surface, indifferent or callous within this same period, yet fanning and manipulating from afar the symbiant's anguish over loss of the relationship because this anguish vicariously expresses some aspect of h/h psyche too. The paradoxical logic here is that a symbiant can inflict a crime of passion only if a countersymbiant allows it for h/h own psychic reasons! Even as cautious a theorist as Shneidman (1970c) has come to much the same conclusion, noting three possibilities when there is murder of a partner: (1) the victim is not knowing, expecting, or wanting h/h demise, (2) the victim knows what may happen but is not consenting, and (3) the victim is consenting and may even participate in the planning or execution. On balance, Shneidman realized that sinister unconscious factors, as outlined by Wolfgang and Meerloo, may be at work in any of the three possibilities.

What would be a countersymbiant's motivation to risk being the target for any sort of crime of passion? This interpretation of the situation makes no sense; there are more reasonable and plausible ways in which a countersymbiant may justify h/h actions. To start with, h/s can point to what it takes to sever a committed union. Although duly recognizing that violent reactions from the ex-mate are possible, h/s cannot afford to be deterred from leaving by signs of violence that amount to blackmail, especially when it is not clear just what will happen. Further, h/s might also be so angry at the point of breakup that hostility cannot fully be held in check, with concomitant lack of concern as to how the symbiant will fare in separation. In addition, h/s may be seen as provocative when retaliating for something the ex has done, feeling such action is a legitimate and necessary defense of h/h own position and rights.

Granted that there is much truth in the preceding assertions, they still remain *conscious* explanations, leaving out of account murky intrapsychic factors that are onerous to admit or face. We will now consider several themes that may be involved at the darker, more irrational level of the countersymbiant's motivation. As noted in Chapter 2, there are always explosive issues of guilt and blame that play out across the blurred ego boundaries of a couple in the throes of separation. By putting pressure on the weaknesses of the symbiant, the countersymbiant can readily show the ex-mate to be precisely the "bad" person from whom h/s had to flee. Thus, at times the countersymbiant's provocations suggest that there may be a need to upset, disorganize, and stigmatize the symbiant. Intertwined with this exposure of the counterpart as *the* problem person, the countersymbiant may also be running from h/h own guilt as a "bad" leaver—projecting much of this onus onto the symbiant but still not obviating all sense of deserved punishment, somehow to be meted out by the ex-mate. Beyond the guilt–blame turmoil, an even more potent unconscious factor is represented by persistent enmeshment in a relationship that the countersymbiant has behaviorally chosen to exit. Yet despite vehement denial of an embarrassing attachment, h/s cannot help but have some remaining investment in the mate. The anomaly of enmeshment while seeking separation calls for *masked statements of symbiotic attachment*—responsibility for making such a statement is vicariously delegated to the ex-mate, in this way permitting disavowal of any lingering emotional involvement. The specific workings of such unconscious dynamics will become clear as we look into boundary issues in various types of crimes of passion.

A COMPENDIUM OF CRIMES OF PASSION

There are two broad categories of physical aggression by the symbiant. First, violence is directed toward the countersymbiant, ranging from reckless endangerment to murder. Second, reprisals are taken against collaterals; homicidal impulses are displaced so that the countersymbiant may be spared but intimate others are killed, such as lover, parents, or children.

Reckless Endangerment

Reckless endangerment involves a threat expressed through a symbiant's action that momentarily places the countersymbiant in jeopardy and at the mercy of the ex. A man held his ex-wife over the edge of their apartment terrace when she sneered at his love making and suggested that she now knew where to do better. Locked out of the house, one man rammed his car through the front door, and another briefly kidnapped his wife. A jilted husband set a fire in his wife's tenement building when she was entertaining a male visitor. A woman caught sight of her husband walking down the street with his new girlfriend; she attacked the pair with her car, sending the woman running and pinning the man against a wall. In all these cases, subsequent sexual contact between former mates occurred, and in two cases reconciliation occurred.

As can be seen, the rage in reckless endangerment is barely contained. The countersymbiant emerges shaken but unscathed: had defiance been manifested, h/s risked getting killed on the spot. The line between terrorizing and injuring appears tenuous, but holds for the time being. The symbiant remains an ever present threat, vigilantly "out there" to extract suitable revenge if the errant partner continues to do wrong. Also implicit in the terror is a cry for help—violent reprisals can be avoided if only the countersymbiant reconciles, or stays celibate, or is at least so discreet as to never be seen in the company of another.

In some of these cases, the collusion of the countersymbiant might be inferred from failure to prosecute, not to mention the retention of contacts with the symbiant, which often involve sex. However, we cannot minimize the factor of *fear* on the part of a countersymbiant so that a dangerous still-involved mate has to be placated and a total break postponed; this certainly must be taken into account. Yet fear alone does not fully explain the confusing and contradictory behavior by certain countersymbiants, including some of the aforementioned cases in which chances to leave and never look back were passed up.

Assault

The next degree of enacted vengeance involves beating the countersymbiant, though such attacks stop short of inflicting permanent injury or death. As in reckless endangerment, the countersymbiant can neither protest nor resist without risking a fiasco, for the perpetrator's view is that the partner must submit to physical battering as quid pro quo for the emotional battering caused by leaving. Such beatings may be wordlessly administered, commencing as soon as the estranged partner is within arm's reach.

A woman lay almost paralyzed in her bed for 2 weeks after her boyfriend left her to be with her best friend. At last, she arose. She went to her boyfriend's office and began pummeling him. She returned every day to do the same, until employees there began warning him of her appearance so he could hide or leave. Then she went to her girlfriend's job, smacked her, and finished off several weeks of mayhem by visiting the apartment where the two resided. There she became violent and was taken away by police. In another case, a man blackened his wife's eye when she told him to leave. Afterward, he often battered her during visits to the children. Even an order of protection did not keep him from the house, but gave him yet another grievance for which to attack his wife. The woman took a lover skilled in karate, and the commotion came to a halt.

In these vignettes, a pattern exists wherein a countersymbiant is terrorized by a sadistic avenger who expects the former partner to accept punishment as h/h due. Still another aspect is that if the former partner cannot "reform," h/s should at least stay out of the symbiant's way, because rage is out of control. The battering forces the countersymbiant to disengage because the symbiant cannot, though it is the symbiant who directs the countersymbiant to do so. The latter's collusion is seen in the initial battering, as guilt hinders remedial action, but the countersymbiant will eventually feel enough is enough and put a stop to the assaults.

Rape

When the countersymbiant is female, there is a risk of forcible rape. Such acting out has little to do with sex but is more a demonstration of male power; indeed, research has shown that this is true of all acts of forcible rape (Brownmiller, 1975). Society has only recently started to deal with marital rape as a criminal act (Freeman, 1985; Whatley, 1993). It is certainly a widespread problem. Russell (1982) found 14% of a sample of 930 married women reported at least one episode. However, the word *rape* is too broadly used to fit many situations (Rowland, 1989). For our purposes, there is a difference when the victim is a stranger as opposed to an intimate of the perpetrator; the usual definition of rape as coercion readily fits the former situation, but in the latter situation an examination of the couple dynamic sometimes points to collusion as well as coercion. From a forensic perspective, yes, a crime has been committed and the word "rape" will be used in framing the charge that a woman can quite rightly bring against her husband. However, from a family systems perspective, resort to forcible sex may occur within an ongoing context of *mutual sexual humiliation,* although resort to violence by the man remains no less reprehensible.

A woman told a friend that she was raped by her ex-husband after she had once again refused to reconcile with him. As her story unfolded, it became apparent that there was much provocation on her part. Thus, the woman had commonly undressed and walked about in lingerie when the man visited and tried to talk to her, offering the rationale that it was spurious to feign modesty after years of marriage. He once entered her unlocked bathroom while she was bathing, and she let him watch, with the silent comment that if he were silly enough to come in there, he might as well eat his heart out. She often allowed him to sleep overnight beside her in what had been their bed, but did not permit physical touching. Yet when she was raped, the woman disregarded the seductive and demeaning tactics she had used and could not acknowledge any hostile teasing or manipulating of the man's feelings. For her, the rape exposed the nature of the man she was rejecting, and she was unforgiving.

While forcible sex in any manifestation is unacceptable, in this instance marital rape was a response from a man who himself may have felt violated by the woman's use of her body to hurt him. Of course, this statement should not be construed to mean that every man who sexually assaults his ex has been provoked into such behavior, nor that a woman who practices "castrating" tactics deserves to be raped. What is at issue here is the principle that a sexual crime of passion may at times best be comprehended by examining the context of the relationship. It may turn out that the parties have taken turns inflicting humiliation all through their history. For the female countersymbiant, treating the male as if he were a nonsexual object may express such factors as manifesting a passive–aggressive determination to even the account for past complaints, fomenting a rancorous interaction that validates her decision to leave, and perhaps having sex with him in the only way she could accept but allowing disavowal of her involvement. For the symbiant male, resort to force may signify a macho reaction to his sexual devaluation, resolve to extract some kind of restitution for past deprivation, and a sexist sense that she remains "his" woman (Goldner, Penn, Sheinberg, & Walker, 1990). Thus, an act of rape between ex-spouses—although criminal—can in some instances represent compliance on the man's part, for reasons of his own sexual dynamics, with the unconscious wishes of the woman to rape and be raped. It is not an isolated event but in context is apt to be part of a sadomasochistic pattern. A notorious Oregon case exemplifies this point. Mrs. Rideout was the first wife in the country to succeed in having her husband charged with rape; but at trial, he was found not guilty and 2 weeks later, to the disgust of many feminists, the couple reconciled (Russell, 1982).

Disfigurement

If rape constitutes a marauding sexual raid, then disfigurement denotes an even more implacable campaign waged against a troubling attraction that makes it hard for a still involved symbiant to let go. Its goal is to ensure that the ex can never again hope to be attractive to anybody else. Further, the penalty inflicted is on the order of a scarlet letter; from the symbiant's viewpoint, the wounds announce to the world: This is a traitor. In addition, the victim must carry a permanent reminder, h/h marred visage, of the former mate. Last but not least, the injuries convey the grim message "You leave this committed relationship at your peril—and will not leave unscarred." A woman's teeth were nearly all knocked out and her jaw broken when her husband learned she planned to go off with his business associate. A man threw lye into his departing wife's face. A woman slashed the cheek of her fickle boyfriend with a razor so she would "leave her mark on him."

An investment in controlling the future of the beloved is always present in the rite of disfigurement, attesting to an element of possessiveness as well as an inability to tolerate loss. The symbiant's fantasy usually is that by engraving a testimonial signature on the face of the ex-partner that makes the latter damaged goods for others, h/s may be forced to return and would be lucky to be accepted back. But even if there is no reunion, the partner is still branded as belonging to the perpetrator forever.

Maiming

In contrast to the facially localized punishment of disfigurement, maiming is usually the result of either a battering that went too far or an attempted homicide that did not go far enough. A woman departing her marriage was punched several times in the body, but cracked her head as she fell, suffering neurological traumata. Another woman walking out on a marriage was hastened on her way by being pushed down a flight of stairs, sustaining serious back injury. A man ducked and dodged a hail of gunfire as he was leaving his wife; one bullet hit him in the knee and he was never again able to ambulate normally. In these cases the symbiant attacked in a blind fury; whatever damage was incurred seemed to be a matter of indifference to the perpetrator. Yet the perpetrator in each instance insisted that h/h intention was only to "scare" or "hurt" the partner, but not to impose permanent disability.

Nevertheless, the degree of injury may not be as accidental as claimed. We are not referring to disingenuous statements made in court to obtain reduction of legal charges; what we mean is that, in general, unconscious determinants regulate the force of attack so that the outcome is not fortuitous. When injury is far worse than consciously intended, we surmise that destructive impulses were more malevolent than the perpetrator can consciously admit. Moreover, when the attack is intended to kill but does not, we surmise that unconscious factors stayed a murderous hand. McDonald (1968) cited a case in which a woman announced her wish to leave, whereupon her man savagely beat her, shot her in the head and arm, and tried to drown her in the bathtub. Somehow she survived, but charges of attempted homicide were dropped after the two married and she refused to testify against him. McDonald considered the case more cooperative sadomasochism than a botched attempt to kill.

Homicide

A forsaken symbiant may resort to terror to let the partner know h/s cannot walk away from conjugal obligations scot-free. But terror is not always enough of a chastisement.

In a case known to us from colleagues, a man was ejected from his home because his wife objected to his seeing another woman; afterward she attacked the rival with a knife. The man rebuffed innumerable attempts on the part of his ex-wife to reconcile and maintained a vindictive attitude, asserting and even boasting that she was getting the separation she deserved. As for his girlfriend, the pair were constantly together over the next several years and they appeared to be an ideal couple. But one night the girlfriend stabbed him to death. Her version of the fatal incident was that he seemed to change all of a sudden, and she speculated that he might have been drugged without his knowledge at the party they attended that evening. When they got home later, she was too tired to have sex. He became angry, started to say something, and then, for the first time in their relationship, he commenced to beat her. After the initial punches landed, she picked up a kitchen knife to make him back off. She did not remember actually stabbing him, but when—to her horror—she saw blood gushing from him, she ran to call for emergency medical services. As her lover lay dying, the last words he uttered to the ambulance personnel when they arrived were: "Don't blame her." The woman was in shock, declaring over and over again how much she loved him, and at the police station called his name repeatedly while slumped in shock and grief.

It is the deceased man's last words that render this case so interesting. His absolution recalls to mind Wolfgang's theory of "victim-precipitated homicide"; after all, he had initially struck blows that set off her fatal assault. Because of his dying words, plus the bruises on the woman's body, the police were able to close the case on the basis of self-defense. She did not spend one night in jail. But the clinical picture is something else again. What the woman did not know on any conscious level was that the man she had just killed was seeing a new lover and was on the verge of telling her that he was leaving her. This key piece of data bearing on his death was available only to his circle of close male friends.

In the light of this information, his final statement takes on new meaning. He was aware that the affair he was about to reveal would be devastating to her. In hitting her that night, he showed that he was unhappy in their relationship, prepared a scene in which he could reveal his affair and depart, goaded her to walk out herself or to lose control in a way that would force him to keep away, and relieved his own guilt by provoking and empathizing with her counterattack. After she stabbed him, "accidentally" going further than intended, she expressed for both the agony of parting. We do not contend that he wished her to kill him, but he did not blame her for it and he wordlessly invited her to *do something*.

As for the perpetrators of homicidal crimes of passion, many display partial or total amnesia for the traumatic situation during which the killing took place (Schachter, 1986). Their emotional state at the time was such as to impart a dissociative quality to their actions; they generally call the police or ambulance and are waiting at the victim's side, not sure as to what happened. Some few wander aimlessly, but it is rare when they do not give themselves up voluntarily. To the extent that they are aware of what they have done, confession is virtually universal—indeed, the murderer often demands to confess and be put to death (Reik, 1959; Blinder, 1985). If capital punishment is not imposed, they often inflict their own death sentence by committing suicide in prison or hospital (Houts, 1970). It is widely acknowledged that solve rates for homicide are higher than for any other class of felony, in part because so many perpetrators literally place themselves in the hands of the law for the execution of justice (Sutherland & Cressey, 1960).

Murders of Collaterals

Either in addition to or instead of the beloved, sometimes others are killed who have some connection to the problems of the relationship. Yarvis (1991) reported a case in which a man not only shot to death his ex-wife but also her father, wounded her mother, and unsuccessfully searched for her attorney to shoot him too. A man was told by a friend that his wife was in the midst of an affair. Upon hearing this he flew into a rage and shot to death not only the rival but also the friend who told him the news! Another man resented his mother-in-law's interference in his marriage; when his wife announced an intention to leave, he bludgeoned the mother-in-law to death. A woman was beaten and abused by her husband. On one occasion, she refused to indulge in sex with a group of his friends at his behest, although she consented to sex with her husband in front of his friends. She finally mustered courage to leave; she took her young child and walked out. Later she was found wandering the street after having strangled the child, remembering nothing of what she had done.

At the extreme, where mass murder is committed, a forsaken mate victimizes passers-by in a frenzy of "world destruction." In such cases the killing orgy is a condemnation of society for being as uncaring as the partner. The assassin no longer values life and, in the language of anthropology, "runs amok" (Arboleda-Florez, 1979). A man killed his wife and went on a shooting spree, killing 14 and wounding 30 from his sniper's perch in a tower before being slain by police (Levin & Fox, 1985).

Nor is this tale complete. A forsaken symbiant may be capable of slaughtering the entire family unit through homicide–suicide. When such an event occurs, the symbiant takes to the grave the family entourage h/s created, away from the pain that they cannot be spared, and which h/s should have been spared by them. As in all love–death rituals, symbiotic reunion is projected whereby earthly separation is nullified. The executioner keeps the family together, beyond disloyalty and breakup, life and death, self and others. It is a paradox of human attachment: those who are loved are killed because they are loved, and in being killed they can no longer kill love.

～ 11

*Psychosomatic Reactions
to Rejection in Love*

One does not ordinarily look to poets for insights into health
care, but Edna St. Vincent Millay . . . expressed a profound truth
when she wrote:

> Love cannot fill the thickened lung with breath,
> Nor clear the blood, nor set the fractured bone,
> Yet many a man is making friends with death
> Even as I speak, for lack of love alone.
> —FUCHS (1974, pp. 51–52)

PSYCHOSOMATIC DISORDERS

According to folk wisdom, illness and death can sometimes be thought
of as physical manifestations of emotional disorder. Hence, we say
someone "died of a broken heart," or we declare that Mr. X passed
away because "there was nothing left to live for." Anthropologists have
documented how primitive man submitted to sudden death under the
sway of psychic stress such as sorcery, spells, or ostracism (Cannon,
1957). Modern man is less apt to be influenced by such supernatural
beliefs but may similarly lose "the will to live" and die when placed in
sufficiently dire circumstances. For example, a Nazi concentration
camp survivor reported that prisoners without "existential purpose"
readily succumbed to malnutrition or disease (Kogan, 1980). Parallel
fates befell those who lost hope in accounts of British and American
prisoners of war who were in Japanese hands during World War II
(Gordon, 1962; Knox, 1981). In brief, a traumatic level of distress has
been recognized throughout human history as a powerful contributor

to many infirmities of the body and even loss of life itself (Dunbar, 1948).

Can divorce bring about serious—even fatal—bodily illness? Medical research has shown that emotional factors, often involving stress around loss, are etiologically significant in many organic diseases. Carr and Shoenberg (1970) listed some of the major disease entities considered to be induced in part by emotional factors, usually derivative aspects of grief: ulcerative colitis, peptic ulcers, thyrotoxicosis, pulmonary tuberculosis, coronary occlusion, heart failure, diabetes, asthma, leukemia, rheumatoid arthritis, multiple sclerosis, pernicious anemia, and cancer. More recent studies simply augment this list; for example, Wolman (1988) addressed dermatologic and gynecologic conditions, and Gatchel and Blanchard (1993) added headaches, temporomandibular disorders, and irritable bowel syndrome. Thus, the medical spectrum is largely covered.

How does this happen? Selye (1976) exposed laboratory animals to unpredictable stressors and described a general adaptation syndrome. Noxious stimuli cause "wear and tear" to the organism over time, leading to somatic decompensation and eventually to a fatal outcome. In short, unremitting stress leads to dread and despair, and from thence to disease and death. As a corollary, research has also shown that stress management has preventive value in maintaining health and that emotional relief from an ongoing stressor fosters recovery from disease (Grinker, 1973). In hospital settings, Cousins (1984) has criticized the medical profession for increasing the stress of patients by an impersonal reliance on technology, adversely affecting how patients interpret their health status and test out on diagnostic procedures. He argued that the consequence of machine-based medicine is typically the initiation of an iatrogenic cycle in which doctors create needless panic, incapacity, or resignation—and the patient stays sick or dies.

The idea that intangible psychic states like grief or lack of will to live can threaten physical survival has been formulated into an empirically testable scientific proposition as follows: *A situation deemed distressing can adversely affect physiological processes, leading to illness and death.* The theory that distress can induce medical illness is called the "psychosomatic hypothesis" and is the focus of this chapter, especially trauma arising from object loss.

WHEN IS ILLNESS PSYCHOSOMATIC?

Before we review data on stress and its medical sequelae, a definition of terms is first necessary because confusion is rampant concerning "psychosomatic" phenomena—the word is used in two very different, even contradictory, fashions, and one can know which is intended only by context. In the sense of "psychosomatic medicine," it refers to emotional factors that cause or exacerbate physical disease, thereby encompassing the entire field of medicine as its subject matter (Alexander, 1950; Dunbar, 1948; Grinker, 1973). A more precise terminology for this first meaning of "psychosomatic" is *psychophysiological reaction*—a nomenclature that the mental health field officially adopted in DSM-II and subsequent revisions.

The other usage of "psychosomatic" derives from the early psychoanalytic literature (Fenichel, 1945, p. 236), where it refers to somatization symptoms without any constitutional basis generated in order to express, as well as to defend against, psychological conflict. Here "psychosomatic" does not apply to the entire field of medicine but only to the specialty of psychiatry. Stoudemire (1991) proposed new terms— "somatothymia" and "somatothymic language"—to remove any psychopathological taint from somatization symptoms, inasmuch as the expression of "bad" feelings as bodily complaints is a worldwide practice, viewed only in ethnocentric Western culture as impaired ego functioning. However, *psychogenic reaction* is the term the field now uses, accepting its inherent psychiatric connotations.

In sum, whereas psychophysiological reactions always include tissue damage or biochemical imbalance of some kind (i.e., real disease), psychogenic reactions involve a hysterical disorder that falsely presents as a medical problem and is interpreted as a psychiatric symptom. What both meanings have in common is mind–body interaction and unity, so that mental distress can readily translate into either real or imagined physical distress.

OBJECT LOSS AND ILLNESS

In psychosomatic research, stress has most frequently been found to be associated with what psychoanalysts call "object loss"—actual, threatened, anticipated, or symbolic separation from a very significant other. Chambers and Reiser (1953) took the histories of 25 patients admitted to hospital with congestive heart failure and found 19 to have suffered some antecedent emotional crises, 4 of which involved a marital separation. Schmale (1958) screened 42 consecutive general hospital admissions and concluded that 14 had experienced real or feared loss of a cherished family member and another 16 had experienced upsetting symbolic losses. An additional 11 of Schmale's sample had sustained suspected psychological deprivation or distress so that, all told, 41 of his 42 medical patients were thought to have undergone emotional upheaval just prior to the onset of illness. So far as timing was concerned, 16 of the 42 cases were hospitalized within 1 day of the stressful event and 15 more within 1 week. A replication of this study with a larger sample was conducted by Imboden, Canter, and Cliff (1963); they found a 25% incidence of traumatic object loss just preceding admission to an acute medical service. These early studies grappled with a cause–effect problem, in that developing medical problems could conceivably trigger emotional embroilment with others, which could later be classified by an investigator as "loss." Thus, object loss was not yet established as a direct cause for disease, but rather as a setting in which disease might well occur.

With the development of family systems theory, medical illness began to be looked at from the perspective of possible function within the dynamics of a family. Citing a study by Henkin (1964) that showed that somatic problems tended to occur or exacerbate in periods of increased marital tension, Grolnick (1972) recommended adjunctive family therapy for certain conditions. Epidemiological research has also indicated that separation from the family is a contributing factor to the onset of disease. Fuchs (1974) concluded that high rates of sickness and death are the lot of that strata of society who have become isolated, and Lynch (1977) found a vast differential in rates associated with such variables as marital status, family cohesion, and type of residence.

Although some investigators are still reserved about designating object loss as an agent in medical illness, others insist that such loss is often the sine qua non—the illness would not have occurred without it. Hutschnecker (1951) cited cases whose course reflected tragic vicissitudes in family or romantic relationships, leading to a generalization that some of these patients died when they wanted to or of diseases they wished to have. Hopkins (1959) asserted that "the chief threat to health . . . comes from a breakdown of some kind in interpersonal relationships." He diagnosed a "stress disorder" whenever any disease began at a time of crisis, its course related to the degree of stress, and cleared when the situation altered. As an example of this psychological approach to medicine, Chambers and Reiser (1953) described a man with previous cardiac problems who was left by his wife and suffered a heart attack 3 weeks later. She did not visit him in the hospital and let it be known to staff that she did not care whether he lived or died. The man did not respond as before to treatment and was doing poorly in the intensive care unit several months afterward when the study was conducted.

In a position paper, Engel and Schmale (1967) argued that if a holistic mind–body approach is taken seriously, a joint etiology must exist for mental and physical disease. They delineated a prodromal state which they held to be a nonspecific condition for the onset of disease, either somatic or psychiatric. As adaptive defenses are overwhelmed by some intense and unremitting stress, resistance gradually withers and the organism will then display what Engel and Schmale call "the giving up–given up complex":

Hopeless and helpless affect. "It's too much," "I can't take it anymore," "I might as well be dead," "I give up."

Loss of control. The person feels unable to maintain the antecedent level of autonomous functioning and becomes desperate.

Object loss. The person feels abandoned by crucial members of h/h network.

Shock. The person feels a break in continuity between past and future; assumptions upon which adjustment has been founded prove fallacious or no longer apply.

Anomie. The external environment appears bereft of "meaning" without familiar social support, roles, and routines.

Flashbacks. The afflicted person tends to revive memories of similar situations in the past, thereby lending a cumulative, synergistic aspect to the trauma.

Engel and Schmale more or less subsume "stress" under the rubric of "object loss," which is the pathogen for either mind or body breakdown—an unconscious "choice of symptoms" determining which pathway is taken. The giving up–given up complex is thus a psychodynamic model to explain any dangerous breach in the will to live, postulating that traumatic separation will precipitate some sort of self-destructive process. However, Engel and Schmale caution that the advent of the complex translates into medical emergency only if the requisite biological predisposition is already present.

Despite the bent in Engel and Schmale's work which makes it seem as if all medical conditions were an outcome of depression, their thesis would be more plausible if presented conversely—that is, that depressed persons are unusually liable to disease. This latter assertion is more readily subjected to empirical verification, and, in fact, considerable statistical data exist to confirm it. Both at-risk mortality and morbidity rates for divorced and widowed people are greatly higher than for the population at large. For example, Chen and Cobb (1960) found that diseases such as influenza, pneumonia, tuberculosis, cirrhosis, and rheumatoid arthritis are far more prevalent among the "never married–no longer married" group as compared with married controls. A demographic study by the Metropolitan Life Insurance Company (1957) found death rates from all causes were higher for divorced people, followed by widowed, single, and—lowest of all—married. Rees and Lutkin (1967) noted a tenfold increase in death rates during the first year of mourning a lost spouse, marking this as the period of greatest risk.

We can offer some anecdotal data, having observed how common it is for physical problems to befall those forsaken in love. Three of our psychotherapy clients suffered a heart attack, gall bladder disease, and pneumonia in the immediate aftermath of being left by a partner. A fourth case involved a male colleague who was found to have an elevated blood pressure. At this point his wife announced her decision to disband the marriage to be with someone else—she had been conducting an affair over the past year. The man soon developed symptoms of spasmodic chest pain, an abnormal EKG, and worse hypertension despite medication. He believed his blood pressure reflected his emotional state and that the initial high readings resulted from becoming unconsciously alert to his wife's growing estrangement. His cardiovascular problems later came under control, despite exacerbations whenever he had a conflict with his ex-wife.

PSYCHODYNAMICS IN PSYCHOSOMATIC REACTIONS

We now come to the issue as to just how distress can make an otherwise healthy person fall ill. Just what mechanisms of action are involved and how direct, immediate, and potent is its impact?

Alfred Adler was the first to link constitutional factors to emotional disorder (Bottome, 1939). As an early psychoanalyst, he argued that some sort of "organ inferiority" led to overcompensating behavior, so that a bodily defect was transformed into patterns of personality that hid or made up for the defect, but at the same time were often socially inappropriate. Freud elaborated on Adler's concept, renaming it "organ neurosis," thereby opening the door to interpretation of medical malady as displaced representation of personal maladjustment (Fenichel, 1945, pp. 236–237). Disease was now regarded as somatization of unbearable anxiety, which allowed the person to unconsciously express aspects of mental life—a view that drew skeptical reactions from many in the medical profession. Alexander (1950) finally established psychosomatic theory on a more respectable scientific basis. He criticized the conception that medical ailments could be seen as symbolic expressions of emotional conflict by drawing a crucial distinction between "conversion" and "vegetative" dysfunctions of the body.

Formerly called "hysterical neurosis," *conversion reaction* refers to a physical incapacitation that has a psychogenic origin, involving no tissue damage in the affected organ and accompanied by a *belle indifférence* (beautiful indifference) to the affliction in that the symptom solves or relieves intrapsychic conflict. Alexander noted that conversions typically involved functional paralysis, blindness, or deafness. These pseudo-medical conditions are thus restricted to neuromuscular and sensory–perceptive organs under the *voluntary* control of the central nervous system. The utility of the symptom is to express a forbidden wish through an unconscious body language, as well as to defend against or punish execution of that forbidden wish. The classic illustration of such dynamics is seen in the combat soldier who suddenly develops a paralysis in his legs that is puzzling but accepted relatively calmly. This symptom encompasses an unconscious compromise between the soldier's self-preserving impulse to run away from battle and his superego demands to be punished for cowardice—an ambivalence that is compromised by his being rendered a "cripple" evacuated to the rear.

Applied to divorce, psychogenic sensory–motor impairment is occasionally found in adults or children during the process of breakup. In one case known to us, a 17-year-old woman, 4 months pregnant, was admitted to a psychiatric hospital with a presenting problem of blindness, although medical examination ruled out any organic basis for this impairment. As if in shock, the woman was apathetic about her plight and disorganized in her thinking. When background information was gathered, it emerged that the patient had married only 2 weeks before, but her husband had volunteered for the Marine Corps prior to the wedding and had just been called to active duty. One day after he left the home they briefly shared, the woman developed her conversion. The woman's sight returned as she faced her sense of abandonment. She felt her husband had never loved her, married her only because she was pregnant, and enlisted in the military to get away from her. Yet this "view" of the matter—that their marriage was over almost as soon as it began—was precisely what she did not want to see.

In contrast, a *vegetative disorder* (the "organ neurosis") involves impairment to a system or organ under the control of the *involuntary* autonomic nervous system. Tissue damage or abnormal vital signs are always involved, so that examination or laboratory tests reveal a genuine disease calling for medical attention. Alexander considered such disease to be devoid of any unconscious content. Instead, he contended that recurrent or continuous stress produced autonomic reactions that eventuated in physical breakdown, but the resultant disease was a *byproduct* of stress, not a direct expression of a latent meaning or message. Moreover, sickness affords no solution to intrapsychic conflict, nor are most patients "beautifully indifferent" to their plight.

As for the etiology of vegetative disorders, Alexander had no qualms accepting the psychosomatic hypothesis, for sufficient scientific data were already available to warrant the conclusion that dysphoric emotion could lead to physical illness. But he kept the mechanisms of disease within strict pathophysiological bounds: severe or repeated stress brings about excessive endocrine activity, which in turn causes a biochemical imbalance that strains and eventually wears out some overtaxed visceral organ. Thus, psychic factors can be only a back-ground cause, and the effective cause is always some sort of somatic hyperfunction.

Following his elucidation of the psychosomatic hypothesis, Alexander (1968) sought to demonstrate a "specificity hypothesis." Audaciously, he would now attempt to predict just *which* disease could be expected to develop in the aftermath of *which* type of emotional conflict! Despite initial favorable findings linking overresponsibility to ulcers as an "executive disease," ensuing psychosomatic investigation has not brought forth data generally favorable to the concept that specific emotional conflicts lead to specific diseases. Indeed, Lacey (Lacey, Bateman, & Van Lehn, 1952, 1953; Lacey, 1956/1957) showed that individual differences in autonomic response mean that the same stressor will not cause wear and tear to the same organ across a population. This means that particular individuals respond to all stresses, from whatever source, by wear and tear on their most sensitive organ. Thus, some react by having a backache when things go wrong, whereas others break out in rashes. Hence, there can never be the correspondence that Alexander hoped to establish between a nuclear conflict and a resultant disease. Any disease can be associated with object loss, depending on the person's autonomic specificity that leads to a particular somatic vulnerability.

The debate over a "specificity hypothesis" continues today. Controversial research leads have been pursued in connection with the derivative idea that distinct personality types will be vulnerable to distinct illnesses—for example, the tendency of workaholics to develop coronary disease (Friedman & Rosenman, 1968). However, a more productive line of research has shown that the immune system is adversely affected by stress (Locke & Hornig-Rohan, 1983). For example, depression appears to lower the white blood cell count, thus weakening the body's resistance to *many* diseases in times of crisis (Bartrop, Lazarus, Luckhorst, Kiloh, & Penny, 1977; Schleifer, Keller, Camerino, Thornton, & Stein, 1983; Wolman, 1988; O'Leary, 1990). Kiecolt-Glaser, Fisher, Ogrocki, Stouf, Speicher, and Glaser (1987) found that women who were recently separated had significantly poorer immune function than married controls; in addition, shorter separation periods and greater attachment to the ex-husband were associated with poorer immune function—results consistent with the known correlation between marital disruption and heightened rates of morbidity and mortality. In a subsequent study of separated men, Kiecolt-Glaser, Kennedy, Malkoff, Fisher, Speicher, and Glaser (1988) obtained even more interesting results. These men too had poorer immune function and more illness than married counterparts. In addition, unhappily married men also had poor immunological function, whereas separated men who were divorce initiators had better immunological function than noninitiators. Although this group of researchers, led by Kiecolt-Glaser, acknowledged that definitive conclusions should not be drawn until longitudinal studies are done that prospectively trace the course of immune function in relation to stress, their research so far bears out the thesis that unrequited love, or even being in a unhappy union, leads to serious decline in immune function and, hence, to increased susceptibility to illness in general.

Given the complexity of psychophysiological disorders, at this time we are still far from knowing just why this particular person with this particular conflict or trait gets this particular disease. But while work on the "specificity" problem is still at a rudimentary stage, the psychosomatic hypothesis is now accepted as valid. *Therefore, unlike psychogenic disorders, somatic disease should no longer be construed as latent, symbolic communications of an unconscious psychological conflict.* The present view is that stress leads to overexertion of vulnerable organs (those organs most central in how an individual processes stress), compounded by the deleterious effects of dysphoric emotion on the functioning of the immune system, leading to susceptibility to many diseases.

THE PSYCHOANALYTIC GHOST OF "ORGAN NEUROSIS" NOT QUITE LAID TO REST

Illness in someone undergoing rejection in love is often viewed with suspicion. In particular, the countersymbiant may react to disease on the part of a forsaken symbiant with concern that this condition is a somatized call demanding reinvolvement. If the mental health literature is consulted, many papers over the years have emphasized psychological aspects of sickness, construing certain medical problems as an unconscious effort to control, punish, and enmesh a significant other.

For example, Sperling (1968) examined the interpersonal style of people who characteristically react to stress with outbreaks of illness. She contended that a "psychosomatic patient" needs a hovering mother surrogate to ward off fear associated with illness. As soon as a customary caretaker (often the spouse) is absent, the patient falls ill, because infirmity has come to be seen as the inevitable consequence of being abandoned. Sperling declared that "an individual with this type of object relationship will react to separation or separation threats . . . with the psychosomatic response, that is, with somatic symptoms. . . . These patients have an inordinate need to possess and control their object at all costs and at all times. They treat people as if they were fetishes" (p. 252). She then compared psychosomatic with acting-out patients and found them similar "in their intolerance of tension and their urge for immediate discharge of it. . . . The acting-out patient achieves . . . discharge of impulses by some actions with an external object in reality, while the psychosomatic patient tries to accomplish this by . . . actions with an internalized object inside his body" (p. 252).

Sperling was maintaining that psychosomatic patients manipulate *organic* disease to "act in" their conflicts and to control critical relationships. The symptoms of their illness supposedly express an unconscious demand: a caretaker cannot be autonomous, because any separation precipitates anxiety about coping alone and therefore regresses the patient back to childhood dependence. Further, she was asserting that the symptoms represented an unconscious attack on the caretaker, displaced to that part of the patient's body symbolizing the abandoning mother archetype. In this paradigm, the recurrence is aggression against the caretaker whenever h/s is not protective enough, binding h/h through induced concern and guilt.

It is intriguing to consider the possibility of repressed rage taking the form of an illness; indeed, exhausted caretakers may at times feel that their charges are in fact using persistent infirmities and complaints as an act of malice, perhaps not all that unconscious. But current psychosomatic theory will no longer permit positing a psychological cause for a psychophysiological disorder. Instead, insofar as there is psychopathology involved in the genesis of a medical condition, it is now attributed to psychic *elaboration and exaggeration* of existing medical problems. Thus, when stressed, a patient may experience an overwhelming despair in which a helpless–dependent mental state is fostered, perhaps deriving from a history in which considerable attention was paid to physical ailments. But this mental state does not *create* medical problems, although obviously affecting treatment and prognosis. For example, if a chronically ill patient contrives to trip off a bona fide medical emergency, say, by overexertion or by noncompliance with a treatment regimen, any resultant illness would still not symbolize a psychological problem—rather, the disease is used to serve ulterior purposes, including opportunities to manipulate or chastise others, and may sometimes lead to such a strong investment in the "sick role" as to become a core facet of personal identity.

A case of "organ neurosis" from the literature concerns an acute illness following rejection in love. Engel and Schmale (1967) argued that psychic conflict can elicit conversion reactions which, once activated, may give rise to physiological complications. They tried to make this sophisticated point by presenting a vignette of rheumatoid arthritis in the ankle of a man with the impulse to kick down the door of his rejecting girlfriend—inhibitions against the chronic flexing of the lower leg in preparation for that momentous kick presumably led to inflammation of the joints. Nevertheless, without clinical evidence of hysterical paralysis of the ankle, the example does not fit and their interpretation of the man's disability may just be fancy analytic footwork.

SECONDARY GAIN: DISEASE AS MANIPULATION

In spite of contemporary efforts to establish psychosomatic theory on a more rigorous scientific basis, the principal reason that intrapsychic meaning and manipulative intention are still attributed to medical disease is the result of failing to make a needed distinction between primary and secondary gain in symptoms.

Primary gain refers to the expression of hitherto repressed emotion through emergence of a behavioral symptom; relief of intrapsychic distress comes from finally being able to release one's forbidden feelings and protest one's social situation, albeit in a disguised and even denied fashion. The primary gain can only be understood psychodynamically, for defense mechanisms keep the self unaware of the significance of the symptom in terms of its underlying affect and import. In short, a symptom permits cathartic release of overwhelming ego-dystonic impulses, which are largely unconscious and still remain masked within its format. The symptom always represents a breakdown in normal functioning—one hurts too much at the moment to carry on as usual.

Secondary gain refers to the social benefits intrinsic to the "sick role." Once physical or mental illness starts to occur, the patient can exploit the situation in ways that have nothing to do with the causes of the condition. As a result of being ill, the patient may anticipate certain advantages—significant others may be compelled to pay attention, offer sympathy, experience guilt, comply with demands, or provide services. Thus, recovery becomes somewhat problematic in that it requires facing issues without the buffer of the sick role. Unlike primary gain, secondary gain may involve conscious aspects in the maintenance of the sick role, although unconscious aspects of the premorbid personality also determine how the individual will handle the advent of symptoms.

Following the work of Alexander, already discussed, the view in psychosomatic medicine today is that primary gain does not exist in organic illness, because medical disorders are not psychological "products" the way psychiatric disorders are. Tissue damage cannot be willed into being according to sadomasochistic intentions—primary gain is not a palpable *biological* mechanism but only an inference about the unconscious *psychological* life of the person. Cases of genuine medical illness with aspects of secondary gain must be sharply differentiated from those in which a patient unconsciously "creates" pseudo-medical psychogenic complaints so that psychodynamic explanations are apposite.

It is therefore an error—although a common one—to treat secondary gain as an etiological factor in the development of *physical* (as opposed to psychiatric) maladies. Exemplifying this error, when Kreitman, Sainsbury, Pearce, and Constain (1965) compared psychosomatic and depressed patients, they found that both wield their distress in a way to coerce benevolent treatment from significant others. True as far as it goes, this observation hardly proves that manipulations of others via medical or psychiatric disease is *why* somebody becomes sick. When Adler (1956) introduced the concept of the "power of the sick," he was referring to the use people often make of infirmity as a paradoxical source of domination—binding, intimidating, and burdening others by means of their very helplessness—but he did not suggest such control is the "cause" of the illness. Turning weakness into strength through force of symptoms is usually the desperate device of somebody already seriously emotionally disturbed, because whatever resources this person possesses may clearly be better utilized in a more adaptive approach to interpersonal troubles. The clinical principle is that secondary gain is by definition only an opportunistic motivation, some sort of solace really, but the unconscious wish for domination of others through sickness cannot in itself bring on medical decompensation.

TO BE OR NOT TO BE

We have shown that although current psychosomatic theory holds that no unconscious determinant of medical illness exists, the stress of object loss can soon lead to serious disease through such mechanisms as wear and tear on the body caused by overextended autonomic functions and immune deficiency associated with depression, in addition lack of self-care is still another precipitating factor. Given these etiological parameters, symbiants are highly vulnerable to breakdowns in health during the crisis of breakup or afterward. Further, because of secondary gain, a traumatized symbiant may wish to be smitten by disease or even come to a modified version of *belle indifférence* if there is an actual onset of disease, on condition that such misfortune can be envisioned as ricocheting through pity and guilt upon the countersymbiant. In this vein, physicians often encounter medical patients who readily neglect the most basic precautions and procedures of health maintenance, virtually begging for trouble, yet readily find a way to proper treatment and ultimate recovery if there is a caring intervention on the part of a significant other. When this pattern occurs in a situation of rejection in love, it is as if the forsaken mate has lost h/h accustomed hold on life, takes perverse pleasure in medical crisis, and wants only to survive if and when the estranged significant other manifests an interest in rescue. But in spite of the prominence of secondary gain when illness strikes in these circumstances, as well as in the frequent fantasies of forsaken mates about falling grievously ill, it is necessary to keep perspective about etiology by remembering that thoughts do not cause disease and, in any case, most forsaken mates somehow manage not to fall grievously ill.

In the end, those who do fall ill will in effect be looking to their professional caretakers to supply not only essential medical services but also some of the concern and commitment they did not receive in their primary love relationship. However, such medical attention is hardly sufficient consolation—it is far better to be healthy and face up to the necessity of letting go. As Dubos (1959) commented on the misguided use of health care providers: "To ward off disease or recover health, men as a rule find it easier to depend on the healers than to attempt the more difficult task of living wisely" (p. 110).

~ 12

Sexual Dysfunction after Breakup

> The biological characteristics of . . . sexual experience include changes in . . . genitalia (in particular [penile] erection and tumescence and lubrication of the vagina), . . . pleasurable erotic sensations, and . . . sexual excitement involving central neurophysiological arousal. [All] this is linked with cognitive processes attending to the sexual meaning of what is happening [so that] the whole gamut of social and interpersonal influences impinge upon our sexuality [in an interplay of] psychological and somatic processes. The sexual experience is par excellence psychosomatic.
>
> —BANCROFT (1989, p. 12)

UNREQUITED LOVE AND SEXUAL IMPAIRMENT

Rejected mates emerge from a shattered union disturbed in their capacity to love, which has an impact on sexual behavior. Problems of a sexual nature may have already existed in the marriage, or even preceded it, but breakup tends to exacerbate long-standing difficulties or usher in new ones. When a relatively serious order of sexual dysfunction appears after breakup, yet another behavioral system is responding to object loss. Traumatic reaction is manifest via genital-based psychosomatic symptoms, which announce in effect: "Listen, I can't love right now—I'm too hurt, mistrustful, angry, and so forth." Such body language communicates symbiotic ties to the former partner that block or mar an equivalent sexual union with anyone else because this would be psychic infidelity. The heart is not the only organ which hath reasons that Reason knows nothing of.

In the field of sex therapy, Bancroft (1989) listed three classes of sexual disorder: (1) *sexual dysfunction*, which includes for men erectile difficulties and for women inability to achieve orgasm, (2) *sexual difficulties*, a heterogeneous category that does not include performance problems, but rather subjective feelings disjunctive to sexual interaction, and (3) *dissatisfaction with the sexual–romantic relationship*, pertaining to assessment of self or consort. A forsaken mate is prone to all three categories of sexual disorder, so such disturbances can be regarded as a common sequel to rejection in love. Months and years after breakup, spurned spouses struggle to reclaim a satisfactory, ego-syntonic sexuality, looking to the libidinal life they once may have had with the beloved as the gold standard against which to measure their current functioning. During this period closeness and commitment to a new lover are more or less precluded by such factors as emotional and sexual limitations that inhibit the forming of fresh attachments, cynicism about any recoupling, and superficial involvements. Thus, an unrequited mate can be so leery of a second emotional investment as to shun any intimate contact with the opposite sex, become impotent or nonorgasmic, or—at the opposite extreme—overindulge in sex so as to make new relationships perfunctory and meaningless.

Risen (1995) drew the classical distinction in the sex therapy field between *primary dysfunction* reflecting a lifelong sexual problem and *secondary dysfunction* reflecting a loss in performance as a result of impairment, conflict, or trauma. Further, a sexual problem may be *global*—present in all circumstances—or *situational*—specific to particular partners or contexts. This chapter discusses sexual pathology that is largely secondary and situational, appearing as symptoms in the aftermath of traumatic loss of the love object. As forsaken mates reluctantly turn into renovated singles, free to do in separation as they erotically please, residual allegiance toward a former partner may be readily translated into sexual "hang-ups" with current lovers. For a time, an unrequited symbiant cannot help but meet the possibilities of the future while still encumbered by emotional fealty to the past. Further, h/s may also treat present suitors as sexual scapegoats to stand in and pay for the antecedent sins of the ex. Thus, the unfinished business forsaken symbiants have with a countersymbiant tends to live on in their ensuing histories with new partners.

As for recovery, as troubling as the sexual pathology may be during its course, in most cases sexual maladjustment tends to remit spontaneously as the letting go process proceeds. However, it should be noted that in certain cases what a clinician may consider a pathological pattern can be an adaptation for the individual because the new sexual economy protects against further traumatic loss. Such a reorganization could last well beyond the causative events, ultimately establishing itself as functionally autonomous.

SYMPTOM FORMATION

Several parameters intersect to determine the type and severity of postseparation sexual symptoms. The most important is undoubtedly the prior sexual history of the individual, which sets a baseline for developments subsequent to breakup. If problematic patterns were present beforehand, whatever tendencies existed are now apt to recur and even intensify, yet still following the well-worn path of character pathology established in early life (Kernberg, 1995). Of course, this aspect of sexual dysfunction cannot be regarded as reactive, so the woes of forsaken mates—despite what may be claimed—should not totally be imputed to the separation.

The circumstances of a breakup also have impact. As Trafford (1992) showed, the period preceding the breakup is often marked by a "shocking degree of sexual starvation." She cited data showing that "more than one-third of both men and women rank sexual deprivation as the major cause of the breakup. . . . A significant number of couples had not had sexual intercourse for three to five years" (p. 203). But whereas the disengaging partner in the relationship has often already developed an outside mode of gratification, the forsaken mate is at first left without a lover, as well as usually blamed for the lack of sex that led to the breakup. Avoidant defenses may come into play in such a situation, so that a forsaken mate eschews any new encounters out of sense of being too unattractive or incompetent as a sexual person. But more often a compensatory reaction formation occurs. Westoff (1977) reported that most women had some kind of affair soon after divorce, turning to lovers to restore self-esteem, as in these examples:

> "After my divorce I had an affair right away. I had to prove to myself that I was an attractive person, to prove I wasn't what he said I was"; and "I knew there wasn't anything wrong with me, as my former husband had made me feel so inadequate. He had said, 'You know you're not sexy and your breasts are too small.' Now there was a renewal of my ego. I found I could be attractive to men and I could enjoy sex." (pp. 30–31)

Thus, the nature of the breakup marks out a direction for compensatory sexual striving to shore up weak areas of the ego most injured by the end of the committed union.

Separation also removes customary controls and leaves forsaken mates vulnerable and drawn to the lures of sexual novelties with unconventional companions. Perhaps for the first time in their lives, spurned adults have no one to whom they must account and are at liberty to permit themselves previously forbidden or unknown sensual pleasures. Trafford (1992) saw considerable benefit in such experimentation, which had a "slightly anti-establishment quality" to heal "sex scars" (p. 198). New experiences help someone emerging from divorce to meet "the challenge of being single" and "to prove to yourself that you are good in bed" (p. 190). But to some extent this opportunity for a variety of sexual encounters also puts the person at the mercy of happenstance—whom h/s chances to meet, the suggestion of friends, the fads of the moment. It is not uncommon to hear a separated person report that h/s is doing sexual things never done before, yet is unsure h/s wants to be doing them. As Trafford acknowledged, "on the negative side, there's an element of self-loathing in frantic sleeping around that matches your depression" (p. 190). In the throes of confusion and without accustomed constraints, forsaken mates may find that they have stumbled into "fortuitous" situations that soon get out of hand. They need time to get their bearings after the shock of breakup.

Of most relevance to our topic of reactive sexual dysfunction is the factor of continued enmeshment with the love object. The more a symbiant still feels bound to the ex, the more unresolved conflict will be highlighted in the symptoms, leading to greater blockage in sexual performance. Thus, insofar as a forsaken mate still feels "married," sexual contact with new lovers is prohibited—monogamous feelings persist and cannot readily be transferred to another object. Yet the forsaken mate may feel a need to go to bed with *somebody* in order to restore a damaged sexual ego, even if an affair with a new lover is also experienced as adultery to be later punished. Hence, a compromise tends to be struck: on one hand, the forbidden wish for a current sex life is granted; on the other hand, new lovers are held at bay so that they do not trespass on the special place reserved for the idealized ex, inasmuch as sexual relations are restricted in the aftermath of separation so that they are not comparable to what was in the marriage, or lovers selected who pose no threat of winning existing loyalties unto themselves. Moreover, needs for self-punishment can be met through dire outcomes in the sexual misadventures typically pursued at this time. All told, despite sexual experiences with new lovers, the devotion owed the beloved may be safeguarded within the confines of a symptom or a pattern that makes sex different from—and less than—what was ostensibly unique about the foregoing committed union. As an illustration, consider the case of a man whose wife left him; afterward, he could not remember the names of the women he had been with in the past year because there were so many. He lamented, "I realized there was no love in my life. Never again will I feel for a woman what I felt for my wife." Finally, he entered therapy and gained control of his sexual promiscuity as he accepted the loss of his marriage. His therapist commented, "It's as though by sleeping with faceless partners he was keeping the space for love open to his ex-wife" (Trafford, 1992, pp. 203–204).

A TYPOLOGY OF REACTIVE SEXUAL DYSFUNCTION

We classify seven types of reactive dysfunction that often occur, briefly or otherwise, in persons who have involuntarily lost their love object. Any one may evolve as a sole reaction, or several may combine at the same time, or they may succeed one another over time. Our list includes (1) orgastic failure, (2) the masturbatory syndrome, (3) multi-partner compensation, (4) ascetic renunciation, (5) paraphiliac reactions, (6) pseudo-homosexual adaptation, and (7) sexual retaliation against the opposite gender.

Orgastic Failure

Orgastic failure is the most common sexual dysfunction after loss of the love object. For a period of time the male is incapable of achieving erection or cannot ejaculate; the female is unable to climax. When there is virtually no antecedent history of orgastic failure, it is clear that such symptoms are secondary to loss, brought on by depression or guilt. Althof (1989) viewed male psychogenic impotence metaphorically ("the penis is attached to the heart") so that such a symptom has adaptive aspects in terms of the mourning process. Despite the panic that may be engendered about loss of sexual performance by orgastic failure, this condition is generally self-correcting: the mediation of a caring, empathic new lover at the right time will work wonders. But a new partner cannot make a difference until some disengagement from the old partner has occurred. It is characteristic of this sort of sexual dysfunction that orgastic inhibition after breakup will be situational and selective. A forsaken mate is initially sexually responsive only to the ex, but then finds that h/s has become too mistrustful to remain so later on with that person. Conversely, although nonorgasmic with new lovers at first, the forsaken mate is likely to recover the ability to be satisfied by a new partner later on.

As Offit (1995) noted, impotence in men "relates to solving power conflicts with women, as the name of the disorder suggests" (p. 124). This particular symptom indicates that the male feels "weak" and subordinated. For example:

> M is a 40-year-old recently divorced man who pursues numerous sexual encounters, seeking to escape his grief and bitterness over his wife's infidelities and eventual rejection of him. In the latter years of the marriage and since divorce, M has been unable to ejaculate during intercourse. Although his stated wish is to remarry, he expresses determination never to give himself so completely to a woman again. (Risen, 1995, p. 49)

Another man tried to have sex with an attractive partner soon after the collapse of his marriage, only to be humiliated by his penis's flaccid response to this opportunity. He had never had this problem before, so he assumed his current lover was to blame. But the same sad tale was repeated with the next available woman. He became so anxious that he could not perform for many months, begging and berating successive lovers to help him get through his trouble.

As for cases known to us of nonorgasmic response in forsaken females, one wife could have no orgasm except with the husband who had jilted her, and after two years not even with him. Recovery of her sexual functioning occurred only after a 3-year period of abstinence and completion of the letting go process. Another wife lay "like a cold woman" with the man she married less than a year after breakup of her sexually satisfying marriage; this frustrating experience told her that she had repartnered "on the rebound."

Heiman and Grafton-Becker (1989) looked at secondary anorgasmia in women from a systems perspective, yet in treating the sexual relationship rather than the symptom, they seemed to overlook that the present system includes not only the current lover but often a still mourned ex-partner whose post hoc influence might be the cause of the symptom. Inasmuch as lack of genital fulfillment after breakup can derive from lingering attachment to an ex, attaining orgasm with a new lover for a time comes too close to emotional acceptance of this person as now legitimately in the role of love object.

The Masturbatory Syndrome

For a time, masturbation is usually the prime modality of gratification for someone who has just lost an accustomed sex partner. In separation's initial seclusion, this activity may be the only available sexual expression, tending to occur more frequently than before. Kinsey found 32% of previously married women age 41–45 masturbated, as compared with only 13% of married controls (Bell, 1975), and Kaplan (1996), a sex therapist, stated that "many patients obsessed with an unavailable object escape from reality into . . . masturbatory worlds of their own making" (p. 34).

But when masturbation is elevated into an elaborate, stylized, and frenetic ritual in order to hold onto the illusion that the beloved is still there, a sexual dysfunction can be said to exist, at least for the interim. In such cases, to the detriment of any possible new relationship, an active–passive split is utilized to assign roles to two people based on different body parts or fetishistic implements, one to serve as the penetrating organ and the other as the receptive other, recreating via fantasy a fusion of the couple. Here, the beloved's image is essential for sexual stimulation, and one may even feel for the moment that some kind of contact has been consummated, although it is recognized that bonding is with an introject rather than with a separate person. Gillespie (1967) has emphasized the role of object splitting in sexual deviations, serving to ward off psychosis around intolerable grief but making allowance for an encapsulated area of compensatory magical thinking. In the masturbatory syndrome, one has not lost the beloved if h/s has been encapsulated via splitting within the sexual apparatus of one's own body or by an adjunctive extension.

A man found himself masturbating about five times a day as his exclusive sex life for 2 years following rejection by his wife. He developed a procedure highly exciting to him: he stole female undergarments from a laundry room, wore these accessories (plus a wig he purchased) when masturbating, and imagined that his overall body was "her" and his penis was "him." His prior sexual history contained no suggestion of fetishism, transvestism, or such a high level of libidinal drive. After he was sufficiently recovered from rejection in love, these rituals stopped and masturbation itself became less and less frequent. He soon had a new girlfriend and resumed his premorbid pattern of heterosexual behavior.

In love making with new partners, a jilted woman became nonorgastic for the first time in her life and resorted to a vibrator to climax in masturbation. For a time she gave up dating, asserting that as long as she had her vibrator, she did not need men. Even after she started going out again, she extended the idea of the vibrator to heterosexual affairs by asking her lovers to masturbate her; she also masturbated herself while asking a lover to embrace her tightly, thinking of her ex-partner as she did this.

Before vibrators became popularly available, another woman used her dog as an aid to masturbation: she smeared grease on her vagina and had the dog lick her there, while imagining during this experience how she could make her ex-partner grovel.

In summary, for a bereft mate, the masturbatory syndrome can defend against unrequited love by incorporation of the object so that one is still a member of a sexually active couple. Fidelity is preserved (even if masturbation is performed by an accommodating lover) because fantasy still belongs to the beloved. However, with letting go, the image of the beloved begins to lose its sharpness and vague perceptions of an ideal but unknown suitor take over. When the sexual object in imagination becomes a person in one's surround—an available object—the masturbatory syndrome breaks down, for it no longer serves the purpose of upholding an internalized symbiosis despite the known reality of a breakup.

Multipartner Compensation

After separation, many people describe a promiscuous stage—casual sex is the only kind of intimacy they can tolerate. In the first year or two, a survey reported that divorced males had an average of eight sexual partners per year; 9% of divorced females were inactive and the rest averaged 3.5 partners per year (Bell, 1975). We call this pattern "multipartner compensation" because, for those rejected in love, it is usually the only time when they are this sexually active and their aim is to cover an inner emptiness. Typical explanations are "It's something to do," "One has to live," "I don't like to be alone," "I can't feel the way I did before about somebody." As one lady said of her nightly attendance at a New York singles bar, "It's better than suicide!" (Blum, 1976). But the procession of consorts does not fill the emptiness. In using sex as a relief in which one lover does about as well as another, these new affairs lack importance so long as passion is still invested in the departed countersymbiant.

In multipartner compensation, the original relationship is preserved as an ideal by not allowing subsequent lovers to combine love, closeness, and monogamous attachment. Thus, quantity replaces quality—or, more accurately, quantity replaces memory of quality. By engaging in numerous affairs, the ex-partner is punished in one's own mind via "infidelities," as well as by making unfavorable sexual comparisons to current lovers. However, given continued investment in the ex-partner, at this point no current lover can be trusted, and grief returns as soon as one is alone. As always, letting go offers the best release from the anguish of rejection in love, but this outcome may be long deferred in cases of multipartner compensation. Insofar as "sleeping around" amounts to a means of denial that there is a loss that must be mourned, the person is running from pain rather than dealing with it. A response to rejection that behaviorally states, "I don't miss you—there are plenty of other fish in the sea," means that working through the trauma of such loss is being denied. The ex-partner is missed, and the sadness of this reality requires recognition.

Nevertheless, in opening up an avenue to eventual recovery, promiscuous patterns may be sorely needed. The affect attached to such behavior is often positive and prideful in certain ways inasmuch as sexual relations attest to a genital revitalization helping to counter depression and improve self-esteem. This is the positive side.

On the negative side, the benefits may prove to be short-lived if the raw sexual contacts do not solve old problems and instead bring new ones. A series of lovers often does little to compensate for loss of the beloved. For example, a woman had sexual experience only with her husband until he walked out after more than 20 years of marriage. She then concluded she had been a fool and commenced to make up for lost time by sleeping with almost every adult male in town. She would sometimes call up her husband to tell him what a lousy lover he had been, now that she had a basis for comparison. Unfortunately, the reunion she wanted did not happen, and she began to feel "like an old whore."

Ascetic Renunciation

In the pattern of ascetic renunciation, a forsaken mate turns away from any sexual–romantic experience, often as a considered policy. Sexuality is regarded as a personal vulnerability, which—if not guarded against—will lead to involvement with another partner who will inflict hurt all over again. To avoid repetition of rejection, relations with the opposite sex are given up and, as far as sex is concerned, one learns "to just leave it alone." The classic instance is the jilted party who carries a torch, thereby enshrining both fidelity to an ex and disinterest in replacement.

Celibacy is not a common pattern among the divorced, so that psychological disorder is usually invoked to explain this reaction. For example, Morton Hunt has suggested that divorced people who no longer have any sexual relations typically have serious neurotic problems (Bell, 1975). Hunt stated that common types of these abstainers were women who had experienced a limited amount of sexual excitement in an unhappy marriage and were even more repelled by sex afterward, and men who had lost potency or desire in the course of a deteriorating relationship and then avoided sex out of a fear of failure.

But blaming "neurosis" can only go so far, for there are cultural aspects involved. Medieval society provided for people severely disappointed in love by making cloisters available as a refuge; both men and women sought in religious orders a way to get over loss, to redeem self-esteem through good works, and to be chastened by abstinence for preceding sexual misdeeds. In modern times many still undergo religious conversion after a traumatic loss, finding solace and self-discipline in their faith, but perhaps in certain cases also using aspects of their church's doctrine in an anti-sexual way to reinforce and rationalize their abstinence. Thus, a man left by his wife suffered greatly for a time, but later moved in with another woman who was still pursuing her ex-husband for a reconciliation. Caught between rejections by the woman to whom he had been married (and for whom he still pined) and the woman he was living with (who pined for someone else), the man turned to his church and ceased "immoral" sexual relations, leading his current partner to ask him to leave. He moved out and continued to live a monastic life as he pursued his religion more strictly than ever.

Very different in method and cultural implications, yet still accomplishing the same result, may be resort to such heavy use of drugs as to effectively obliterate libidinal drive. For example, a woman lost her lover and spent the next 4 years thinking about him, hoping he would reappear, apologize, appreciate her steadfastness, and beg to remain with her ever after. The price of preserving an unswerving devotion to the long-gone lover was the absence of any sex life and a growing reliance on alcohol to manage her depression and fill up the evenings that she routinely spent as a recluse.

A forsaken mate may also become socially isolated by finding other pursuits in which to invest, such as career or child care. For example, when she was still in her teens, a woman was deserted by her boyfriend immediately after the birth of their son; she never dated again but became a workaholic and a motheraholic. Twenty years later she insisted that she did not miss relations with men and felt she had done the right thing by her son.

In ascetic reactions, the tail wags the dog. Celibate stances attributed to extreme religiosity, abuse of mind-numbing chemicals, or self-imposed isolation from the opposite sex do not command abstinence; rather, it is abstinence that commands immersion in an asexual surround. Of course, it may be that loss of the partner was only a precipitating event in someone with predisposing schizoid or hyposexual traits. If so, the breakup solidified already existing tendencies to avoid intimate or sexual involvement. But in all cases of ascetic reaction it can be safely said that after what postdivorce abstainers have seen of the ephemeral nature of love relationships, they protect themselves by sexual renunciation. Yet, though alienated from their own sexuality, they still preserve their original attachment to the love object, for their monogamous investment remains sealed over time. This can be interpreted as a perverse testimonial to the proposition that "love is forever."

Paraphiliac Reactions

Soon after separation, an individual's proclivities may take on new forms in which formerly forbidden modes of gratification are now overtly expressed. Some of these forms have been labeled "sexual perversion," but this term has now been officially replaced by the more euphemistic "paraphilia."

Travin and Protter (1993) attributed motivation for sexual perversions to disturbed childhood attachments and desperate object seeking: "The attempt to engage sexual objects centers around the themes of searching for the inaccessible, accommodating to meet expectations, or escaping from or rebelling against an impinging . . . [parent]" (p. 108). Such core themes are always present in human sexual activity, but are pronounced in sexual perversions in the dialectic between visible and secret, available and unavailable, and rebellion and guilt. In a similar vein, Ackerman (1995) contended that perversion is a defense against intimacy: "Instead of facing the vulnerability and complexity of a real relationship . . . one invents a fantasy that is violent and taboo enough to be erotically exciting, but where people are dehumanized. . . . The sexual theater is exciting, not the partners. . . . Most often, unknown to the players, this is a revenge drama" (pp. 247–248). Stoller (1975) too emphasized vindictive aspects intrinsic to perversions, looking at such behavior as unconscious symbols of revenge against hated parents. Money (1980) believed perversions represent a kind of internalized "mastery," eroticizing painful childhood experiences at the hands of adults. Kaplan (1996) has summed up the regnant psychodynamic viewpoint in one succinct sentence: "Paraphilias (perversions) represent the turning of childhood trauma (tragedy) into (sexual) triumph" (p. 36).

This concise formulation applies to global rather than situational dysfunction. In the special circumstances following romantic loss, a modified formulation for reactive paraphilias substitutes the former loved–hated partner for the abusive, noxious, seductive parent. Thus, in reactive cases, a sex object is related to on the basis of a particular paraphilia, with the new object standing in part as a replica of the original partner but also as a caricature of a love that is being simultaneously mourned, repudiated, and replaced. Again, the sacrosanct nature of the lost love union is actively safeguarded against any encroachment of new involvements. The sex object is shunted into a different, deviant category of sexuality, with the paraphilia proclaiming in behavioral language to an intrapsychic ex that "there will never be another like you!" In this double entendre, no one else will ever get a chance to betray as the beloved did, nor will anyone ever be loved as the beloved was. The unwillingness or incapacity to restore "normal" genital expression after breakup is a damning commentary, for it accuses the lost partner of crimes against love. It is also a damning commentary on the paraphiliac's mental health, pointing to preexisting sadomasochistic tendencies as well as more emotional turmoil than the other syndromes we have so far reviewed.

When a paraphilia first occurs in the aftermath of breakup, deflection of libidinal impulses into some aim-inhibited channel reflects temporary disorganization. The new sexual pattern does not usually give erotic satisfaction equal to the old relationship, and may ultimately become vexing, if not alarmingly alien. The ego damage incurred by loss of the partner is embodied in acceptance of a socially disapproved, "inferior" type of relationship, as well as in shame were this erotic behavior to become known. In the end, the new sexual adjustment will often be seen as a problem rather than a solution, although sometimes such erotic activities wind up being defended as justified by past abuse.

A man began touring the neighborhood looking in windows after his wife walked out; he masturbated during this act, fantasizing about being able to take any female he wanted. Considering how angry he was at the woman who left him, he regarded this behavior as harmless because it was so impersonal. Another man fondled his 4-year-old daughter while she sat in his lap and he masturbated thinking of his ex-wife; he too saw no harm in using the girl as a wife surrogate. Still another man tried to satisfy himself with the family female dog, whom he cursed for being "a hard-to-get bitch, just like his ex." A divorced woman, very proper in her marriage, insisted that new lovers beat her so she could arrive at orgasm—this was how she dealt with her guilt about extramarital sex.

In these cases, the disintegration of the marriage prompted a forsaken mate to react along idiosyncratic lines, becoming aware of and behaviorally enacting what may have been largely repressed and forbidden sexual dynamics. As already noted, if such behavior is purely reactive, it tends to disappear as the letting go process is accomplished. However, there are some for whom the breakup has turned into a chance to engage in erotic gratification antithetical to traditional marriage and who never return to the sexual status quo ante. In many instances, such proclivities existed during the marriage and may have been indirectly responsible for the breakup.

Pseudo-Homosexual Adaptation

The rates of homosexuality after divorce is indicated by data from Kinsey (Bell, 1975). In a sample of female respondents, about 6% of divorced women were involved in homosexual relationships as compared with 0% of married controls. Unfortunately, these data do not differentiate between those who left their marriages to pursue an exclusively homosexual life style and those who only temporarily engaged in homosexuality in the aftermath of divorce. When a marriage breaks up because one of the partners wishes to "come out of the closet" in terms of preferred sexual orientation, this is not a reaction but rather the emergence and self-acceptance of hidden or denied aspects of sexual identity. In contrast, the sudden switch from a heterosexual to a homosexual orientation *as a result* of breakup follows different dynamics. Without the breakup, in all likelihood the forsaken mate would never have become involved in a homosexual relationship, despite vague inclinations along these lines. Ovesey (1969) has called the latter pattern "pseudo-homosexual adaptation"; for men, he interpreted it as a product of a transient sense of castration. Thus, a man who had been exclusively heterosexual until his woman left him for someone else suddenly fell in love with a long-time male friend. At first exhilarated by the discovery of his new-found identity, within a year he resumed a heterosexual orientation.

In a very different outcome, a woman "turned lesbian" after both her first and second marriages fell apart; she steadfastly rejected any further sexual contact with males. In this instance, a homosexual adaptation proved to be viable, serving to accommodate not only her new-found satisfaction and safety in relations with women but also her experience-based fear of and contempt for men, which may have been an undercurrent in her failed marriages.

Sexual Retaliation against the Opposite Gender

The pattern of sexual retaliation against the opposite gender involves a predominantly hostile reaction to breakup, in which the main purpose of sex is to hurt or humiliate any new lover. Perhaps anger at the opposite sex is present to some extent in many other sexual dysfunctions, but here it is the salient motivation. For the time being, sexuality becomes a way to manipulate, degrade, and torture lovers, providing revenge in the form of sadistic gratification. According to Stekel (1935), in the sexual aberration of sadism an object is valued precisely because h/s has become a foil for the discharge of hostility—love is redefined so as to incorporate the choosing of a partner for cruel treatment. A sexual sadist need no longer distinguish between love and hate: hate is love, love is hate.

The relations between the sexes have always had ingredients of sadism, and trouble within any given relationship can sometimes be traced to bedroom maneuvers in which one or the other spouse uses sex for dominance or vengeance. Millet (1971) contended that men in a sexist culture have used sex as a weapon to keep women in an inferior status, citing well-known male authors to show how men think they are conquering, taming, or controlling women by the act of "fucking" them. Millet concluded that all sexual relations in our society are tainted in some measure by male "sexual politics"; in every heterosexual union she saw oppression of the female because of masculine power games. Millet's stance was partisan, and she deliberately fanned the flames of intersexual combat in the ordinary relations between male and female (Lasch, 1977). However, although male sexism is indeed a serious social problem, women too can have recourse to sexual politics, most commonly by withholding sex to avoid, manipulate, or punish their partners. All told, sex can become an avenging weapon for either gender.

In the male version of retaliation against the opposite sex, power is expressed through calculated seduction with the idea of exploiting and then abandoning the female partner. In more severe cases, violence or rape occurs in interactions with a "bitch" who is getting what she "deserves." Through hostile acts, the man disowns dependent yearnings for comforts that were supposed to be provided by an ex. He will now opportunistically seize what he requires.

In the female version, retaliation against the opposite sex usually takes a somewhat different tack. Sex is an asset wielded by a woman to seduce and castrate men who must "pay" for what has been done to her by a man. She often crowns the insult by making sure that her suitors never actually receive sexual rewards anything like what they were promised. The point is to demonstrate the woman's power; like her male counterpart, she no longer wishes to feel dependent on anyone. Using sex as a resource, she gets what she wants, with the male suitor seldom catching on to what she is doing until it is too late. At the very extreme, some women become very calculated and mercenary after breakup in order to vent their rage at men. No longer will such a female "give it away for free."

A man whose wife had left him visited a prostitute for the first time. He took this woman by force, without paying, and then robbed her. He considered his ex-wife a "whore" because of her interest in an affluent man and stated he lost control when he was with a woman who was like her. A woman "led men on"—she was drawn to passive and needy types, but once they appeared to fall in love, she stood them up, sent them away, and found a new lover. She explained that it was not yet possible for her to get over the loss of her alcoholic husband to someone else.

Pathological extremes of retaliation against the opposite sex after breakup surely raise questions as to whether there were at least latent aggressive or psychopathic traits in these individuals prior to breakup. Probably so, but such examples also highlight sexual politics run amok, for sexual pleasure now comes from discharging aggression vis-à-vis the opposite sex rather than from the sex act itself. The guiding idea is to visit agony upon a current object by making love in a spirit of emotional detachment and contrived brutality. In so doing, a posthumous revenge is inflicted by turning an unfortunate new lover into a scapegoat to make amends for what the former partner has done. If anger at rejection abates with time, hostile symptoms will recede in intensity and eventually fade away. In retrospect, it becomes apparent that the foremost victim of retaliation against the opposite sex was always the perpetrator, still caught up in passions unresolved so long as dispassionate torture had to be imposed on others.

Values and Current Sexual Relations between the Sexes

It is obvious that our conception of sexual health mirrors the traditional Freudian notion of "genitality" defined as orgasmic functioning within the context of a love relationship. But significant segments of contemporary society do not share this viewpoint and posit a counterideal: sexual organization is deemed optimal when no psychological inhibition unduly deprives or disturbs one in the pursuit of libidinal fulfillment. If that perspective is correct, multipartner compensation is but one variant of sexual normality. We have stepped into the midst of a momentous clash of values within our culture. Contrary to how we have organized this chapter, perhaps the description of sexual dysfunction in divorce should have come after discussion of just what is "normal" nowadays in erotic relations. After all, social values change and thus sexual behavior perceived by mental health workers as pathological also changes. For example, during this century American psychiatry has made major shifts in assessment of the normality of masturbation, oral sex, and homosexuality (Travin & Protter, 1993).

In the period of the Great Sexual Revolution, an attempt was made to broaden the scope of normal sexuality. Comfort (1974), a prominent sexologist, defended the practice of what he called "recreational sex." He predicted that the average person will have two lifespans as a result of increased longevity, with an intervening identity crisis at about age 40. Thus, in early adulthood people will sleep with many partners for experimentation and fun, finally marry someone for the procreation of children, and then, as offspring approach adulthood, break up the first marriage and forge a second with a more companionate partner or, as an alternative, return to the premarital pattern of recreational sex. Within the institution of marriage, he maintained that sexual exclusivity will not hold up as the keystone of commitment, so that recreational sex with third parties will also become normative.

Comfort approved the weakening of the nuclear family when he maintained that mounting divorce rates, nonmonogamous marriage, and recreational sex all exemplify survival-of-the-species adaptations. He traced the Great Sexual Revolution to enlightened social policy that made second marriage or affairs within marriage acceptable because we each must now deal with much longer life expectancy. He also argued that society must keep procreative unions relatively time-limited in order to control population explosion. Thus, Comfort saw the current state of the culture as reflecting the ineluctable workings of Darwinian evolution. Looking back on his contribution, his brand of sociology seems farfetched, because the culture was not *mandating* more permissive sexual mores and, even if it were, society still does not take the view that marital breakup and recreational sex promote its survival.

But Comfort's writing did provide an apologia for midlife divorce and the casual affairs an ex-couple tends to pursue once they are out of their marriage. As we have seen, the forsaken mate is generally capable *only* of recreational sex in breakup, and it may not have all that much to do with *fun*. In separation, most ex-marrieds cannot form a committed attachment for several years; sexual dalliance may be the best level of relatedness they can manage. As Offit (1995) observed about "hypersexuality" (her word, but which she did not see as morally or psychologically deviant), "There are times in people's lives when sex is likely to be the most common and sometimes the best defense against isolation or trouble" (p. 149). True, but this does not mean that isolation or trouble is being dealt with (other than momentarily) or that there is no problem with it. In the wake of breakup, recourse to successive liaisons is often a sign of at least short-term distress and perhaps of long-term characterological disturbance—it is not necessarily a socially harmless "adjustment." Such movement from lover to lover may indeed be a temporary aid to self-esteem, but at the same time this behavior clearly expresses despair about the permanence, worth, and reciprocity of one's sexual dealings.

After loss of a primary relationship, forsaken mates today are seldom continent while the sexual ego heals. Chastity seems almost medieval, whereas Comfort's prescription of hedonism tends to be accepted as a way to fast relief. Instead of intoning, "Get thee to a nunnery!" members of one's social network now may urge, "Get thee laid!" However, as Freud (1912/1925) pointed out, much is sacrificed when the culture assigns to sex an absolute value in itself, without regard to the human context in which it occurs:

> In times in which there were no difficulties standing in the way of sexual satisfaction, such as perhaps during the decline of ancient civilizations, love became worthless and life empty, and strong reaction-formations were required to restore indispensable affective values. . . . The ascetic current in christianity created psychological values for love which pagan antiquity was never able to confer on it. (pp. 187–188)

May (1969) also saw difficulties with advocacy of unrestricted sexuality as if this were a solution to emotional problems. He accused American society of overemphasis on sexual proficiency, leading to the quixotic result that erotic experience has become more and more mechanical, ultimately anxiety ridden, and even antisexual. May was addressing the overall social scene of the day, not directing his comments to the special situation of postdivorce adjustment. However, in so doing, he poignantly called attention to the alarming state of relations between the two sexes. For example, he recounted the story of one of his psychotherapy patients who was applying ointment to anesthetize his penis so as to defer orgasm for hours and thus prevent what his female partner regarded as "premature ejaculation." According to May, the man appeared to have no idea that it was a loving relationship to the woman that mattered—not all-night erections, simultaneous orgasms, or other criteria of sexual prowess. Rather than trying to fortify the patient's potency as many therapists might have done, May advised the patient that "his penis, before it was drugged senseless, seemed to be the only character with enough 'sense' to have the appropriate intention, namely to get out as quickly as possible" (p. 55). In another case reported by May, he treated a medical student for sexual impotence. In a dream, the patient asked his therapist "to put a pipe in his head that would go down through his body and come out the other end as his penis. He was confident in the dream that the pipe would constitute an admirably strong erection" (p. 56). May remarked of this case, "What was missing in this intelligent scion of our sophisticated times was any understanding . . . that *what he conceived of as his solution was exactly the cause of his problem,* namely the image of himself as a 'screwing machine'" (p. 56).

May's view supports our thesis that sexual dysfunction after breakup is a psychosomatic communication reading, "Danger—Beware of Any New Involvement!" The symptoms are a disturbed but quasi-adaptive response to object-loss: a simultaneous lament and protest against an environment devoid of love and trust. All too often the problem underlying the symptoms becomes incorporated into one's own sexual behavior and is simply perpetuated by being passed along to an unwitting other. The ultimate cure for sexual dysfunction requires an overcoming of ungiving and uncaring attitudes. It will not avail much in this respect to perfect one's sexual technique or to engage in a steady pursuit of a variety of lovers or pleasures.

In conclusion, we observe that forsaken mates have much to contend with in reaffirming their loveability. Temporarily injured in their capacity to love, they often follow cultural prescriptions—"Forget your troubles and have a good time!" Although acutely wounded and emotionally disorganized, these people are encouraged to enter a sexual carnival to make a "new life," as if they were without history or recollection. Despite the insensitivity of the culture, most of them will find one way or another to recover their capacity to love, yet precious years will probably have to be spent in the process of regeneration. But true healing is accomplished psychologically—by learning to care and trust again. In our view, it is not accomplished by running around the community looking for what Erica Jong (1973, pp. 14–15) celebrated as the "zipless fuck"—sex as instant, efficient, and impersonal as possible. If this were to be the new "therapeutic" adjustment to conditions in the modern world, the remedy is more alienating than the disease. We would argue that sexual dysfunction after breakup does far more credit to the individual than does transformation into a well-functioning sex machine oblivious to feelings, relationships, and the social matrix that converts sexuality into enduring love.

∽ IV

The Nuclear Family in Fission: Effects on Children

Introduction

> In many ways, the family [as traditionally conceived] is the most
> conspicuous field of conflict in the culture war. Some . . . argue
> it is the most decisive battleground. Pessimists view rising trends
> in divorce . . . as symptoms of [cultural] decline [while] optimists
> regard the change as . . . positive or benign [inasmuch] the
> American family is not disintegrating [but] adapting to new
> social conditions.
>
> —HUNTER (1994, p. 537)

Glick (1994), a family demographer, has argued that marriage is in
decline: since the 1960s, American society has moved away from
familism toward individualism. In 1962, 400,000 divorces were recorded; this figure increased steeply over the next 10 years, then leveled
off at an annual one million cases (Cohen & Jones, 1983). The rate has
passed the 40% mark every year since 1965 (Hetherington, 1979), and
it now stands as the highest in the Western world, doubling that of the
next highest countries (Bjorksten & Stewart, 1984). Nearly one-half of
marriages today involve a second or more marriage for the bride or
groom, with about 60% of these too ending in divorce (Glick, 1994).
Thus, second marriages have a much higher divorce rate, with each
successive failed remarriage tending to be shorter in duration (Bell,
1975).

As the divorce curve has climbed upward, more children are affected; about 60% involve offspring (Glick, 1994), averaging slightly more
than two per family (Norton & Glick, 1979). Thus, families undergoing
divorce each year amount to roughly 5% of the population. In 1976,
Kahne projected that we were reaching the range where 34–46% of all
children under age 18 will average 5 years growing up in a single-parent

home, mainly as a result of divorce (Tessman, 1978, p. 30). This prediction's upper limit was soon established as the more accurate estimate (Norman, 1980). Still upgrading the rate, Weitzman (1985) found that whereas 82% of American children are born into two-parent homes, demographers now forecast that at least 60% born since 1983 will witness their parents' breakup before turning 18. Indeed, remarriage has become so commonplace that one child in seven under 18 currently lives in a stepfamily, although a more precise figure may be one out of three when allowance is made for children whose parents have not yet remarried, as well as those whose parents' second marriage had already collapsed and so were not counted (Glick, 1994). Visher and Visher (1993) have pointed out that when remarried adults plus former spouses are added to the number of children, one-third of Americans are in a steprelation; by the year 2000 there will be more stepfamilies than nuclear families. In short, exposure to divorce is fast becoming a modal experience for the American child and can be considered normative in contemporary society (Walsh, 1993).

These statistics indicate that American households, more and more, are composed of single-parent or remarried families; in the latter case, clinicians speak of a "blended" or "binuclear" family. Such terms are misleading: a blended family is only seldom as integrated as implied, and a binuclear family usually has disconnected or conflictual centers. Perhaps a more descriptive term is Elkin's (1994) "permeable family," referring to the ease with which transient nonblood members (such as live-in lovers) and paid professional child care people are incorporated into American family systems these days.

As for the children of divorce, the rule in most cultures (and in our own until a generation ago) is that it is the parents' duty to stay together "for the sake of the kids." Social punishment—disrepute or ostracism—was meted out to an adult who jeopardized the care of youngsters by leaving a marriage. Contemporary American society continues this injunction against divorce in families where there are children, but modifies its basis by shifting emphasis from penalties based on moral–religious grounds to concern with possible psychological damage to the child. Thus, objections to the breakup of parents are currently expressed in the fear that divorce will cause suffering to the offspring, making them vulnerable to emotional disturbance. In a very real sense, children's problems are now seen as the modern punishment for a separating parent.

The sympathy and solicitude of the parting couple's social network are accordingly directed to the children. In the past this concern was often pushed to its limits for purposes of sparing youngsters the rigors of divorce: parents should sleep in separate beds, or take lovers, or whatever, but at all costs should refrain from breakup, at least until youngsters were old enough to be on their own. In line with this view, adults were accused of irresponsibility if they did not compromise their conflicts or live together despite them. The central idea in this "traditional" approach is that, except for the most grossly destructive marriages, the home must be maintained as a two-parent unit for the well-being of children.

But hypocrisy was evident in urging unhappy parents to remain together, presumably to provide an optimal environment for child rearing. In the 1960s, an alternative "progressive" conception took hold that has maintained its dominance ever since, but has not totally driven out the traditional conception. This new view promotes a contrary set of beliefs about the impact of divorce on children: they are resilient; being with unhappy parents is worse for them than divorce; and the parent who rejects a spouse does not also reject them, who are loved as much as ever. Claims that divorce need not cause emotional damage to children and may even be in their best interest are now as firmly implanted in our social thinking as the "stay together" principle used to be.

In the process of breakup, controversy between traditional and progressive principles first plays out at the intrapsychic level in the mind of a nascent rejector. This person must debate whether the desire to leave should be subordinated to children's need for a two-parent home, or whether they would fare better with a parent who functions without resentment emanating from felt marital entrapment. If the person opts to end the marriage, the controversy moves up to an interpersonal level: countersymbiant *qua* progressive and symbiant *qua* traditionalist now will clash over disparate expectations as to how children will fare in separation, as well as often divergent opinions as to how children should be raised. At the next remove to the cultural level, the disagreements reflecting the parents' incompatibility are cast in ideological terms with both parties seeking support from the mental health literature, itself polarized in terms of opposing values and recommendations within a divorce-ambivalent society.

Chapter 13 deals with traditional versus progressive theories on how to protect children from a parental cross fire by offering very different models of visitation rights and custodial disposition in divorce. Each side can call on experts who cite different social science data, leading to contrary conclusions.

In Chapter 14, we attempt to counter the view that divorce need not harm youngsters if only parents "cooperate where children are concerned." According to this truism, parents who did not stay together "for the sake of the kids" will now be enjoined to work together in separation "for the sake of the kids." The fallacy in this commendable—but utopian—prescription is that the conflict between estranged coparents may be unavoidable because, as we have repeatedly noted, their conflict has psychological functions to perform. Indeed, most divorcing parents try hard to cooperate in the care of offspring but tend to fall into quarrels anyway over such matters as custody, child support, visitation, styles of child rearing, and loyalty of offspring, because these issues are usually extensions of their struggle around the divorce itself. The feelings of divorcing parents toward children and toward each other when children are involved unfortunately cannot be decreed by fiat. Instead, the real divorce most children know encompasses acrimony between parents, or the eventual withdrawal of one parent, or both. In general, parting parents can only sporadically cooperate where children are concerned, because divorce is not about cooperation.

In Chapter 15 we take issue with the premise that divorce will be nontraumatic for children if they are sufficiently prepared and the divorce is properly managed. We argue that it is not feasible to divorce children from the divorce: parents and their progeny are too enmeshed for one segment of a family system to be immune to dysfunction in another segment. Youngsters cannot readily adjust to divorce because they have trouble integrating identifications with two parting parents who don't get along. Hence, expecting a child to accommodate with relative ease to fission within h/h nuclear family is akin to demanding a "civilized" reaction from an adult to separation. When applied to offspring, this philosophy requires that negative feelings should be buried so that parental divorce (and subsequent remarriage) can proceed smoothly.

Despite the many problems for children posed by divorce of their parents, it should be pointed out that clinical evidence bearing on what happens to children in this situation is sobering, but not bleak. Most children eventually work through their initial distress, and most coparents ultimately find ways to cooperate enough to let children settle down. Nevertheless, high at-risk rates for many kinds of problems have been reported for children of divorce, and this aspect has raised alarm—as well it should. After all, there is nothing automatic in divorce about the subsequent adjustment of children. It is not time that heals their wounds, but rather the commitments of both parents to parent after breakup. Yet too often this does not happen, as one or both parents are unwilling or unable to carry through this responsibility.

~ 13

Children of Divorce in the New American Families

[In a family therapy meeting, a social worker] said, "I sat there . .
. listening to studies about THE family, arguments about THE
family, until I couldn't stand it any longer. I got up and said,
'What on earth do you mean . . . THE family? There is no such
thing. There are two-parent families, one-parent families,
no-parent families, three- or four-parent families, families
without children.' There was a burst of applause when I
finished."

—WESTOFF (1974, p. 3)

If . . . diversity is taken into account, one can no longer
speak about "the American family," but . . . about "American
families." . . . Note that the *empirical fact* of diversity is here
quietly translated into a *norm* of diversity. In other words,
[traditional] values . . . are simply bypassed by this definition.
Put simply, *demography is translated into a new morality.*

—BERGER AND BERGER (1983, p. 63)

PROVISION FOR CHILDREN IN SEPARATION AGREEMENTS

In divorce involving children, controversy often swirls around provision
of care for youngsters. The specific issues are: (1) *physical custody*—
whether offspring should be in single-parent custody with either
mother or father, or shared in joint custody, or assigned to different
parents in split custody; (2) *child support*—the financial contribution
levied on the outside parent; (3) *visitation*—the access the outside parent
should have to children. These parameters have to be negotiated and
eventually formalized in a separation agreement, but they have been

261

pragmatically dealt with from the day the couple parted company. Usually, the legal settlement ratifies whatever arrangements are already in effect.

But current child care arrangements can be challenged or changed at any time. In a Wisconsin study, 52% of divorced people with children were back in court within 2 years (Wheeler, 1980). Maccoby and Mnookin (1992) found that single-parent custody usually remained stable over time, but within 3 years half of their joint custody cases experienced a de facto shift to single-parent custody. Moreover, even in single-parent custody, children may be sent to the opposite parent many years after divorce. Alterations in the initial plan may be the result of unforseen circumstances, but more often parental reversals in attitude occur as strategic moves in an ongoing separation tug of war, for issues of custody offer a convenient forum to fight out the divorce. As an added complication, children too can induce reconstellation of custody as they request to live with the outside parent, or run away from home, or become disturbed enough to force a change in environment. All told, custody will not necessarily be settled for long by a signed agreement, court order, or existing practice.

Each parent comes to custody with a point of view. Typically, the countersymbiant believes that breakup will ultimately not harm the children if custody arrangements are cooperatively carried out. In contrast, the symbiant tends to assume that breakup has already harmed the children and is often not ready to cooperate with a coparent who did not protect the children from this harm. Parents who cannot agree on custody then turn to experts for counsel, seeking to learn what disposition is best for their situation. But, as we shall now show, the experts themselves are similarly polarized.

DOES DIVORCE HARM CHILDREN?

Up until about 1960, professional literature on the "broken home" pointed to empirical findings that divorce produced higher rates of juvenile delinquency and other forms of social pathology (Glueck & Glueck, 1950, 1962; McCord & McCord, 1959). A rather dim future was forecast for children reared by mother alone, particularly young boys deprived of a "father image" in the home. Except for very disturbed marriages, the prevailing social science doctrine was that parental separation was injurious, leaving children at risk to psychopathology, especially antisocial behavior. This *traditional* position regards the nuclear family as the natural, legitimate, and optimal unit within which to raise children, aligning itself with anti-divorce social forces that nowadays rally under the banner of "THE American family" and "family values."

A review of fresh data by Goode (1964) indicated that children from single-parent homes were often notably higher functioning than those from "empty shell" families where the facade of a working marriage was kept up by the two parents. This finding was received as something of a revelation, confirming a theory just coming to attention by Despert (1953), a child psychiatrist, who viewed "emotional divorce" between parents as the noxious agent that harmed children, as opposed to the broken home per se. Despert's conceptual approach to divorce has held sway ever since, more or less supplanting the earlier concept of the father image as presumed to be a crucial developmental need of children. We label this new doctrine the *progressive* point of view because it forms part of a pro-divorce ideology, making a single-parent or stepfamily unit just as valid and viable a home in which to rear youngsters as the idealized but sometimes problematic nuclear family. Clinicians of the progressive persuasion adhere to the position that the idea "that the nuclear family is 'normal' while that of divorce is 'pathological' is absurd" (Calvin, 1981, p. 100). Instead, they tend to identify alienation between parents as the malignancy that harms children, whether this disordered domestic reality is hidden or not. Despert's lead is also followed when she argued that for children the least detrimental course was evident when their emotionally estranged parents conducted an honest and mutually accepted divorce, one in which they cooperate to ensure that each adult has access to children afterward. In a recent reformulation of this position, Ahrons (1994) declared, *"Children benefit when the relationship between their parents– whether married or divorced–is generally supportive and cooperative"* (p. 126, italics in original).

Subsequent to the publication of Despert's theory, several research projects have empirically examined the impact of divorce on children. In a British study of nearly 5,000 youngsters over 23 years, Douglas (1970) reported significantly higher rates among those from broken, as compared with intact, homes for the three variables he studied: delinquency in boys, out-of-wedlock pregnancy in girls, and childhood enuresis in both sexes.

Hetherington, Cox, and Cox (1976) conducted a longitudinal study of 48 Virginia families, with a matched control group of 48 intact families. As compared with parents in intact families, divorced parents made fewer maturity demands of their children, communicated less well with them, tended to be less affectionate, and showed a notable inconsistency in discipline. In this sample, after 2 years the custodial mothers had made substantial gains in their ability to relate to their offspring, but noncustodial fathers became in many cases markedly more detached from youngsters.

In the best-known investigation, conducted in the "divorce capitol of the United States" (Marin County, California), Wallerstein and Kelly (1980) probed the reaction of children ages 2 to 18 to the divorce of their parents, interviewing youngsters 6 weeks and 1 year after legal dissolution of the marriage. Their conclusion was that divorce is a traumatic occurrence in a child's psychic life, especially for preschoolers. No child under 13 wanted h/h parents to divorce, and all dreamed of reconciliation. After a year many of the children had come to terms with divorce as an inevitable but sad necessity for their parents; however, 35 of the 89 children under 11 years of age were showing increased mental symptoms. Thus, more than a third of nonadolescents did not readily adjust. In addition, a 10-year follow-up by Wallerstein (1984b) indicated that such pathological patterns still persisted in this subgroup, as did a 15-year follow-up (Wallerstein & Blakeslee, 1989), with the index children of the original study now adolescents or young adults.

Wallerstein's results have been criticized as exaggerating the long-term problems, because many of the families were enrolled in her study when they came to a child guidance clinic for counseling, already had extensive psychiatric histories, and there was no matched control group of nondivorced families (Furstenberg & Cherlin, 1991). Nevertheless, support of her findings is afforded by Isaacs, Montalvo, and Abelson (1986), who investigated whether maladjustment of mothers and children is established so strongly early in the breakup that it endures long afterward. In their sample, about 80% of mothers and 70% of children improved from the first to the third year "and in fact resembled a normal population" (p. 269). However, the mothers and children who were initially more disturbed by breakup remained relatively more disturbed at the 3-year mark, suggesting that maladjustment tends to persist for those who are most emotionally distressed by divorce. Further confirmation of the Wallerstein and Kelly conclusion about the long-term effects of divorce on children was provided by Hetherington, Law, and O'Connor (1993). They cited studies using clinical cutoffs on standardized tests that found that 20% of children from divorced homes were at extreme levels of deviant behavior beyond the crisis period of divorce transition, as compared with 10% of children from intact homes. Although these investigators' rates, based on paper-and-pencil measures as opposed to clinical interviews, are lower for long-term disturbance, the studies they cited did have control groups.

In a review of current research, Furstenberg and Cherlin (1991) stated, "Researchers agree that almost all children are moderately or severely distressed when their parents separate and that most continue to experience confusion, sadness, or anger for a period of months or even years" (p. 67). Yet no study can indisputably prove that divorce is harmful to the emotional maturation of children, because there is no practical way to set up a truly satisfactory control group. If the question is whether children whose parents are unhappily married would be worse off if their parents separated, it is impossible to do an experiment in which such a child could be examined both under conditions where the parents parted and under conditions where they remained together. Research can only compare children from intact versus broken homes—probably apples and oranges. However, despite intrinsic limitations to the validity of the data, the cumulative weight seems to indicate that there is a correlation between divorce and psychological distress in children, which can endure into adulthood in up to one-third of the cases. But it still remains an open issue as to whether this is caused by the separation of the parents or by the way particular parents handle separation. In a third possibility, the issue may be moot—children of an unhappy marriage may be liable to emotional damage whatever their parents do about their marriage; hence, any conjugal decision on behalf of offspring may be merely a type of damage control.

It must be also be understood that statistical generalizations can be misleading in individual cases. Extraneous factors (like sexual abuse, addiction, or violence in the home) that affect a child's later adjustment are seldom addressed in divorce research. Further, children react differently to their parents' breakup. Despite the finding that they generally oppose divorce, some youngsters—often teenagers—have reported to investigators that they were relieved or even glad when their parents finally separated, with improved functioning as a result. There were also some children who stated they had become closer to a noncustodial parent in spite of, or perhaps because of, separation. To go beyond generic data and obtain a more refined picture of how divorce impinges on various families, we must invoke clinical observation to discern patterns.

DESPERT'S VIEW OF THE "GOOD" DIVORCE FOR CHILDREN

Despert startled the field in 1953 when she proclaimed that children are most damaged where an "emotional divorce" exists in a so-called intact family, or where an emotional divorce is not allowed to run its course because one of the partners engages in a futile endeavor to hold onto the marriage, even after breakup:

> Even a very young child . . . responds to the true feelings of his parents for each other and for himself, however carefully this may be veiled. This is not speculation. A clinical observer finds the same patterns of emotional disturbance in children of parents *who do not divorce,* though they have failed at marriage, as in children of divorced parents *who have not made their peace with divorce.* (p. 9)

This thesis delivered a pulverizing blow to the conventional wisdom that divorce is inherently destructive to the mental health of children. Indeed, Despert insisted that the reverse was more often true, asserting that a concealed emotional divorce was far more harmful. Children can validate their intuitive sense that something is amiss in their family only when parental alienation comes to the surface as an authentic, avowed, and decisive separation.

Despert started from the psychoanalytic truism that "neurotic individuals seek neurotic mates, make neurotic marriages, and beget neurotic children" (p. 151). She initially sounds anti-divorce, much like Bergler in *Divorce Won't Help* (1948), but Despert argued that divorce would at least help children. Given collaboration by parents in visitation and custody, she was optimistic about their prospects, with psychotherapy available if needed. At a minimum, the parents had made the best of a bad situation.

As the key to Despert's approach to custody, she advocated that disposition must be harmonious, because the marriage was not. Her position was that despite divorce acrimony, a youngster still needs both parents, so adults must cooperate to ensure mutual rights of access. In her own way, Despert paid homage to the import of a "father image" by insisting that offspring may be subject to emotional damage after breakup if the custodial mother effectively blocks the outside father from contact. In a seminal family systems conception, she was establishing a cooperative model for custody in which both parents would have to accept the divorce as an immutable fact of their daily lives. To her, "making peace with divorce" did not mean that the ex-couple had to be friendly, but they did have to recognize that the marriage's end did not also mean the end of parenting, in that each adult's relationship to the child continued. Despert's ideal was that parents were to put their children's needs before their own—that is, by letting them benefit from what the other parent offered, not vindictively withholding access, and accepting that youngsters might have to deal with an ex-mate's new mate.

The bulk of Despert's clinical presentation concerned 6-year-old Mary (pp. 151–185), who lived in circumstances far removed from Despert's ideally-conducted divorce. Mary had "three Mommies and three Daddies." Mary's Mommy #1 and Daddy #1 had two children and separated when Mary was 3. Mother remarried immediately (Daddy #2), bore her third child, broke up with her new husband after two years, remarried again (Daddy #3), and produced her fourth child. Meanwhile, Mary's father also remarried after a time (Mommy #2), as did her first stepfather (Mommy #3). Obviously, Mary had much to deal with by way of traumatic loss and family upheaval. She reacted by developing psychiatric symptoms that included temper tantrums, fighting, school problems, nightmares, and obsessive recitations of her complicated genealogy. These symptoms began right after Mommy #1 informed Mary and her sister that Daddy #1 had left and would not return. Mary screamed, "Daddy cannot go!" and demanded that the family relocate in order to join him. Despert was critical of how both parents managed their breakup: the father left without telling the children until he had set up his new residence in a distant city; the mother delayed telling the children the truth, shortly left home herself for 6 weeks to file for divorce in Reno, and within a few days of her return moved a new husband into the house as Daddy #2. Despert found these actions destructive because they left Mary alone and without explanation at a crucial time; in addition, the parents were too self-absorbed to take care of Mary, resulting in a disturbed adjustment. But the damage was done, and Despert now recounted her work as a psychotherapist to assist Mary's recovery.

Mary's case illustrated how Despert thought parents should *not* handle their children in divorce, but did not involve custody issues. However, she presented other cases (though in less detail) that exemplify how she approached custody as a psychiatric expert.

Jerry's father walked out when the boy was four; years later father remarried and tried to get custody of his son. He went to the extreme of withholding child support payments to force consent from Jerry's mother; he also accused her of turning their boy into a "sissy" and blamed her for Jerry's sporadic acting out in the neighborhood as well as his academic difficulties. The mother countered that the boy was always upset after he visited his father and new wife; she wanted to cut down on weekend visitation as a way to help Jerry. The father brought a lawsuit for custody when his ex-wife did not voluntarily give up the boy. The court's decision hinged on a psychiatric recommendation, which was that the parents were equally culpable for creating the child's disturbance and that the boy would be best served by living with neither of them! Despert defended this recommendation (p. 219) inasmuch as parents were in the wrong for trying to impede the other's access to Jerry.

Despert also discussed a celebrated 1951 case, *In re Bologna et al.*

(pp. 205–207). Mrs. Bologna quit her marriage, abandoning her children "with no concern for their future welfare"—as the undisputed testimony went—to the sole care of Mr. Bologna. The father worked and tried to care for them with the assistance of housekeepers, but the children were unhappy and maladjusted and at one point had to be placed in a boarding school. After some years, Mrs. Bologna changed her mind and wished to assume custody. She used a legal gimmick: because she knew that as the deserting parent she could not win a custody suit under laws then existing, she had her lawyer declare the children "neglected" by the father. This maneuver threw the case into a special division of family court where psychiatric input would routinely be arranged and probably decisive. In the psychiatrist's view, the overwhelmed father was more emotionally unstable than the mother, whereas her behavior was diagnosed as an "anxiety reaction" because her husband pushed her close to breakdown and caused her to flee. The mother was awarded custody. Despert approved this decision too, noting that lines of communication had been restored between mother and children.

As we assess Despert's contribution, her resolve to protect children from the strife of parting parents shines forth. She established a standard of psychiatric intervention that ensured the child's right to see both parents; by the same token, she was not impressed by the qualifications of any parent who thwarted the other's relationship to the child. When emotional disturbance in a child of divorce was found, she either blamed the parent who denied access, or attributed responsibility in equal measure to parents fighting over children, resorting to a "plague on both your houses" if they did not cooperate "for the sake of the kids."

But in our view, it is doctrinaire to make granting access the single most important criterion of "good" parenting in divorce; access may have to be curtailed because of how it is used—perhaps by frequent failure to appear as promised, or by abuse. Moreover, it is naive to indiscriminately blame both parents when there is fighting. Sometimes one parent has no choice but to stand up to the other on behalf of the child. For example, when a custodial parent is neglectful or a noncustodial parent withholds child support, a "lack of cooperation" is to be expected. Guarding against the failure of one parent is not ipso facto an equivalent failure by the coparent; when there is trouble over sharing the child, equal condemnation of both parents may be a bias in its own right.

All told, there will often be a natural justice to the claims of one parent over the other, based on their commitments, proven in action, to the child. Mrs. Bologna could have left a bad marriage with her children in hand (as most women in such situations do), yet she blamed her overburdened husband for the problems of their children when she just walked away, provided no support, and found fault from an uninvolved distance. Jerry's father did not consider the mother unfit when he left his son with her, but did when he remarried. It is adding insult to injury for a man to leave wife and child, go find a new wife, and then demand custody when opportune. In Mary's case, her father's sudden departure had to do with the evident fact that her mother was replacing him in the home with another man. It is too much to demand proper parenting from a father in such a devastating moment (though soon afterward, he arranged for Mary and her sister to spend every summer with him). Spreading culpability around in equal measure may be democratic, but it is neither sound law nor sound psychiatry. Parents will not each do their promised share, their respective shares may not be equal to begin with, and fighting may be provoked.

Despert categorically dismissed any possibility that partners unhappily married can still be "good enough" parents (Winnicott, 1965). Instead, she admonished those who are tempted to break up their marriages to do so quickly—before children are hurt by their staying together—so that by dint of leaving they become good enough parents. Her stance gives carte blanche to those who seek their identity outside marriage at the expense of a family unit; it also lends an air of respectability to unrealistic entitlement as parents, such as in the disruptive reclaiming of children after desertion (Mrs. Bologna), introduction of a new mate into the home right after breakup (Mary's mother), or stopping child support to compel a custody change (Jerry's father). Her theoretical outlook projects the "progressive" view that parting parents must cooperate no matter what the issues, inasmuch as divorce has no right or wrong.

The fallacy in Despert's reasoning is the supposition that children can be spared dissension in divorce by parents who readily exposed them to this dissension during marriage. If parents could actually have done this, they need not have divorced. In any event, people hardly ever behave better in divorce than they did in marriage. As Myers (1989) said, separation "when there are children is usually so calamitous that it is hard, if not impossible, for parents to be civil and fair, as much as they would like to be" (p. 175). Thus, parting parents usually move from an "empty shell" marriage to a "hard-core" divorce. Despert is preaching to those who may want to accept her ideas but are likely not to live up to them in practice.

On the positive side, whatever her preconceptions, Despert dealt as best she could in her role as child psychiatrist with tragic situations. She was justified in asserting the principle that children want continued and untrammeled contact with both parents. She urged parents to give their children this crucial opportunity, providing a model of a "good" divorce for children by setting a realistic standard toward which estranged parents could aim—to wit, if they are cooperative about rights of access, the youngsters will fare better in the family breakup. However, at the same time, Despert did not glorify divorce; she realized that even without strife over children, parting parents will still fight.

THE DIRTY SECRET OF MANY DIVORCES

By vesting custody mainly on the basis of which adult best fosters access, Despert treated the two parent–child relationships as if they are always compatible and productive. She plainly did not want to make invidious comparisons between parents. Nor did she want to deal with the impact of romantic triangles on custody and visitation. Nor did she relate to the vexing problem of whether visitation rights are compromised when child support has not been paid. Her clinical contribution overlooked a major aspect of fighting over children: it may be that one parent is a far less involved or responsible caretaker, but still makes presumptive claims and invokes parental "rights." For example, in the 1979 film *Kramer vs. Kramer*, Mr. Kramer was hard-pressed to cope with his wife's sudden exit. He had to find a housekeeper to care for his 4-year-old son while he struggled to make ends meet (it did not occur to either parent that she should pay child support). He later fended off Mrs. Kramer's custody suit after her absence for more than a year without contact or a forwarding address. Against this backdrop, her calm demeanor during the court proceedings made a better impression on the judge than Mr. Kramer's agitation on the stand, although we think his distress was more suitable than her composure. Mrs. Kramer actually won her custody suit in court, but on the day she arrived to pick up her son, she reneged and tearfully went away alone. In the novel (Corman, 1977), she admitted that she was reluctant to assume single-parenting duties as Mr. Kramer had done; in the film, however, she stated she could not bear to part the boy from his father. Undoubtedly, Mrs. Kramer cared about her son and was upset about not having custody. Yet she put her son through an ordeal while she worked out her "identity." She could not be in the mother role so long as she was caught up in "finding herself," but she also would not relinquish claim to being a responsible parent. Meanwhile, her son's world was turned topsy-turvy as she tested out her priorities without regard for his need to have a stable family unit. In this breakup, her rights of access were never an issue—it was her commitment as a parent.

In Despert's cases, the common denominator is that the partner less committed to the marriage is also the less committed parent. We do not think this is a coincidence. Contrary to the prevailing dictum in the divorce therapy field that "a parting parent leaves spouse but not children," our clinical experience has been that a partner who becomes emotionally estranged from the mate within the marriage may often manifest similar interpersonal difficulties in closeness and attachment to children. Thus, the one who emotionally leaves the marriage generally emotionally leaves the children as well, despite promises and intentions to stay as loving and involved as ever. Even if this parent had been a good caretaker and provider before the breakup, afterward such qualities seem to become increasingly subordinated to more pressing personal needs for autonomy, sexual–romantic fulfillment, and self-development. In brief, *just as divorce represents a breach in commitment between conjugal mates, there may be a subsequent–but denied–breach in commitment between a countersymbiant parent and the children of the marriage.* At times this breach is only temporary, lasting as long as it takes for the countersymbiant to become established out of the marriage, but it can last long after the crisis of separation has passed.

Our personal observations about emotional estrangement of a countersymbiant parent from children after breakup constitute an iconoclastic inference that members of the mental health community adhering to the "progressive" ideology will adamantly contest. But our reading of the divorce literature is that case histories tend to confirm our thesis, as we have already indicated with Despert's clinical material. We will now cite others in the field who have reached generalizations from their data congruent with our own.

Vaughan (1986) noted that "in order to uncouple, some divorce initiators also begin to separate from their children . . . by spending less time with them, redefining them in negative terms, finding an alternative family, or taking other actions that neutralize the commitment and loss" (p. 54). When the father is the noncustodial parent, Myers (1989) described a common "negligent" type: "These men have been unhappily married for years and felt very constrained in their marriages. Their pursuit of the 'good life' and their egocentricity in its pursuit seem to be a reaction against a sense of inner deprivation" (p. 205). When a mother is the noncustodial parent, Hodges (1986) found that "involvement of the ex-wife with another man was a common description of fathers with custody and rare in noncustodial fathers" (p. 106). Thus, though mothers seldom relinquish custody voluntarily, wives who ended their marriages because of a new romantic involvement were more likely to let their children go to the father, and even if they originally had custody, they were more apt to give it up later.

Gersick (1979) mentioned the case of a father who cried, "I gave her a choice: [little] Billy and me or the other guy—so she left." He also knew of seven settlements in which such mothers left custody up to the children, who then chose paternal care. In a *reductio ad absurdum* of willing loss of custody, Wheeler (1980, p. 51) pointed to a case in which a mother sought not only a divorce in court but also a decree that compelled the father to take custody. According to West and Kissman (1991), "the noncustodial mother who is neither child-free nor a mother in the conventional sense" typically reported little or no problems, other than being "relegated to deviant status" (p. 236).

Even when the mother retains custody, she may still leave her children emotionally. Hetherington et al. (1993) have identified a

> small cluster of egocentric, self-fulfilling women who threw themselves into self-improvement programs . . . and sought out new stable intimate partnerships. However, their success came at the expense of their children's well-being. They spent little time with [them] and were preoccupied with their own . . . activities. These children were among the most dysfunctional in our study. (p. 217)

These investigators' subset of divorced women were countersymbiants in that they were happy to be separated, reported no self-esteem problems, and had adapted remarkably well (perhaps too well) to their new situations.

THEORIES OF CUSTODY: SINGLE-PARENT DISPOSITION

After the revolutionary contribution of Despert, books showing how children can adjust to dissolution of their nuclear family have become increasingly didactic, detailed, and reassuring, offering advice to separated parents who are raising youngsters. In general, the new publications paint a more sanguine picture of divorce than Despert did and cover areas other than rights of access. Thus, in the "progressive" camp, professional attention is devoted mainly to the couple's conduct of the separation as the causative factor for emotional disturbance in offspring. Given that clinicians of the "traditional" persuasion still consider the harm to youngsters to emanate from the divorce per se, we once again find polarization of views within the divorce therapy field such that controversy has arisen over what constitutes a "therapeutic" custody arrangement.

From the traditional side, let us start with the position of Goldstein, Freud, and Solnit (1973), who proposed codification of judicial disposition in foster care, adoption, and divorce cases where custody was being litigated. They held that custody suits are so damaging to a child's mental health that it is essential to give a judge power to make swift and irreversible decisions. In contrast to Despert, they thought custody should be awarded to that claimant who has distinguished himself or herself as "the psychological parent," leaving the other claimant's involvement with the child to the discretion of the more invested parent. Goldstein et al. justified this position with the observation that former spouses seldom get along, tending to use children in their attacks on one another; since the divisiveness of divorce may preclude cooperation in raising children, only one parent should have complete and exclusive control over every aspect of custody in order to undercut such strife. At the very least, vesting authority in a sole parent avoids confusing children about who is in charge and prevents cross fire. For Goldstein et al., single-parent custody makes organizational sense: when parents no longer function as a team, one of them should more or less drop out as a partner.

As can be seen, the visitation rights of the outside parent are here dismissed as of little value, to be dispensed—or not—by the custodial parent. In their design of a therapeutic custody arrangement, Goldstein et al. said they were following the "least detrimental alternative," salvaging as much as possible for the child by placing h/h with a constant parental figure who can be effective only when not undermined by the demands and incursions of a potentially hostile or uncongenial coparent.

The merit of Goldstein et al.'s position has been recognized in its application to foster care and adoption cases, but their stand on custody in divorce has been sharply criticized. To begin with, their assertion that single-parent custody makes the best of a bad situation immediately raised hackles among joint custody proponents. But the brunt of the outcry has been to condemn their curt rejection of Despert's maxim that the outside parent's rights of access must be honored. Almost the entire divorce therapy field stands against them concerning their disregard for preservation of the outside parent's relationship to children. For example, Gardner (1976) evaluated their position in a caustic passage:

> [Goldstein et al.], in an otherwise excellent book, have recommended that the custodial parent be granted full control over visitation arrangements. It is like placing a lethal weapon in the hands of children or incompetents. An enraged parent, at his or her whim, may unilaterally decide to cut the children off completely from the ex-spouse for reasons that may be quite frivolous. (p. 335)

Gardner doesn't say "vengeful," which is far more to the point than "frivolous." Taken to the extreme to which Goldstein et al. go, the single-parent model of custody readily becomes punitive: it faces those who leave spouse and children with the possibility of being "defrocked" as a parent. Using the threat of loss of access as a deterrent to breakup, the nuclear family will not be shored up in this manner. Nor will the outside parent necessarily accept and submit to such a court ruling after breakup. With the stakes an all-or-nothing relation to children, separation strife can only become just that much more ruthless, generating even more numerous custody suits and child abductions (Calvin, 1981).

Further, it is not always clear just who is "the psychological parent." Sometimes both parents in divorce are equally emotionally engaged with youngsters, in which case Goldstein et al. recommended that custody be determined by a coin toss! Moreover, their model is too inflexible, for each parent may take care of the children in different ways or excel during certain developmental stages of a child but draw back at other stages; or one parent may be closer to a particular offspring, whereas the coparent relates better to another. In short, what Goldstein et al. have done is to treat *all* custody disputes in divorce as if one parent departed with insufficient concern for the welfare of youngsters, then making this situation the mold for judicial disposition in every case coming before the bar.

A final criticism is that Goldstein et al. implicitly advocated a "therapeutic" exorcism of the noncustodial parent from the psychic realm of the child—as if this were possible. Even a rarely seen parent is hardly forgotten, and may be idealized (Tessman, 1978). As for the outside parent who is regularly seen, it is conceivable that this adult may become more of a "psychological parent" over time than the custodial parent—and be barred for just that reason.

The ideological position taken by Goldstein et al. has seemed to nearly all professionals, ourselves included, as unduly harsh, impractical, and unfair. They overidentify with the forsaken wife who cannot bear to acknowledge parental claims of an ex-husband who quit the home for greener pastures. Their proposal seems like a moralistic throwback to the traditional attitude that a parent who leaves is automatically irresponsible and deserves ostracism.

Yet despite the many problems of single-parent custody, the vast majority of parting parents opt for this disposition. Prior to the advent of joint custody statutes, nationwide statistics showed that mothers obtained custody in 90% of cases, fathers in 7.5%, and others in 2.5% (Hodges, 1986). Since then, Maccoby and Mnookin (1992) found that in California mothers received sole custody in 67% of cases, fathers in 9%, others in 4%, and joint custody in 20%.

However, although there is more joint custody and single-father custody, the typical disposition is still the single-mother home: when people "vote with their feet" in such numbers, compelling reasons must exist. First, single-parent custody is not necessarily problematic, as research has indicated that such domiciles have been unduly maligned in previous literature and are generally adequate places for raising children (Brandwein, Brown, & Fox, 1974). It has also been shown that over time the well-being of the child is more closely associated with the adjustment of the custodial parent than with the rights of access of the noncustodial parent (Hetherington et al., 1993). In many cases, there may not be much choice: within 2 years of separation, visitation by the noncustodial parent tends to drop off precipitously (Seltzer, 1991). Still another factor in favor of single custody is that the outside parent's "right of access"—considered absolute by Despert—is not supported by current research as necessarily good for children when parents are in constant combat. About 25% of ex-couples are hostile far beyond the usually stormy first year or so of separation (Garrity & Baris, 1994), and Maccoby and Mnookin (1992) found that without cooperation, "evidence supporting beneficial effects of contact with non-resident fathers was thin and inconsistent" (p. 164).

All told, it must be concluded that single-parent custody, despite its obvious limitations, is popular as the solution of choice (or is perhaps the only available choice) when the outside parent is—or becomes—effectively uncommitted to caretaking.

DOWN WITH SINGLE-PARENT CUSTODY: THE TWO-HOME SOLUTION

An alternative "therapeutic" conception of custody is advanced by proponents of the joint custody movement. In view of the extent of mother-only custody, this approach has been particularly favored by advocates of fathers' rights (Warshak, 1992). Roman and Haddad (1978), both noncustodial fathers—wrote their sarcastically titled *The Disposable Parent* to protest the draconian implications for the outside parent in Goldstein et al.'s position. Roman and Haddad noted that single-parent custody already may make visiting arrangements so artificial and demeaning that rather than bringing father and child closer together, such a format may actually drive them apart; eventually, the father might stop visiting or paying child support. Like

Despert, they maintained that the child of divorce still needs both parents as emotional resources; a therapeutic custody arrangement can only be one that promotes such a goal. But how to accomplish this in practice? Roman and Haddad emphasized that the joint custody formula of "two homes" is a pragmatic device to guarantee the child foolproof access to both parents. (As an aside, we should mention that a "bird's nest" variation of joint custody also exists, whereby children stay in the original home and the separated parents—each with h/h own outside home—take turns living there, thus involving three homes. Ahrons [1994, p. 139] reported with approval several such three-home cases, including one in which a Michigan judge awarded the family house in a custody dispute to the young children of the litigating couple, ordering the parents to alternate living in the residence each month.)

In joint custody, Roman and Haddad envisioned a solution whereby children are shared so that rancorous competition for their affection is neutralized. At worst, if parents cannot stand each other, joint custody does not require them to communicate or cooperate, except to set a plan prescribing times and places for the transfer of custody (e.g., by picking the child up at school). Thereafter, they need not ever cross paths. Hodges has noted that "joint custody has been surprisingly effective, even when there is a significant level of parental conflict" (p. 119). In more ideal circumstances where parents can get along, they can discuss children regularly and even reconvene the former family unit as they wish, sometimes including new spouses. In all cases, whether or not parents are cooperative, the two homes are separate, equal, and fully autonomous units; where necessary, they duplicate—accepting the extra expense for dual sets of furniture, clothes, toys, and so forth. Neither parent has reason to interfere with the other because the joint custody format permits avoidance of contentious issues such as differing values concerning child rearing, expenditure of funds, implementation of visitation, or with whom the ex-mate is living. Each parent maintains control in h/h home, and the child learns to adjust to each setting. Roman and Haddad insisted on as nearly "equal time" as possible, with a minimum of one-third time necessary to qualify a coparent for joint custody status. The schedule can be apportioned as suits the needs of the two adults.

In Roman and Haddad's concern for the preservation of a child's ongoing contact with the parent who departs the home, they were more thoroughly Despertian than Despert. For them, joint custody by definition eliminates a "disposable" parent, thus doing away with the very concept of custodial and noncustodial parents. They parried well such familiar disparagements of their position as "the parents will not be able to get along well enough to coordinate," "the logistics are too cumbersome," or "children need a consistent home base." They believed that joint custody turns a divorce into a kind of rearrangement of the old nuclear family, now spread out over two households but with the same cast of characters in essentially the same relationships. Indeed, new mates can now be added in (or later subtracted) without upset to the overall design. So long as the child has h/h set of two parents, albeit the relationship to each is independent, the child will be emotionally protected from what they regard as the most lasting damage of divorce—the loss of the noncustodial parent. If such loss is prevented, Roman and Haddad held that the child can become a fuller human being than would have been possible in either an unhappy intact family or a single-parent family. In accord with their view that joint custody fixes what is most destructive in divorce to children, they interpreted statistics showing that divorce harms children as the result of the prevalence of single-parent custody: "As long as custody is an either/or arrangement, the great pain of loss that children and fathers suffer and the equally great pressures . . . the responsible mother must feel will continue to show up as the damaging aftermath of divorce. The terrible pity . . . is that it need not be this way" (p. 83).

As extreme in their own way as Goldstein et al., Roman and Haddad lobbied for joint custody as the mandatory legislative presumption in all cases of divorce that involved settlement of custody, unless outright unfitness can be proven against one parent. As of 1984, their approach has now been enacted into law by eight states, requiring judicial bias in favor of joint custody such that any alternative has to show cause (Hodges, 1986). Yet although joint custody seems to be an excellent technology, it has a unique handicap in terms of image: joint custody is perhaps too reminiscent of King Solomon's plan to settle a custody dispute by offering to hack in twain the contested child. Thus, Roman and Haddad saw enlightening the public as the advocate's first step: later it would become obvious that divorce need no longer hold terror for children because joint custody would render parental separation only temporarily upsetting, and our society could continue sustaining high divorce rates without fear of adverse impact on the next generation. Some proponents have even argued that joint custody would itself promote parental cooperation and reciprocal support (Moreland, Schwebel, Fine, & Vess, 1982). In short, this vision of divorce without pain for children has been so enrapturing that Calvin (1981) predicted that joint custody would become the norm of the 1980s. As we now know, this did not happen. What went wrong?

All advocates of joint custody as the "presumptive" solution to divorce custody disputes glide over psychological issues in a nonpsychological way. To start with, one cannot be so quick to blame single-parent custody for the behavior of outside fathers who do not visit their children or pay child support. Further, most separated parents know their quarreling is injurious to children, but they consciously or unconsciously cannot help but quarrel, and precisely over the children who are the living incarnations of their former union. And they are likely to quarrel over joint custody too! If parents need to fight, sooner or later there will be accusations that agreements are not fair, or should not be so rigid, or that one of the parents is not around when h/s should be or merely turns children over to a surrogate, or neglects them altogether. From her own experience, Ephron (1986) learned that commuting youngsters between two separate households is an intricate game that has no rules—"nevertheless, each player is convinced that the other is not playing by them" (p. 68). She complained that a new but incongruous version of the extended family is created by joint custody. A reviewer of her book (McFadden, 1986) noted that Ephron's title, *Funny Sauce,* implies that joint custody is a sauce never meant to be mixed. Thus, deciding when children should be in each home can turn out to be a crude, mechanical way of putting two homes in order. For the child, the primary problem often is that *there are two homes.* In fine, custody is not simply a matter of social engineering, and no disposition can be considered a prophylaxis against the ill effects of divorce or lack of involvement by an outside parent. Even Warshak (1992), a staunch proponent of shared parenting, acknowledged that joint custody is no panacea: "[It] does not release parents from the obligation to create a positive environment for their children after divorce" (p. 195). Thus, how a joint-custody father conducts his end of the arrangement is more crucial than simply having it.

In summary of this section on joint custody, we agree with Despert's stance that the child ordinarily needs both parents after breakup and that the outside parent's rights of access should not be hindered by parental malevolence or judicial decree. Joint custody implements these ideals. However, Despert's two-parent involvement does not literally call for joint custody. Roman and Haddad go far beyond what she had in mind by urging presumptions in an effort to legislate the attitudes adults should uphold toward coparenting in divorce. But ideals can never be imposed unless the requisite psychological foundation exists. No matter how appealing joint custody may seem on presentation, we wonder whether most families in breakup can think of it as a feasible and appropriate solution in their circumstances. In many cases, a shared custody arrangement is not a viable alternative, given the absence or disinterest of one parent, and even when it is enacted, all too often such a pact unravels in short order. As with any arrangement, the couple will swiftly sort out *through experience* which of them really wants responsibility for children and which of them does not. If both do their parts, a shared custody format works and may indeed be the best arrangement. But if one parent spends less time with the children than the format mandates, the other parent—voluntarily or not—must spend correspondingly more. Joint custody then turns into an "empty shell" facade that is only disguised single-parent custody. Furstenberg and Cherlin (1991) have concluded that in families in which one parent provides nearly all the child care, voluntary joint custody soon breaks down to single-parent custody, and that court-imposed joint custody is rarely beneficial in that ongoing conflict is invited. In our view, each parent's comparative involvement is what eventually determines the actual distribution and quality of custodial responsibility, not the formal agreement.

In practice, most estranged parents find the single-parent format most suitable, often with the countersymbiant electing to be cast in the instant or ultimate role of "odd man/woman out." Although countersymbiants usually want some involvement with youngsters, they tend to gravitate toward peripheral participation in the life of the young, frequently taking up residence apart from both spouse and offspring or neglecting children in their home in favor of vocational or romantic projects. Even when a countersymbiant later fights for full or joint custody, it may only be secondarily in the service of gaining greater proximity to youngsters. The motivation may have more to do with egoistic needs to project a self-image as a "good" parent. Thus, in the course of a "love entitlement quest," the reactions of a countersymbiant are often to eschew custody in spite of verbal or litigious protestations to the contrary. Witness the final decision of the tormented Mrs. Kramer. Witness the man who told a divorce mediator that he wanted joint custody and would take his children every weekend, but added that he planned to hire a baby-sitter when he had them because he expected to be out on dates. Or note the plight of the mother who received distraught phone calls from her son begging to "come home" when the child was ostensibly with his father according to a joint custody protocol, but was routinely deposited for entire stays with the new wife while the father was away on business (Gillis, 1986). Consider the puzzling cases cited by Tessman (1978, p. 279): the father seeking custody who repeatedly rejected his son's attempts to make plans to see him, the mother who won custody of her four children but then shipped them back to their father, or the woman who sued for custody but told her youngsters not to call her "Mother" any more because she had her own life to live. And what about the "false custody" battles

Hodges (1986, p. 92) warns against? In these trials, rage leads to such strange outcomes as the one in which a woman won a bitter lawsuit, then promptly turned the children over to their father, boasting that she had proven she could beat him in court.

Countersymbiants may demand joint or full custody, litigate for their rights as parents, and speak of the justice of their claims. Yet, if such a parent is in an identity crisis or otherwise preoccupied, h/s may not be able to do more than sporadically fulfill the material and psychological needs of children. Instead, a countersymbiant is often prone to count on the other parent to provide for children and will often withdraw to an outside role on h/h own initiative. Further complicating the situation, it should be added that the children themselves can intuitively sense with which adult they are most secure and then spontaneously close ranks with the parent who is most consistently invested in their caretaking. Indeed, older children can veto any visitation or custody protocol through their reluctance or outright refusal to be with a given parent; in this way, they flag which one of their elders they perceive to be emotionally absent.

Roman and Haddad (1978) took a psychological truth—that children of divorce fare best when they have ongoing relationships to both parents—and tried to make it a statutory presumption that both parents will stay more or less equally engaged with their children. There is nothing inherently wrong with joint custody; all families in situations of separation should give it serious consideration. Nevertheless, even in the Los Angeles mediation court, heavily oriented toward joint custody, only some 20% of its cases were closed out with a plan for joint custody (Dullea, 1980). Theory and reality evidently do not jibe that well.

As has been typical of many suggestions to take the acrimony out of divorce, the proposals advanced by Roman and Haddad are quite rational, forgetting that people are not always rational and that the "rational" itself is not always rational (Yapko, 1997). Custody conforms more to emotional commitment than to legal prescription. Courtroom standards are needed to safeguard the rights of children, but still cannot shape the passions of adults who share coparental duties. What about the woman left to raise children alone while an ex-husband proves to be unreliable in visitation or child support? What about the jealous spouse whose stomach turns at the thought of seeing the children with an unfaithful partner and h/h new lover? Are these parents with bitter grievances against an ex going to agree to joint custody? Or if joint custody is imposed on them by court order, will it work? And what about marital partners who go off on a consuming identity quest that leaves little time or money for children—is it not worse for children if such parents obtain a joint custody they cannot handle at this point in their lives?

Hugh McIsaac stated the avuncular doctrine of the joint custody movement when he said, "We are beginning to realize that divorce is not the death, but the reorganization of the family" (Dullea, 1980, p. 46). Instead of characterizing divorce as both product of and contributor to the chaotic social conditions of today, McIsaac euphemistically redefined it as a stabilizing reorganization in a fluctuating world. The blind spot of the proponents of joint custody is not their promotion of a formula that compartmentalizes management of the child (neither parent interfering with the other's "internal affairs") and hence "normalizes" division within the family unit. It is not even the oversell of the "two homes" or "binuclear family" concept as a way for a parent to feel guilt-free as h/s divorces, perhaps remarries, and perhaps redivorces. What we find most objectionable is the complicity of these experts in the notion that families can readily afford to dance to the tune of divorce because a "quick fix" technology will save them—adults and children alike—from having to pay the piper. All in all, this is an attempt to "civilize" custody disputes in divorce. Presumably, if children spend equivalent time in their parents' homes, then nuclear relationships continue unchanged and new mates can be incorporated or not as each parent wishes. But it is a mistake to suppose that most families can or will comply in the execution of a polygamous dream which, were it to be believed, would render joint custody an ideal system for the upbringing of children.

CUSTOMIZED CUSTODY FOR
EACH FAMILY OF DIVORCE

In the final analysis, there is a need for diverse modes of custody to suit specific families. Where a departed parent takes minimal notice of children, or is destructive to them when present, or is fickle in terms of involvement, absolute control by the custodial parent is what makes most sense. It is imperative for youngsters to know that there is one adult who continues to have responsibility and authority for daily care. At the other end of the spectrum, where capacity and willingness to nurture are about evenly distributed between parents, joint custody offers a viable and effective disposition. The vast majority of cases will fall in between, with children staying with one "home" parent and having some schedule of visitation with an "outside" parent. Since it is usually the parents who fashion and implement a custody plan, *each tends to be involved with offspring to the extent h/s wants to be.* Legalities seldom hold them back for long or propel them forward. It is a fiction to view modern-day parenting as an innate "instinct," a forensic "right," or a "civic obligation." For better or worse, parenting is simply a human commitment. As such, tragic though it may be for some children and, by extension, for society in general, this commitment will not always be honored.

~ 14

How Feasible Is "Cooperation Where Children Are Concerned"?

> Our recommendation for developing ex-spouse . . .
> cooperation suggests [that] some form of joint custody or
> co-parenting is the optimal post-divorce arrangement.
> Although such agreements are not without potential
> problems . . . the literature justifies taking the position
> that cooperative co-parenting is a legitimate goal.
> —MORELAND ET AL. (1982, p. 643)

> Almost everyone [in our study] wished that he or she was
> on better terms with his or her ex. When we asked them to
> describe *an ideal divorced parenting relationship,* even the
> fieriest of foes mentioned the importance of open and
> frequent communication.
> —AHRONS (1994, p. 7)

CALLING FOR COOPERATION IN THE MIDST OF CONFLICT

In a study involving 98 divorced Wisconsin couples, Ahrons (1994) found that many more coparents worked together in the care of their young than one might expect from a generally discouraging divorce literature. She divided her sample into four categories: *perfect pals* who remained platonic friends after their divorce, *cooperative colleagues* who were able to manage their occasional conflicts so as not to involve children, *angry associates* whose occasional conflicts infused all family relationships, and *fiery foes* who could be violent or fought over custody.

283

She found that the first year was usually rife with crises but coparents later settled into one of the four types, which then carried on even when second marriages occurred. Almost half of her sample were in the first two categories; thus, they were said to be conducting a "good divorce." Ahrons also noted that some ex-couples in the last two categories still sometimes developed parallel cooperation where child care was concerned: they might not be able to deal directly with each other but were able to reach some accommodation. Based on this survey's data, Ahrons held that a "good divorce" was possible for most couples, especially if professional intervention was available during the critical first year. But, as for the quality of their postdivorce relationship, her criterion for a good divorce mainly seemed to be cooperation in child care.

Ahrons's book exemplifies a major tenet of the "progressive" movement: the injunction that parting parents must cooperate where children are concerned. If this tenet is met, it is assumed that youngsters will adjust to divorce. Elsewhere, we have discussed other progressive tenets assuring adults of similar prospects, so that the old myth whereby people marry and live happily ever after has been replaced by a new myth—that people now divorce so that they and their children can live happily ever after. To accomplish this feat, however, one is urged to remember that the ex-couple must conduct their breakup *properly*. Insofar as the rearing of offspring is concerned, this specifically means no fighting over children, no vilification of the other parent in front of children, and no use of children as pawns. According to the progressive approach, the issue at hand is whether adults are able to isolate their marital conflicts from their roles as parents (Calvin, 1981); if not, the divorce fails and children are harmed.

Despite the best of intentions on the part of parents, there are two glaring problems with what appears to be eminently rational guidelines to shield children from the stress of family breakup. To begin with, *it is unlikely that most coparents will cooperate as well or better in divorce than they did in the working marriage.* Parting parents usually fight, and indeed some of the fighting is over these very children, often with the aim of enlisting them as allies on their respective sides in the separation strife. The second problem is that *children frequently have adverse reactions to divorce*: they tend to develop (at least initially) some type of behavioral disturbance as a way to remonstrate against what is, to most of them, a frightening disruption of their security. The symptoms of a child will make even the most pacifist parents argue over which of them is responsible and what each should do about it.

In sum, "cooperation where children are concerned" is a worthy ideal, but it is frequently not practicable because it mandates that parents must rise above their own feelings to make divorce benign for offspring. The current emphasis on harmonious coparenting despite breakup makes divorce seem a more controlled process than it is, as if ongoing acrimony could stop abruptly whenever children are affected. The actuality is that divorce must run its course in accord with the degree of loss and rage experienced by the parties. Although parents engaged in an acrimonious breakup can be made to feel guilty when their strife hurts children, they are still likely to fight directly or indirectly over progeny who personify their union. It is true that potential for a tragic situation exists when children are "caught in the middle," but contrary to hopes for a cooperative divorce, how can a caring parent avoid conflict with a coparent if as often happens the welfare of a child is at stake? Moreover, is such conflict necessarily a bad thing?

WHEN PARENTS PART IN ACRIMONY: CO-FOES

In breakups, the bonds of coparents are chiefly preserved, justified, and expressed via their dealings in regard to children. Their young embody the love that once united them, but at the same time, whatever was the conflict leading to separation will be carried over to conflict about how the children are to be raised, by whom, and with what loyalties and values. In acrimonious cases, it can be expected that the issues of breakup will be ineluctably woven into their separate and often clashing efforts to bring up their offspring.

To highlight the ex-mates' commonly seen oscillation between concord and combat, we call them *co-foes*. Not all parting parents alternate between the polarities of "co" and "foe," but even when cooperating well, there is always potential for sudden changes in an ambivalent partnership. Interactions sometimes become inconsistent: one day the coparents avow their solidarity and reciprocity; the next day they are locked in intransigent dispute. The term "co-foe" is meant to convey the inherent contradictions of divorced co-parent relations. Although an ex-couple remain interdependent and tied through their children, their breakup also implies segregated, nonaccountable, and at times incompatible arrangements set up by two adults with disparate agendas. Hence, fluctuations in the quality of their partnership merely reflect an innate confusion in the divorce process. Once living apart, parents simultaneously share and do not share responsibilities for children.

Parting parents ordinarily start on a note of collaboration. They agree that mutual restraint is to be exercised where the well-being of their children is concerned, but determination to work in unison at the outset does not always prove feasible for long. One reason that breakdown in collaboration may occur is that there is competition for the predominant loyalty of offspring. When fought over in this way, children of divorce are placed in the untenable role of arbiters of which side is "right" or which parent is "better."

Besides the emotional pulls emanating from two needy parents, the child is also "partitioned" according to some custodial formula worked out by parents. If rivalry precludes ex-mates from agreeing on a division of responsibilities, a contested child may wind up jammed into "an ill-fitting custody suit," in the memorable phrase of Tessman (1978, p. 277). Indeed, according to Wheeler (1980), it appears that as many as 10% of divorcing couples go to the drastic extent of litigating aspects of custody in court. A majority of the rest still fight over children, wrangling over their care, the money to pay for it, and the access and influence each parent will have. These dealings, not adult intentions or promises, are the actual measure of their level of coop-eration.

Where competition to be the "good parent" is an issue in some divorces, self-removal of a parent becomes a reality in others. In this situation, where rivalry for the children's loyalty does not occur because one adult has voluntarily forfeited h/h parental role, cooperation is impossible. By withdrawal, one parent disregards the emotional and material needs of offspring, leaving the other parent burdened in that h/s is forced to make up the difference or to watch offspring do without (Weiss, 1979a). Such an overtaxed adult tends to be enraged at what is seen as an unforgivable malfeasance; this anger is to be expressed if ever the two parents' paths cross again.

In fine, there is both positive and negative potential in divorce coparenting. The optimal side is seen when ex-mates labor to avoid either the extreme of destructive vying for the love of children or the "dropping out" of either parent. They take conjoint measures to protect their children—each stays involved and wants the other to stay involved, recognizing that families do best when fathers as well as mothers are providers (Furstenberg, 1994). They tolerate constructive criticism from each other. In times of crisis, they can put differences aside in order to be at their cooperative best.

On the minus side of the ledger, children are symbols of the marriage and their very existence makes breakup of the union that produced them tragic. Further, because of the children, parting adults still have to maintain a parental and financial partnership and cannot just deal with their conflicts by going their separate ways. In addition, any problems of children that can be attributed to the breakup instantly create blind rage at the coparent. All told, the hateful side of an ambivalent co-foe partnership will then trigger episodic confrontations, and these encounters will find the two adults at their cooperative worst.

COOPERATION QUICKLY STYMIED:
ECONOMIC WARFARE

The lofty principle that coparents should cooperate where children are concerned often crashes as soon as translated into the palpable currency of *cold cash*. Parents have a joint responsibility to underwrite their children's upbringing, but in separation their budgets are totally independent, which sets up a clash of vested interests. Even if there was adequate income before breakup to support the family unit, monetary distribution after breakup may not be equitable. Men and women are not necessarily equal wage earners, nor are financial requirements of custodial parents the same as noncustodial parents. Thus, in many separations, economic conflict quickly makes a mockery of the ideal of cooperation.

As a didactic example, consider the case of a mother seeking child support from a man himself in precarious financial straits:

> When we were first separated I had to apply for welfare because he was in arrears with his check. Then he was paying again and I went off welfare. Then he was in arrears again and I had to go back to court. And going into court, he said, "Look what you are doing! You are taking me to court! What a wonderful inheritance you are giving your children!" And I said, "Well, you're showing your boys that they can get married, have children, leave them, go their merry way. . . . And you are showing [your daughters] when they get married their husbands can walk out, and the hell with the kids." (Weiss, 1979a, p. 153)

In this example, the father maintains he is being fiscally assaulted by an ex-wife who humiliates him by dragging him into court like a criminal; according to him, the mother is modeling vindictiveness to youngsters. Conversely, the mother maintains she is being financially deprived by her ex-husband and feels indignant about having to resort to legal proceedings; according to her, he models irresponsibility. Both parties here are short of funds, but they blame their predicament on the greed and other failings of the coparent. Each lays guilt trips, criticizing on the grounds that the other's behavior hurts the children. Each hopes to get the children—and court—to validate h/h position as victim of a selfish ex. They are fighting out their divorce, including their images in the eyes of the children, through the medium of fighting over money.

Is there a mercenary edge to their claims, trying to get as much as they can for themselves at the expense of the counterpart? One lawyer stated, "It's an obscenity, but a lot of these cases are really about money instead of the children" (Wheeler, 1980, p. 27). And so indeed it might seem in the context of divorce litigation. But psychologically speaking, parents fight over money, custody, or anything else as part of their ongoing separation strife, and many have been known to willingly bankrupt themselves in the process of so doing. The novel *Kramer vs. Kramer* (Corman, 1977) is one such example—the husband is ruined for years to come by defending against his ex-wife's custody suit (her costs are nil because she is represented by her new boyfriend, an attorney). Abrahms (1983) gave the contemporary cost of a custody suit as about $40,000; Sheresky and Mannes (1972) have decried the costly folly, economic and otherwise, of many ex-couples who turn to the courts to settle moral and self-esteem issues in the guise of property or child-related disputes.

Beyond the acrimony over money, the preceding anecdote also draws attention to the fact that divorce is expensive. Legal costs aside, two households now have to be maintained on the same resources that supported one. The outside parent needs h/h earnings to set up a new life and usually sends a fixed, affordable amount to the home parent. Hence, the latter must supplement for lost funds by undertaking a higher level of employment, going on welfare, or depending on the generosity of h/h family of origin or a new mate. Making ends meet is a daily and very stressful concern. Demographic data make clear that custodial mothers are among the most disadvantaged groups in the country (Mednick, 1994; Arendell, 1986). A Michigan study over 7 years showed that the dollar income of divorced men and women declined by 19% and 29% respectively, whereas a control group of intact couples saw a rise of 22% (Weitzman, 1985, p. 337). It is plain from this study that both sexes suffer a diminution of assets in divorce, though females more so. But the situation is far worse for women than at first appears, according to Weitzman. In terms of current purchasing power as compared with what they had in marriage, men's economic position actually improved by 17%, but women lost 29% of their disposable income. The disparity occurs because, even with less absolute income resulting from support payments, men were better off economically in divorce than in marriage because they now had but a limited fiscal liability for their children, often covering only a fraction of the costs of raising them. For example, their obligation to pay support usually ends on a child's 18th birthday, putting the burden of college expenses mainly on the mother (Rowe, 1991). Weitzman also cited a California study (p. 339) that showed an even greater gender difference: men made a 42% improvement in their postdivorce standard of living, whereas women experienced a 73% decline—a gross disparity she attributed to a no-fault divorce statute recently enacted in California. Weitzman concluded that divorce was creating a "two tier society" in which men, and the women and children who live with them, are the upper tier and the former wives and their children are the lower tier. In sharp disagreement, Victor and Winkler (1977) held that "the question of who gets raked over the coals in a divorce settlement is, oddly enough, not as explosive between men and women as it is between women and women. Resentment . . . runs high among second wives who . . . upon marrying, find . . . their income going to support first wives' 'middle-class comfort' " (p. 86). Thus, in divorced families either first or second wives, or both, may be struggling, but first wives with no husband tend to be worse off.

Social scientists are greatly concerned at present about the "feminization of poverty" (Pearce, 1978), which refers to the link between single-parent mothers and a minimal standard of living, if not destitution. Contrary to popular belief, most female-headed families are not the result of out-of-wedlock births but of divorce (50%) or separation (31%). In 1982, 21% of American children were living below the poverty line with mothers who were mostly on welfare. As for single-parent mothers not on welfare, even with full-time jobs only half earned enough to support two children without needing help from an ex-husband or the government. Arendell (1986) found that 56 of 60 middle-class women in a California sample were "declassed" by divorce, being instantly pushed below the poverty line or close to it—in most cases irreversibly, with only 4 of the 60 able to establish a standard of living 4 years after divorce close to what they had when married. At one time, almost half of Arendell's sample contemplated suicide, saying financial stress was a prime factor in this desperation. Thus, economic injustice, falling disproportionately on women, compounds the high cost of divorce; it can be concluded that in breakup children tend to be where money is not. Weitzman remarked that festering anger must occur when fathers fly off to a Hawaii vacation while the ex-wife and children are pinching pennies, working menial jobs, or doing without (p. 353).

Another point raised by the Weiss vignette is the reality many women face in divorce whereby child support can be obtained only through onerous personal and legal efforts, not to mention that in any event such payments cannot be counted on. Eckhardt (1973) found that 42% of Wisconsin men did not pay mandated child support after 1 year, rising to 81% after 10 years, and that an additional 20% were in partial arrears after 1 year and 8% after 10 years. A U.S. Census Bureau survey in 1981 reported 25% noncompliance where the custodial mother received nothing and 30% where there was partial payment; Hetherington et al.'s (1993) more recent estimate of the combined total puts the figure at 70%. Moreover, Weitzman (1985) noted many allegations of underpayment because husbands hide their assets from ex-wives. All told, as a result of underassessment and nonpayment, women frequently have to petition the courts to ask for enforcement of the legal principle that a husband cannot separate from wife and children with little or no provision for their material survival. A man too can petition the court for a reduced contribution if he should suffer a loss of earnings, but rather than engage in still more litigation, he can also become ever more stinting—and may even "disappear," address unknown, to avert further disbursement.

Despite the gravity of the financial situation, weight must be given to psychological factors that so often underlie economic conflict. Different motives drive parents to fight over money, and these factors have to be looked at from both sides of the breakup. *Entitlement* is one such motive. For example, in the aftermath of leaving, many identity-seeking rejectors will expend fiscal assets as a "free spirit" to fund long-deferred projects impossible to fulfill in the marriage, as well as to pay for the expenses incurred in separation. Funds must somehow be found for these purposes, so old obligations may be neglected and even regarded as impediments that threaten the new life style. In refusing to be constrained by the material needs of ex-mate and children, the warrant to make oneself the foremost financial priority expresses the fury felt for being tethered to a family, functioning for others at cost to self.

Revenge is the other most common psychological factor involved in fights over money, mostly pertaining to those who feel they were unjustly treated in breakup. Women who have been left can be avid to obtain as much as possible of their ex-husband's resources, in part because of a wish to secure their children's future, but also to leave the man financially strapped. Men who have been expelled from their homes may have their own form of vindictive reaction, feeling justified in not paying someone who has opted to do without them. Such a refusal can be overt, as in the case of a man who refused to pay a bill for orthodontal work urgently needed by his son. But, as the ex-wife said, "By making me suffer, he made his child suffer too" (Arendell, 1986, p. 40). Or the refusal may take a devious route—for example, the surgeon who deliberately lost most of his practice, preferring to be virtually unemployed rather than provide the money that would make it easy for wife and children to manage apart.

The issue of control through money frequently comes up. Feifer (1995) presented the personal account of Jocelyn, whose divorce from David, a wealthy man, was rancorously contested around finances:

> The money's a symbol and more than a symbol. In David's case, it was probably connected to his deepest emotions. He took it out on me by faking poverty, hiding assets, not paying what he promised. *I* took it out on *him* by saying I wanted a total end to our relationship and therefore insisted on a lump-sum settlement; no alimony because I didn't want him writing monthly checks or failing to write them. . . . That was the worst thing I could ask for because it was the kind of control David couldn't give up. (p. 104)

Jocelyn lived austerely while David hired a battery of lawyers to prevent a settlement satisfactory to her. But he was not happy:

> Just last month he said I should come to Europe and we'll discuss things over a glass of champagne. "You'll pay my ticket?" I bristled. "But that's obscene. You won't pay for health insurance, your son and I have been two years without health insurance. Yet you want to fly me over there to drink champagne? How dare you do that to your children?"
>
> That started him raging. "You don't know what *I've* been through! . . . You cost me over $250,000 in legal fees alone."
>
> "Really, $250,000?" I asked. "Then you're an idiot. . . . I wasn't worth that much!" (p. 105)

In short, economic deprivation is accepted by both parties as a legitimate weapon in co-foe combat—when wielded against the other. From a legal perspective, Wheeler (1980) has noted that some men demand more visitation than they truly want, aiming to extract pecuniary concessions, and Lonsdorf (1991) described "blackmail custody" in which a husband threatens to sue as an intimidation to reduce child support, as well as behavior by a wife in which financial leverage is used for retaliation. Ultimately, cooperation ceases as soon as demands are made for wherewithal the ex cannot or will not spare.

At worst, an outside parent sends no support, leading ex-spouse and children to believe that an adult who does not provide does not care. This criticism is usually merited, for withholding money constitutes manifest rejection of the child (Weiss, 1979a). In the following vignette, the speaker is a mother seeking a monthly allotment from a man looking to society to support his family:

> We had this argument about money, where my husband said, "Well, I have to live." And I said, "You get as much a month as I do. And you're single. You have no responsibilities. Your girlfriend cooks for you. She does your wash. Stop spending so much money taking her out! Then you will be able to give it to me for the kids, so they can eat!" So he said, "Go get food stamps." So I said, "What about their medical expenses?" And he said, "Go get Medicaid." And I said, "No, that's still your responsibility." (Weiss, 1979a, p. 152)

Even when the outside parent is forthcoming with funds on a generous basis, bitterness around material matters may still exist; nothing could make plainer that fighting over money is not just over money. Thus, acrimony can still occur when ample support is given and the child is showered with gifts, trips, private education, and so forth, so that a munificent parent is involved but leaves all the routine or unpleasant aspects of child rearing to the other parent. In one case, a woman commented about the hefty stipend she received from her former husband for the care of their son:

> I'm getting a certain fee . . . for raising Elliot. . . . [My ex-husband] has none of the responsibilities for taking care of Elliot twenty-four hours a day, taking him to the hospital every time he needs stitches, which is often, taking him to the doctors, getting him shoes, all of these things. He's bringing Elliot up by check. He pays the check and I do all the work [and] I don't think that's fair. (Weiss, 1979a, p. 153)

THE OUTSIDE PARENT'S "RIGHT OF ACCESS": USE AND ABUSE

It has been noted that visitation, despite its importance, is not always what it should be. A shortfall between real and ideal is as true today as when Goode (1956) stated:

> The husband is likely to have exaggerated notions about how much visiting he *can* do. . . . Consequently, he may make promises, to himself and possibly to the children, to visit as often as permitted. Nevertheless, in general these promises are not oriented to the realities of time, energy, and money, and visits will probably become less and less frequent with time. (pp. 314–315)

Gardner (1976) added, "At times a parent may demand far more visitation than is reasonable so as to reduce guilt over separation. . . .

Such enthusiasm is usually short-lived as it is based on guilt rather than genuine affection" (p. 335).

It is clear that outside parents—usually men—often fail to visit their children regularly in divorce, no matter what they promised on the eve of departure. A sample of divorced mothers reported that only a quarter of children saw their fathers once a week or more, whereas more than a third saw their fathers a few times a year or not at all (Seltzer, 1991). Arendell (1986) found that two-thirds of fathers in her study saw their children less than five times a year. She commented, "Ironically, these mothers did not 'feel divorced' from their husbands in ways they had expected, but they came to believe that their children 'felt divorced' in ways they had not expected" (p. 109). Wheeler (1980) reviewed research by Wallerstein in which it was found that "only" 30% of divorced fathers rarely or never visited their children—a much lower rate than that reported by other investigations—and then wondered whether the rate was so low because "the fact that they knew they were being studied had made the men in Wallerstein's sample somewhat more conscientious" (p. 58). Indeed, Wheeler's cynicism proved to be quite justified, because the Wallerstein researchers did provide services in their sample to keep fathers involved with children.

Furstenberg and Cherlin (1991) asked why is it so difficult to maintain fathers' involvement after divorce. Their answer pointed to inadequate social preparation of males for child rearing, plus the predivorce history of divorcing couples:

> Many men don't seem to know how to relate to their children except through their wives. Typically, when married, they were present but passive. . . . When they separate, they carry this pattern of limited involvement with them [because they are] uncomfortable and unskilled at being an active parent, marginalized by infrequent contact, [and] focused on building a new family life. (p. 74)

However, Furstenberg and Cherlin recognized that the trauma of the separation process itself was also a factor in poor postdivorce parenting by fathers.

In connection with this latter factor, Kelly (1981) reported data that showed that "the father's attitude and feelings about the divorce more often took precedence in determining visiting arrangements than did the quality of the predivorce relationship with their children" (p. 345). She showed that depressed or guilty fathers tend to visit less often. But Kelly also addressed the mother's role in fostering nonvisitation by the father, especially when an "embittered custodial parent, opposed to the divorce, attempted to severely limit visits, or failing that, to sabotage those that were legally scheduled" (p. 345). Kelly illustrated this in the case of a woman who scheduled her children for medical appointments or parties with friends during planned visits. The ex-husband of this woman became angry, accusing her of preventing visits or turning the children against him for not "being around."

Dudley (1994) wanted to hear directly from men who had little or nothing to do with their children after breakup. He found that 33 of 84 such men from Philadelphia viewed the former spouse as the obstacle to visitation, either by hindering their access (often with support from the courts) or by saying such damaging things to the children about them that a negative attitude was inculcated toward visitation (one father was said to be gay and a second was falsely accused of child abuse). Another 22 men gave personal problems as the reason they did not visit: several stated that job, health, or addiction problems were involved, and 2 worried that they might jeopardize their current romantic relationships (e.g., "The woman I love requires a lot of time and attention. I know I would lose her if I spent more time with my kids"). Most of the remaining men in the sample referred to distance problems: either the ex-wife had taken the children far away (sometimes to get away from the husband and in one case to hide from him), or the father himself had pursued an opportunity elsewhere. Dudley concluded that there was no simple explanation for infrequent visitation, but that conflict with the ex-wife was the most important single factor.

However, research utilizing interviews and questionnaires can only go so far because these instruments are limited by what respondents choose to reveal, as well as by the level of their conscious awareness. If we wish to penetrate more deeply into motivation, clinical methods must be used. One pattern mentioned in the preceding chapter is that identity-seeking rejectors often become so caught up in sexual–romantic, career, or other self-actualizing needs (for which they engineered the breakup) as to be unable to keep prior promises to children once out of the home—and they are not apt to say this to a researcher. Also not likely to be reported, motives of revenge can lead a divorce-resistant outside father to neglect contact with his children. Thus, when a husband has been ousted from his home, he may feel so attacked in his manhood that he strives to punish the wife even if it means also harming the children. One such maneuver is to not visit his offspring *on principle*. The message to the wife is that because of her asking him to leave, she and the youngsters will have to operate in future without him. However, left unsaid is a more malevolent communication: "By depriving our young of ongoing contact with me, they will be hurt, and this I do in order to hurt you, the mother." To be sure, such a tactic will indeed punish the mother; one woman was outraged by her ex-husband's behavior along these lines:

> There was nobody that was a better father than Wally. So I said, "What happened, . . . Wally? You don't even call the kids up. They call you up; you could care less. . . . You're rejecting them. . . . What happened to this father?" And he said, "He died." I looked at him and all of a sudden I'd like to give him a kick in the ass. I said, "You fucking bastard. What do I owe you for the coffee?" And I got out of that place so fast. I had no sympathy whatever. He was drowning in self-pity. . . . He called me up in half an hour and he said, "I'm sorry." I said, "I don't talk to dead people," and I hung up. (Weiss, 1979a, p. 151)

Even when visitation is regular or frequent, there may still be problems when ex-mates meet in the context of being coparents. An out-of-the-house male may view the children as instruments in the pursuit of unfinished business with the former mate. Such men "visit the kids" at their convenience, in many cases appearing at the house without advance notice, expecting to be welcomed and fed during visits, and wanting to make love to the ex after the children go to sleep. The woman can only suspect that he is really visiting her, using the children as an excuse. She particularly resents this behavior if the man is an undependable father, concluding that his interest in the youngsters is as a conduit to her.

A woman too has ways to take advantage of a father's relation to offspring, using visitation as an opportunity to make her points about the divorce. Picking children up in the former home makes men keenly aware of the woman's activity; the female can utilize this fact to humiliate the male. Thus, the ex-wife can arrange to be conspicuously in the process of getting dressed for a date. Many an ex-husband will be upset, suspecting that the woman is using his baby-sitting services as an aid to her romantic trysts (Kelly, 1981). Indeed, if a woman wishes to flaunt her new sexual freedom, as the father steps in the door to call on his children, she can introduce him to her own gentleman caller. Worse yet, the mother can move far away, letting him know that she does not value his parenting enough to care whether he visits.

In addition, children are subject to scenes in which parents seize the occasion of visitation to discuss pending matters, thus sometimes turning their contact into a flashpoint for rancorous quarrels. Not coincidentally, these fights tend to occur right in front of the children. An example is provided by Arendell (1986): "He always wants to argue because he blames me for kicking him out; the kids are usually crying before he even gets out of the house with them. And he still threatens me in front of them. I can't keep him away from the kids even when he's been drinking" (p. 115). As can be seen, the children stand by, impatient for their visitor to spend time with them and in pain over parental conflict. It may happen that whole visits pass by with the parents locked in tense discourse, or perhaps the visitor storms out at some point, in either case demonstrating that the parents' involvement with each other takes precedence over concern for the children. Next time, the youngsters will try to get the outside parent to leave with them immediately, but they do not always succeed in forestalling another embroilment. Hence, for some children, the visitations they look forward to can become events they learn to dread as well.

ARE VISITATION RIGHTS CONTINGENT ON PAYING CHILD SUPPORT?

As a generalization it can be said that men often fight in separation by withholding money, whereas women tend to fight by withholding access to children. Among the most contentious issues in a co-foe relationship is whether to allow visitation when the man falls far behind in his child support payments or, conversely, whether the man must still make such payments if his visitation rights are grossly hindered. As a rule, courts have held that two wrongs do not make a right—parents do not forfeit prerogatives in one area even if they are derelict in another (Wheeler, 1980). Moreover, courts emphasize the *noncontingent rights of the child*— hence, the outside parent's visitations cannot be lost because of financial dereliction (Hodges, 1986) nor is this parent free of financial liability if visitation is withheld (Weitzman, 1985).

But abstract, court-promulgated "rights" can seldom impress co-foes. The law's philosophy seems contrary to common sense: the court reinforces noncompliance with the rights of children by disallowing aversive consequences. Thus, a custodial mother is not likely to let chronic fiscal delinquency go unanswered while she petitions a court in the hope of eventual redress, although she realizes that cutting off visitation means depriving her children of access to their father. Similarly, an outside father is rarely going to keep sending funds while turning to a court in the hope of eventual visitation, although he knows that not providing support means hardship for the children. Such impasses between co-foes make a mockery of the cliché "cooperation where children are concerned." Every proposed solution to these conundrums, including the current standard in legal practice, is disquieting, because children will lose out whether either parent retaliates or turns the other cheek.

THE "NO VILIFICATION" RULE

Because faith in their parents is an essential psychic need of children, comments are always decried in which one parent devalues the other in the children's eyes. Nevertheless, it still happens:

> Over and over the advice is repeated: "Refrain from voicing criticism of the other parent. It is difficult but absolutely necessary for a child's healthy development. It is important that the child respect both parents." But vilification of the noncustodial father is widespread. (Victor & Winkler, 1977, p. 89)

Everett and Everett (1994) recently repeated the same advice, extending it to both parents: "If the children want to complain, tell them to talk to the other parent . . . not you. Don't get pulled into judging or criticizing the other parent's decisions. . . . You have enough to work on with your own parenting" (p. 109).

Of course, disparaging the other parent in front of offspring is not a good idea, as would also be true in intact marriages. But in divorce, things are not so simple as the "no vilification" rule suggests. Breakup has already made obvious the fact that parents cannot get along. Even if they hide their mutual criticisms from offspring, it is impossible to entirely conceal negative opinions. Indeed, sometimes a parent will have no choice but to deal with this issue because a child may specifically ask about h/h attitude. What the parent can reveal becomes a question of what a particular child can understand and bear, as well as how existing arrangements will be affected. On one hand, there is no doubt that parting parents tend to be biased and invidious in what they say and may do great damage to the other's image in the child's mind, meanwhile worsening relations between themselves. On the other hand, it may also be appropriate to validate what a youngster has observed or concluded about the other parent's conduct. Moreover, referring children back to the other parent with their complaints runs the risk of leaving them unheard and unprotected.

Simon (1964) assessed the no vilification rule from her own personal background as a stepchild and, later, a stepmother:

> Intellectually the parent gets the message: [both emotion and critical opinion] must be swallowed in colossal repression; better the parental

> stomach be ulcerated than the psyche of the child. . . . Whether all
> parents can follow these instructions is a question mark to the prag-
> matist; whether they should is a moral inquiry rarely raised. The . . .
> injunction is so firmly established in divorce mores that to challenge it
> is almost heresy. (p. 109)

Thus, beyond human limitations as to whether "no vilification" is
realistic, Simon struggled with whether or not the rule should be
honored. She decided on a middle ground. Yes, children should not
be exposed to divorce antagonisms born of personal hurts or be
encouraged to form a negative stereotype of the other parent. But they
eventually have to know where their parents really stand on crucial
issues and what the consequences of those stands have been in their
family's history. Accordingly, in answer to her own query whether "lip
service to the sterling qualities of the absent parent, the practice of
ersatz friendship with the person one could not bear to live with, and
the parroting of aphorisms from how-to books, is not more a vice than
a virtue," she replied, "If the child cannot know the truth as his parent
sees it, he cannot understand the divorce. He must assume that it had
no solid base, in which case there was no respect for his childish needs"
(pp. 109–110).

As we see it, good parenting in divorce means restraint and
fairness in criticism of the coparent, but such regulation cannot mean
silence or evasion when children ask delicate questions about the
breakup or when they suffer from what the coparent is doing. Such
parental self-censorship shows children "pseudo-mutuality" (Wynne,
Ryckoff, Day, & Hirsch, 1958)—the same false facade long regarded by
clinicians as harmful in intact families. Further, enjoining "no vilification" can be construed as literally forbidding moral condemnation of
anything the coparent does in relation to youngsters, leaving a concerned parent with nothing to do except practice toleration as in the
"Why can't they be civilized?" approach. But adults do not parent in a
moral vacuum. They may quite validly insist that it is their duty to
protect children, even—if need be—from each other.

CONFLICT ARISING FROM THE UNEQUAL
ROLES OF SEPARATED PARENTS

After breakup, each parent must cope with either new parental functions or the loss of old ones; many problems are caused by "the ways
in which the wife is *shut in* with the children and the husband is *shut*

out" (Calvin, 1981, p. 114). Such imbalance in itself creates tensions, often leading to strife between an overwhelmed custodial mother and an underinvolved noncustodial father.

The Mother's Side

Whether or not the initiator of breakup, a custodial mother's life is beset by augmented responsibilities, financial pressures, the task of finding a new mate, and closing down the relationship to the former mate (Arendell, 1986). Her children are bound to feel the impact of this overload. Single-parent mothers usually push their children toward early self-sufficiency, but this resource can only go so far. Because children cannot fully care for themselves, their mother usually needs adult assistance, so she may return to live with her family of origin, or let a new mate live with her, or try to get her ex-husband more involved, even though each option has its price. So long as the custodial mother is largely on her own, either because adjunctive support is unavailable or too costly, she tends to become overtaxed and then depleted. She has difficulties satisfying the ongoing clamor for more of her time from children looking to her to compensate for their absent father. Youngsters may make trouble, especially about sharing her attentions with a new man in her life—someone she needs in order to replenish herself emotionally to keep on giving, despite entailing temporary unavailability to children. When there is not enough of her to go around, her offspring may come to be seen as voraciously demanding; at the extreme, a vicious cycle can ensue between an increasingly exhausted mother and an increasingly symptomatic child. Such symptoms compel more attention, until the mother realizes she is losing control and cannot parent well enough any longer. Child in hand, she may then appear at the door of a psychiatric facility, stating that her youngster needs help—which is also a way of stating that the mother needs help.

This description is considerably mitigated when the custodial mother has personal or financial resources so that her children's developmental needs can be balanced with her own. Not every woman is pushed to her limits. And even under very adverse conditions, a single-parent mother can still do an outstanding job of raising youngsters. But it is vital to recognize that such a woman must cope with much stress to function as an adequate parent. Meanwhile, she cannot but keenly resent that her colleague in this responsibility—the noncustodial father—seems to have a less burdened existence. This resentment will enter into her feelings toward him, sometimes exploding in episodic expressions of contempt or hostility.

The Father's Side

"While it is frequently asked, 'What effect will father absence have on children?' it is rarely . . . asked, 'What effect will child deprivation have on a father?' " (Victor & Winkler, 1977, p. 72). Separated fathers often suffer painful loss of contact with children; indeed, research has shown that some fathers who were close to their children prior to divorce have a difficult time maintaining contact afterward because the loss is so painful (Kruk, 1991). Fathers may also be limited in their access by what the custodial mother will allow, the workings of the court system, and geographical moves by either party. Moreover, much as men may miss their offspring, a new "visitation" arrangement seems awkward and contrived, for a father must in effect set up dates with his children. In the course of taking them out, he must establish a more intimate relationship to older children than he had before; with the younger ones, he may have to learn to relate on his own—finding places to go, things to do, and if he takes them overnight, mastering cooking, cleaning, and getting them ready for school.

Although some men have said that they eventually enjoy new dimensions in their contact with children, others have problems taking care of offspring alone and accordingly turn to a woman for assistance. In separation, the father takes the children out for a specified period, but often he has lined up a female with whom to deposit them while he retreats to the sidelines or, in some instances, leaves the premises altogether. In this manner, Dad may bring children "visiting" him to his mother's or sister's house. He also can ask the current lady in his life to take charge of their care—a practice that may have destructive repercussions coming from ex-wife or children, or possibly even from girlfriend.

The limitations of the noncustodial father can also extend to the spirit in which he approaches his new role. He may be grandiose and appear at the old homestead in a heroic guise, lavishing goods and laughter so as to be accorded a royal welcome when he chooses to come. Or he can pop up without notice or invitation, using his involvement with the children to get next to Mom. Or he can begrudge every penny and every minute he has to spend with people who make him uncomfortable. Or he can elect not to appear when expected, or ever. All in all, there are a multitude of ways to go wrong. But men who take their parenting seriously seldom go to such extremes. They utilize the part-time schedule of visitation to be as caring a father as they can be. Even so, the noncustodial father has an unnatural role; he feels largely cut off from his family to the point where intermittent access to children generates rage at the mother for her ready contact and centrality in this respect.

CONFLICT ARISING FROM THE USE
OF CHILDREN AS PAWNS

Although offspring are harmed by adult machinations in divorce for ulterior purposes, this phenomenon is fairly pervasive, varying mainly in degree and style. Of course, all parents deny using such tactics.

Messengers

At the lower end of the scale of using children as pawns is their delegation to carry messages. When parents are not talking, children are often their best channel of communication. Youngsters can be charged with various missions to "the other side," such as conveying information, negotiating arrangements, or passing along a point of view. They may also be allowed to witness things that they are sure to report on their own initiative to the other camp. A child has access to each parent's home, which allows intimate glimpses into what is going on there. Thus, the child can transmit vital data to make it possible for parents to see how the breakup is working for one another, but, by the same token, a child can also be used to relay a given image through disinformation so as to mislead. This is not to say that parents put on a show for their children, but each adult definitely tries to control what children know and will report, much to the other's irritation.

Spies

Children are transformed into agents of espionage when they are pumped for data concerning the ex-mate's sexual–romantic status. Men are apt to want to know who is visiting the home to see Mom, when she goes out, and whether she speaks to a certain person on the phone. Women will question children about the person Dad is seeing and how this female interacts with him. Younger children are more susceptible to unwitting recruitment as spies, for although adolescents are much better informants, they detect and resist the parent's motives in posing such queries. Yet, even without being asked, it may suit a child to volunteer information as a means to check out one parent's reactions to the doings of the other, or for attention. All told, the negative aspects of such spying far outweigh any benefits. The child feels like a traitor to the opposite parent and, to boot, seldom wants to be too aware of a parent's sex life. However, wars of any kind cannot be waged without intelligence, and intelligence gathering is always a dirty business.

Custodians

Most women accept constant involvement with their children as inherent in the custodial role. They feel uneasy about leaving home overnight, bringing a lover into the home, or getting close to a man the youngsters do not like. Thus, most custodial mothers voluntarily accept limitations on freedom, but at the same time they are also aware that single-parent status has put them in a position where they are controlled by virtue of being a mother. A father can take advantage of this situation by refusing to take the children overnight, using his absence to make the mother stay bound to the children. He thereby makes youngsters the custodians of the custodial parent, keeping her chained to a domestic post and often soliciting reports if she falters in her duties. The mother may seethe with rage but seldom can do much about this situation.

Magnets

Parents sometimes regulate their relationship with a child to influence their relationship to the ex-spouse, using offspring to attract or repel the coparent. Thus, an outside parent may too "busy" or say "it is too painful" to see the children. Such behavior makes the custodial parent angry and leads to further estrangement. In contrast, an outside parent desirous of reconciliation will try to make up to the children in order to make up to the former partner.

A custodial parent also can use children in this fashion. The special events and developmental landmarks of offspring can be opportunities to invite the outside parent back into a reunited family circle. Or the outside parent can be extruded from the family unit so that when either an emergency or celebration occurs, h/s hears nothing about it until the event has passed. For example, a woman did not mention that a child had won a prestigious scholarship; another did not inform her ex-husband that the house had burned down and the family was living elsewhere. The message in these cases is that the outside parent, seen as being irrelevant or unhelpful, is excluded from participation in the family, even though the children will lose whatever contact they would otherwise have had. Oddly enough, this tactic can sometimes have the paradoxical effect of bringing the ex-mate closer by pushing h/h further away than is comfortable.

It may be impossible to fix accountability as to which parent is using children as magnets. An outside parent may "forget" from time to time that there are children, and a custodial parent can "forget" from time to time that children have an outside parent. To be sure, such forgetting on either side is a closeness–distance dance carefully choreographed. When the co-foe relationship is what matters, the children tend to lose significance in their own right.

Custody Suits

At the upper end of use of children as pawns, we come to custody disputes. However, not every custody suit in divorce is motivated by malice; there are instances in which children are too neglected or unhappy to be left where they are. Yet, many—perhaps most—custody litigations are fueled by a desire to injure the custodial parent by stripping the children away on grounds of "unfitness." Filing a custody suit is an act that not only disparages the custodial parent's public image, but also attacks the children's faith in that parent. Where the purpose is to humble the custodial parent, the child is exploited—not saved. The psychic damage to the youngster can be enormous. The custodial parent is under legal and moral siege, the parent–child bond is threatened, and for a period the child is placed in a contested no-man's land. At times the outside parent is even hoping to set up loss of the children to compel the custodial parent's return to the marriage, but such tactics can only backfire.

Child Kidnapping

Even the cruel aspects of a vengeful custody suit pale alongside the expedient of kidnapping a child to a site beyond knowledge or reach of the custodial parent. In such cases, hatred for the custodial parent may be too great to show compassion or play by any rules. Not counting teenage runaways, about half the missing children in the United States have been abducted by their fathers or mothers (Hyde & Hyde, 1985). Despite the fact that statistics are hard to come by because cases are not recorded by police unless there is a legal separation agreement, Abrahms (1983) has estimated that there is one child kidnapping, however brief, per 22 divorces in this country. She mentioned one egregious example in which the children were snatched six times, three by each parent. She also noted that as fathers receive more custody awards from the courts, women now tend to be the parent-turned-kidnapper about a third of the time. However, Victor and Winkler (1977), who are divorced father advocates, defended some abductions on the grounds that they were from an unfit mother whose custody rights were being protected by the court, or from a foster home or institution where offspring had been placed rather than letting them be cared for by the father.

CONCLUSION: CAN PARTING PARENTS COOPERATE?

Research has shown that parting parents can indeed cooperate where children are concerned, particularly after the first year. However, it is clear that co-foe acrimony is typical in the first year and tends to endure far beyond that in about half of divorces where children are involved. And there is good reason for this: unsavory behavior occurs as the parents reenact in conflicts over children many of the issues of their breakup. Mental health workers can accomplish little when they make parting parents feel ashamed because they are not "cooperating" with each other as they should. Rather, it must be recognized that each adult is operating within a psychological universe which, in an evolving polarization, has precipitated first marital conflict, then breakup, and ultimately acrimonious dealings in separation. Cooperation does not come from an act of will or a clinician's intervention; it flows from respective capacities of coparents to create a genuine partnership. Put plainly, *without mutual consideration, there will likely be no cooperation.*

In the final analysis, we cannot support "cooperation where children are concerned" as a noncontingent standard. We agree that it is a pro-social, useful, and generally valid rule to protect children from the fighting of their parents. But when posited as an absolute rule, regardless of context, it is assumed that the threat to the welfare of children in divorce comes from such fighting and not from the derelictions of one parent toward coparent, children, or both. Thus, such an injunction automatically favors the less committed or more problematic parent, declaring by fiat that the h/s is not to be challenged or impugned as an equally involved and effective parent. *Yet, not to challenge or impugn what amounts to "bad" parenting by one parent would itself be bad parenting by the other.* In philosophy, an "antinomy" occurs when two valid moral imperatives clash. Applying this to divorce, cooperation where children are concerned is one such imperative, but so is parental protection and emotional validation of children. In the antinomy that results from this clash of categorical values, each parting parent must find h/h own balance as the divorce unfolds.

∾ 15

The Fairy Tale Divorce for Children

[When I announced I was leaving the marriage] my husband asked how he was going to raise a [three-year-old] daughter by himself. "You'll have to pretend I died," I said. . . . [Then my daughter asked], her voice breaking, "Mama . . . when will I see you again? Will you be glad to see me?" I told her I loved her very much.

—SULLIVAN (1974, pp. 230–231)

As if reciting a memorized poem, [children] repeat what their parents said when they separated: "Parents may get divorced, but they never divorce their children." Or, "Mommy and Daddy may stop loving each other, but they always love their children." Any child who is told these lines will [both accept and doubt them] because the words don't make sense. If Mommy and Daddy can stop loving each other, they can stop loving their children. These kids have friends whose parents have divorced, and, in some cases, one of those parents took off, rarely, or never, to be heard from again. . . . It's understandable why parents say these things, even if they're not true. They are desperate to comfort their children.

—EPHRON (1986, pp. 176–177)

LOSS OF INNOCENCE

One premise of this book is that in divorce the symbiant's passions of involvement are now seen as problematic because such reactions infringe on the countersymbiant's autonomy. Similarly, the passions of children must be stifled until they too learn to "adjust" by being more accommodating and philosophic about their parents' decision to separate. To survive in today's society, youngsters are required to learn that

305

marriages do not necessarily last, that one parent can leave the household, and that their elders may take new partners who become stepparents. Further, children must not make trouble for the new relationships and must cope well with their parents' divergent life styles. Any offspring who protests too much may be viewed as "difficult" or "disturbed" and sent off to either therapy or another relative (usually the outside parent). Children of divorce get along best if, instead of hostile attitudes or self-injurious behavior, they cultivate a precocious cynicism, which has adaptive value for their circumstances—children in these families grow up faster (Weiss, 1979b). Indeed, children of divorce can frequently be recognized by their worldly wisdom, which makes their peers from intact homes appear naive in comparison.

> In an overheard telephone conversation, an astounded adult listened to two 9-year-old girls discussing a weighty problem. As one of the girls, from an intact family, was making a midnight trip to the bathroom, she had seen her father having intercourse on the living room couch with a neighbor. She could not decide whether to tell what she had seen to her father, mother, both, or neither. Her friend, whose parents were divorced, counseled confronting the father. The girl hung up and spoke to her father on the spot. She then called back and reported that her father had denied everything and insisted his daughter was terribly mistaken. The friend became angry, saying, "You have to face reality. Your father was lying. If my mother were to do that, and I saw her, she would tell me the truth." Evidently, this child of divorce could size up a marital problem too well to be subjected to the usual parental obfuscation.

> Two 13-year-old boys, both from divorced homes, shared how the departure of their fathers had hurt them. One noted that he did not even know his father was leaving for good, since he had stated he was "just going out." The other boy exclaimed, "Wow, are you a jerk!" The more sophisticated youngster considered his friend foolish for not being alert to his parents' impending breakup by not realizing that each time his father inexplicably went out the door, it could mean the dissolution of the family unit.

Ephron (1986) described her role as stepmother to two children of divorce in joint custody. One day she approached her latency-age son to tell him she was going to New York. Never looking up from his television program, he asked, "To live?" (p. 177). Ephron was shocked. Since she was only going on a brief business trip, she interpreted the boy's overreaction as a fear of abandonment. He was reflecting his experience that parents can precipitously leave, and children must not be too surprised or get too emotional about it.

In contrast to skeptical detachment, there are children who make an issue of their disapproval when parents separate. An 8-year-old girl was brought to a mental health clinic because she was so upset by her father's departure that she refused to learn in school "until Daddy comes back." Her therapist began play therapy, and she was given some paper upon which to draw whatever she liked. The young girl immediately produced a picture of a broken egg lying at the foot of a wall, remarking, "It's disgusting what they did to Humpty Dumpty!" In a family session, she was able to express such feelings to her parents. She chided them for being irresponsible: "It's fine for you to fall in love and get married. It's fine for you to have children. And it's fine for you to decide you're not in love anymore and separate. But what am I supposed to do?" This girl was not cynical, but she viewed her parents as being childishly self-centered, while expecting that she would manage like an adult.

Offspring have become almost incidental to the course of modern marriage that now exists to serve the psychic needs of adults. As Hetherington (1993) noted, "The decision to divorce is usually made on the basis of the possibility of improving the life situation of parents, in many cases with little or no consideration for the concerns of the child. . . . Adults whose parents divorced when they were children, unlike those from intact families, report that childhood was the most unhappy time in their lives" (p. 222). When parents part, children are soon caught between the demands of their elders for readjustment and their own internal reactions to loss. Although divorce is nearly always unwelcome to children and costs them dearly in many respects, they need time to work out whether it is more congenial in their circumstances to be bitter or blasé.

HOW TO MAKE THE CHILD PERCEIVE THE BEAUTIFUL RAIMENT OF DIVORCE

The rationale of the "good" divorce for children is that they will benefit later on, after parents have taken care of themselves so that they can be better parents. To many children, this is an adult-imposed myth, on the order of the tale of the emperor's new clothes. Although the divorcing parents may be naked, a child will often be admonished not to perceive things this way.

Enter "progressive" ideology. It is now presumed that there is nothing to fear—parental cooperation and, especially, joint custody are regarded as measures that can shortly immunize children against the potential pathology of a family rift. In addition, much of the current literature proclaims that edification, reassurances, and sensitive management will help a child transition through divorce with minimal traumatization, soon thereafter to be well adjusted.

To more closely examine this approach as to how children can be disposed to take divorce in stride, let us start with the work of Gettleman and Markowitz (1974). They concluded that divorce is a bad experience for both adults and offspring because it has a bad name! Instead of the family breakup per se, Gettleman and Markowitz blamed cultural bias against divorce as the factor that causes traumatic reactions in youngsters. Disputing research data that showed that children from "broken homes" are prone to psychopathology, they insisted that these data both reflect and foster "anti-divorce indoctrination." Because children are unprepared for the possibility that their parents may separate, those who find themselves in that situation readily think they were deceived and dealt a low blow. Gettleman and Markowitz proposed to take the shock out of divorce by urging that children be disabused early on of the illusion that marriage is forever. Thus, if breakup occurs, such enlightenment will render it a less dismaying prospect. It seems that these authors believed that parents should sit a young child down and introduce the concept of divorce analogous to the way that the "the birds and the bees" commences sex education: "Honey, do you know what divorce is? If we should split up, would you rather live with Mommy, or Daddy, or take turns?" They go on to say:

> If divorce is handled maturely by parents, their children can experience it as a relatively non-traumatic event: as adults they may then be able to accept *with equanimity* [italics ours] its possible occurrence in their own lives. . . . Children of divorce have a unique opportunity to experience a variety of family styles, including the one-parent and the multi-marriage family. Exposure to new adults . . . can enrich children's lives by providing them with a chance to break away from *excessive dependency on their biological parents.* (pp. 86–87, italics added)

Gettleman and Markowitz are mental health professionals who viewed children as small adults who can rise above developmental needs ("excessive dependency on their biological parents") and adapt to any change, with the proviso that parents handle their separation "maturely" so that everything is suitably explicated beforehand. They are right when they state that a child will make some type of accommodation to the new family constellation, and they are right too when they argue that the dissolution of the nuclear family unit is not always the unmitigated catastrophe the child may initially apprehend. But they go too far: it is hardly a worthy or workable ideal for anyone to accept divorce "with equanimity," and it staggers the imagination to read a serious suggestion that the child's sorrow is not caused by loss but is the result of a public relations campaign against divorce. As Wheeler (1980) commented, "In their effort to point out the silver lining, Gettleman and Markowitz seem to have ignored the cloud" (p. 92).

Taking the trend represented by Gettleman and Markowitz a step further, a vast array of books now detail how parting parents can manage their children's feelings, assuaging much of their pain by timely interventions. Some of these books are by expert clinicians (e.g., Everett & Everett, 1994); others are in the pop psychology genre (Richards & Willis, 1977; Turow, 1978; Spilke, 1979). At whatever level, the common theme is that divorce must be carefully explained to children and their emotions handled with tact and comfort. Thus, the texts consist of practical advice conveyed to both parents and children on coping with situations that regularly come up. For instance, it is recommended that children be informed directly by parents of the decision to separate, with oft-repeated pledges that each adult will continue to love them as before. Or, when the custodial mother invites a date over for dinner but her children are less than enthusiastic about her new friend, they need to hear that no man will ever take their father's place. Or it is put to youngsters that should they prefer living with Dad but are afraid to ask for fear of causing Mom apoplexy, they might phrase their wish as an "experiment," avoiding unflattering comparisons.

Nevertheless, it is clear that when diplomacy is so sensitive, the reality can only be that much cannot be said, because at least one parent cannot tolerate the child's feelings. Thus, instructions that are intended to ease readjustment may represent cosmetic soothing just when it is important to get issues out into the open. In the preceding examples, it is unlikely that the outgoing parent will be involved with the child as before; it can indeed be that Mom's new "friend" is usurping Dad's role in the family; and it is all but inconceivable that mother will graciously accept the idea that her child prefers to live with father. Moreover, although how-to manuals humanely attempt to reduce the troubles of children, at the same time they intimate that divorce could be made almost easy if only parents were skilled in spotting and preventing trouble. Once again, the devil–divorce is denied its due: a child can be rescued from the stresses of breakup, given the "right" social engineering (such as joint custody), the "right" cultural attitude (no anti-divorce indoctrination), and now the "right" verbal interventions.

And the "right" children's literature—Westoff (1977) held that youngsters could deal with divorce better if bedtime stories were refashioned. She called for a new image of divorce in their books, lauding the ingenuity of a baby-sitter who sent her charges from a multimarriage family to bed with this modified fairy tale: "Once upon a time there were three bears. There was the Papa bear, the Mama bear, and there was the little bear from an earlier marriage" (p. 70).

But Westoff forgets that animal counterparts of stepchildren seldom survive in the wild. Such absurdity may be amusing at first, but youngsters cannot be inured to an upsetting and implausible reality in this manner.

The "right" public relations attitude must also be inculcated in respect to stepfamilies. Visher and Visher (1993) saw the use of bland synonyms such as the "reconstituted," "blended," or "remarriage" family as ways to counter ancient stereotypes about living with a "the wicked stepmother." They awaited the waning of "the influence of old fairy tales, the negative bias toward divorce and remarriage, and the idealization of the nuclear family, so that marriages other than first marriages will be accepted as positive, albeit challenging, life cycle stages" (p. 236). We do not doubt the value of stepfamilies, but children of divorce often enter such situations with ambivalent or even very negative emotions, so that it is a new fairy tale to depict the transition as just a "positive . . . life cycle stage."

All told, "progressive" thinking seems to assume that youngsters are sufficiently rational, malleable, and resourceful to be fitted into almost any family structure, largely ignoring developmental limitations. Not only is a youngster greatly affected by a parental separation, but more important, the child's faith in the parents—the foundation of h/h emotional life—is also affected. Hence, a child's feelings cannot be sufficiently controlled by cognitive manipulations so as to pass through divorce more or less unscathed.

MORE ON WHY THE CHILD CANNOT BE DIVORCED FROM THE DIVORCE

By their being, children are symbols of the love that connects parents. Just as love for the mate produced the child, love for the child encompasses love for the partner with whom the child was procreated. From the parent's point of view, the child is not quite an independent entity, but "flesh of our flesh and blood of our blood." Although the child is a separate person, feelings for the child and coparent tend to merge together in a family symbiosis.

Indeed, symbiosis makes a family more than the sum of its members. Youngsters draw crucial aspects of their identity from parents, and progeny are seen as extensions of the parents into posterity. For each generation, such identifications are entailed in normal human development. But when a marriage ends in acrimony, loving the mate through the child soon becomes problematic. Tender feelings remain for the partner of the time the child was conceived and raised, but the estranged coparent of "now" may be seen as the destroyer of the mate of "then." Once the coparent is deemed to betray the dreams one had in creating the child, the reciprocal is suspect as a parent (biological claims aside) since h/s may fail the child much as h/s failed the mate. In short, fair or unfair, a "bad" mate can readily become characterized as a "bad" parent too.

Taking the process another step, how the coparent treats the child greatly affects the relationship between two estranged mates. When h/s is nurturing to the child, a tone is set for affection, and even rapprochement, despite separation. Conversely, when h/s is neglectful or abusive, the bonds between parents are suspended and a tone is set for militancy in defense of the child. In sum, how the child is treated becomes a litmus test for the quality of relationship possible with the ex-mate. Behavior in this regard speaks louder than any words, financial transactions, or legal claims. Love or hate for the child (an extension of "me") is love or hate for me.

At the next step, an adverse relationship to the coparent can also affect the relationship to the child. If the child seems to defend a hated coparent, then the child too begins to elicit the same negative associations and is soon regarded as a reprehensible "chip off the old block." Having the character traits of the co-parent may also lead to a child's being lumped in as "just like h/h Dad (or Mom)," as well as factors such as physical resemblance the child cannot control. Sadly, it is possible to come to hate the mate-in-the-child and, therefore, the child. In divorce, relating to a child without contamination from conscious or unconscious resentment held toward a coparent must stand as a necessary goal, but it is one that in bitter breakups is often inconsistently realized.

Moreover, in bitter breakups, children caught in a cross fire are not equally liable to harm. Youngsters are not just pawns of parents, they are also active agents who after separation seek to sway events in accord with personal needs to structure the family unit they want to have. Different children may agitate in favor of different needs, depending on such factors as preference for one or the other parent, concern about protecting the more vulnerable of their elders, or practical issues such as their own schooling, housing, and economic support. Thus, of their own volition they may choose a side, and the side chosen is fateful for them. In our clinical experience, we have noticed that the child who identifies with the outside parent is generally more at risk of psychological disturbance than siblings. We have coined the term *proxy child* to describe a youngster who defends the behavior and reputation of the outside parent, communicates with and represents h/h interests in absentia, and even adopts some of the outside parent's attitudes toward life in general and toward the home parent in particular. Moreover, the proxy child tends to accept, cooperate with, and even like the outside parent's new mate and, thus, in the situation of a triangle, breaches the "defilement taboo." The proxy child will then be quickly told by the home parent that h/s acts too much like the outside parent by being ungrateful and opportunistic. In brief, the proxy child cannot avoid—or even invites—the home parent's displaced anger, which really belongs to the ex-partner. In fights with the home parent the youngster may threaten to run away to the outside parent, or may be taunted to do so if things are so much better "over there." If the proxy child actually does want to leave, h/s will not always be offered sanctuary by the outside parent, or may be sent back shortly if any problems develop. In contrast, siblings who side with the home parent may incur the displeasure of the outside parent, but the latter has less leverage to inflict damage.

All mental health authorities agree that what reproduction has joined together, divorce cannot and should not put asunder—the family symbiosis continues after divorce. One consequence is that children cannot be exempted from tensions between parents just because the adults have now separated. Despert (1953) pointed out many years ago that children are harmed by parental conflict, even when this conflict is hidden in an "empty shell" marriage. If Despert is right in the context of marriage, her principle applies equally well to divorce. Conflict here is unmistakable in view of de facto separation, even if parents cooperate. The child cannot really stand outside the divorce, to be treated as an "innocent bystander" rather than as a participant in the family drama. Nor can the child be shielded from separation strife by being expressly accorded neutral status by combatant parents, for two reasons. First, even when coparents strive to keep children out of the strife, this status will not always be accepted as truly impartial, particularly if a child's support is deemed essential by one parent. Second, as modern history teaches, neutral territory is not long respected if it lies athwart a powerful belligerent's urgent axis of advance.

THE CHILD'S IDENTIFICATIONS
WITH WARRING PARENTS

Tessman (1978) described how the child's personality is formed through a series of identifications, the most significant of which are with parental figures. However, after breakup identifications become conflicted—the child may even be pressured by one parent to disavow psychic bonds to the other. This is particularly true when the outside parent gets a stigmatizing label from the home parent, such as "mental patient," "alcoholic," "homosexual," "womanizer," "whore," and so on, which then "explains" why the child is largely cut off from this parent's company. (What Tessman doesn't say is that the absent parent can utilize a similar explanation to justify why h/s had to leave.) Explicitly or implicitly, a child may be encouraged to regard divorce as the fault of that "bad" adult—with salvation represented by this "good" adult.

Tessman traced how the child is inevitably thrust into intolerable loyalty choices between contending parents. Internally, the loyalty conflicts are translated into disorganization and self-hatred. The child's need for security rests on having strong parents, and the child strives to preserve this confidence in both caretakers. If either parent is criticized, that parent's alleged moral shortcomings bid fair to be understood by the child as a reflection not of adult "badness," but of the child's own "badness." Tessman showed that a young child is peculiarly susceptible to the fantasy that if h/s had been a better person, the absent parent would not have left. Such guilt feelings can persist, even when the departing parent insists that the child is not responsible for the breakup.

Tessman held that a child of divorce needs both parents, not only as sources of love and security, but as resources for building an integrated self-concept. Only through continuous contact with both elders can the child determine who the parents really are, acknowledge them for what they have contributed, learn from their failures, and slowly start to differentiate from them. If, however, one of the parents takes on an onus as "no good," then a derivative part of the child is shamefully felt to be "no good." Tessman therefore opposed any stigmatizing bans on contact with the other parent as destructively divisive, engendering psychic fission in the mind of the child to match the parental fission in reality.

Tessman went further than Despert in that she did not see rights of access as nearly enough to save the child of divorce from psychopathology. She wanted the divorcing couple to take care not to tarnish the image of the coparent in the child's eyes. Here, it seems to us, her policy contradicted her theory. She had argued through her psycho-analytic study of identifications that you can take the child out of the nuclear family, but you cannot take the nuclear family out of the child. The child is so enmeshed with h/h parents as to make divorce an inherent trauma: one or both parents must be "bad" if they do not love each other, or the child must be "bad." Tessman sought to counter childish logic by insisting that parents not only demonstrate that they did not divorce the child, but also that they never criticize each other to the child. As we know, the "no vilification" rule is valid to a point, but divorce cannot be totally sanitized by outward parental adherence to a well-meaning principle, as if a youngster were not exquisitely tuned into h/h family dynamics through innate identifications. A child's rent in self-esteem is not brought about solely by one parent's derogation that blemishes the other parent's "image"; rather, a fission in the psyche of the child cannot be avoided, because there is an undeniable fission in the family. Moreover, the child has needs to reality test h/h family situation and in many instances is encountering problems with the same type of behavior in a parent that contributed to, or even caused, the divorce. In trying to maintain an unsullied image of the other parent for the child, the coparent must thus withhold validation of the child's personal experience—an empathic failure that can be more harmful than confirming what the child has probably already surmised.

In summary of Tessman's work, she devoted her clinical talents to enable the child of divorce to believe that parents are gods who have not failed. But our understanding of the situation is to the contrary: the vision of many children of divorce is that parents are gods who have indeed failed (the route to cynicism) or gods whose children have failed (the route to emotional disturbance).

SYMPTOMS OF EMOTIONAL DISTURBANCE IN A CHILD OF DIVORCE

The most potent arsenal at the disposal of children, when they feel their security has been menaced by the fact and conduct of a parental breakup, is symptomatic behavior. Oppawsky (1991) observed the following pervasive behavior patterns in children that seemed to be divorce-specific: denunciation and emotional distancing from parents, a secret or open wish for reunification of the family, a fall in academic grades, and the seeking of solace from peers with similar experiences. In addition to such quasi-universal reactions, Oppawsky noted that some children develop maladjustment—for example, they become un-manageable at home, act out with drugs or sex, engage in delinquency, or develop psychiatric disorders. When symptoms of behavioral disorder occur, they serve notice that the child cannot function under current conditions—family upheaval has done such damage that desperate, often masochistic acts are a last resort.

When disturbed behavior occurs as a reaction to a parental breakup, no coping skills exist that would give the child channel for protest and compensation other than the development of symptoms. Such symptoms include the following primary dynamics: to mourn an absent parent, to express anger at the breakup of the two-parent home, to turn anger at parents onto self so as to preserve idealization, and to expiate guilt for somehow having driven the parents apart. As for secondary gain, such symptoms include conscious or unconscious manipulation of parents—specifically, to get solicitous attention from adults who seem caught up in their own needs, to punish by inducing guilt, to create pressure for reunion of the family, and/or to set up possible removal from a noxious environment.

The child who must resort to symptoms in order to remonstrate against h/h situation is waging a losing battle. The guilt that both parents eschew (and assign to the other by way of blame) usually winds up in the child's lap. In the triangle father–mother–child, only the latter is ready, through love and need, to accept blame for the family breakup. With their limited cognitive capacity, younger children in particular tend to maintain crucial identifications with both parents by taking responsibility for their failings, as well as giving and getting punishment via symptom formation (Jacobson & Jacobson, 1987). There is also the desperation factor: because the child's basic developmental needs are at stake, something drastic must be done to compel change. In many of these cases, it is only a symptomatic child's dysfunction that brings parents into contact around common concern for h/h welfare. But the parents' reaction is often not exactly what the child might have hoped, inasmuch as h/h woes are a symbolic comment on deprivations the parental breakup has imposed, and this is a truth that adults may not be able to stand hearing. Parents may therefore negate the child's communication by regarding the youngster as "disturbed" and sending h/h off for treatment. For such parents, the problem is seen as *in* the child—not in what is happening *to* the child.

PSYCHOTHERAPY: TREATING THE CHILD
TO SAVE THE DIVORCE

To make divorce nontraumatic, the child needs the "right" therapy too. Of course an emotionally disturbed child requires treatment. But to focus only on the condition of the child is apt to miss its meaning. Without ever making etiological connections, parents may want their child's impairment remedied by means of therapeutic intervention: the child must adjust so that the divorce carries on. And the child too has motives not to explore beyond the mechanics of symptom relief. Whatever the diagnosis, the child's need is to protect parents from h/h own anger, deflecting such anger onto self through "bad" actions so that h/h parents are not "bad." Thus, in the midst of separation strife, the tendency of the symptomatic child to be a voluntary scapegoat interlocks with the tendency on the part of parents not to want to catch on to the symptom-message that represents a living rebuke to them.

In a case example (Beilin & Izen, 1991), a 10-year-old girl became unable to walk, to speak in a voice louder than a whisper, or to attend school; no physiological basis was found for these symptoms. At the time, the parents were locked in divorce acrimony, but with the advent of the girl's symptoms, the father brought a suit for custody, in effect blaming the mother. The mother hired an attorney to contest the suit, blaming the father for the plight of their daughter. On referral from the school, a social work agency threatened to place the child in foster care and also arranged for divorce mediation. After treatment, the custody dispute ended; the girl's condition improved and within 4 months she was singing in the school choir. The clinicians involved said that it took a major decompensation on her part to make parents and school recognize that she was not adjusting to divorce and needed "to maintain the family as a fantasized, internalized whole" (p. 309).

Tessman (1978, pp. 171–174) presented the case of 4-year-old Sean, who came to treatment because he had suddenly lost his sunny disposition and said, "I wish I were blind." His parents had recently separated. Several days before, Sean had witnessed his father crying when, during an unexpected visit, the man came upon the boy's mother and "uncle" together (this uncle was really the mother's lover). What is a therapist to make of the situation? On one hand, the child is unconsciously wishing to control his parents' lives through a masochistic wish to give up his vision. But is his mother to have no male companionship after breakup, or his father to stop being jealous, or the parents to reconcile to save Sean's "sight"? No child can be allowed to be this powerful. On the other hand, the boy cannot bear what he beholds. His symptom is the device he uses to force the parents to consider his needs. Although the child's needs are influenced by his father's wish to have his estranged wife's fidelity and his mother's wish to have her ex-husband accept the breakup, the boy still must have an emotionally intact father and a mother whose attention is not diverted away. As Tessman also noted, Sean did not want to see that his father was the excluded, injured party in the family unit, so instead he presented himself as deserving to be the injured one.

Young Sean was exhibiting a "depressive equivalent"—the boy wanted to be bereft of vision not only to protect his parents from his own criticisms, but also to turn the reason for his upset into a physical problem. But his wish for a psychosomatic disability expressed a sorrowful accusation without words. He was damning his mother for putting his father out, and damning his father for making it painful to live with his mother if she was with someone else. Enough of what the boy was feeling was grasped to have him rushed to the nearest therapist to be "adjusted," thereby silencing the symptom. And Tessman did her job well; she worked with Sean for 2 years to help him overcome his grief at his parents' divorce. Her approach was to show the boy that he was needlessly afraid his mother would leave him as his father had, that he need not punish himself for being happy with mother and "uncle" while the father was unhappy, and that he was a lovable child. Through treatment, Sean learned that neither mother nor father had abandoned him, that their separation could not be undone no matter what he did, and that his parents (certainly his mother) had to have this divorce. The boy eventually accommodated to a binuclear family. His symptoms disappeared, and he got along well with his mother's new partner and, later on, his father's new mate as well. With his problems resolved, nobody any longer had to see what the "blind" boy saw.

In another case of a child who saw too much, an 8-year-old boy came upon his mother in a compromising position with a male neighbor and told his father. The father promptly walked out on the marriage, taking his son with him. He began divorce proceedings, meanwhile denying the mother any rights of access. When finally worked out, the divorce decree stipulated that the father would retain custody and granted the mother weekly visitation. But the father still refused the mother access, and she was obliged to go back to court for an order allowing her to be in the company of her son. It was almost 2 years after initial separation before mother and son at last made contact, and then only for half an hour, supervised by father. The ex-couple could hardly look at each other and spoke in icy, hateful tones. The same sort of scene was repeated at every visitation over the next several years, with the mother coming less and less often. The boy, who had inadvertently started all this by reporting an observed sexual event, developed in adolescence a voyeuristic problem, constantly peeping in at the sexual activities of his father. But no amount of replay of his original "crime" (this time perpetrated against his father) could overcome his inner conviction that he was responsible for the divorce of his parents and his mother's subsequent outcasting from the family. At age 21, he became so disorganized in his thinking as to need a psychiatric admission. His hospital therapist was at length able to arrange a meeting with the long-estranged parents. When they arrived, each contended that the earlier history had nothing to do with their son's current illness. Their reason for coming was to learn whether there was any medication that might correct his disorder.

Although psychopathology is multidetermined and frequently of uncertain etiology, we interpret the symptoms of the youngsters in the preceding three cases as related to the breakup of the family unit. An "emotionally disturbed" child from a divorced family seemed to be ambivalently dealing with a *forbidden perception* that could not be integrated with love and dependence on both parents, nor were the parents able to abide what the child perceived. Simon (1964) has noted the singular clarity with which a child may express h/h actual losses and emotional needs in divorce, rashly exclaiming that the emperor has no clothes, in contrast to the egocentricity and defensiveness of the parting parents: "The child sees what adults don't want to see, that a man can have a new wife, a woman a new husband, but that he, the child, cannot have a new parent. There is no such thing as an ex-mother or an ex-father" (p. 132).

Parents who are being held accountable by a child will often go to astonishing lengths not to hear what the child has to say. For example, when the child states negative feelings about one parent to the other, Beilin and Izen (1991) showed how that offended parent, when told by the other, gives several possible explanations to disqualify the meaning of the statement: (1) the child is afraid of telling you the truth—but not me; (2) the child is manipulating us, playing both ends against the middle; and (3) you—the other parent—are lying and being manipulative yourself. Beilin and Izen then pointed to the clinical consequences of such invalidation for a boy they had treated. The youngster dealt with what each parent wanted to hear by dissociative compartmentalizing:

> For as long as this boy could remember, his parents, step-parents, and other powerful adults (including the psychologists, mediator, and attorneys) who spoke to him about himself could be satisfied by his recounting one or another set of feelings and thoughts. His clue as to which to present was which parent introduced the adult into his life. This was a matter of holding two discrete realities, and surviving by experiencing and telling one at a time. (p. 311)

Over and above the usual stresses in divorce for children, when parents and society are also invalidating the forbidden perceptions and communications of children, it is not surprising that psychiatric disorders proliferate. All experts concur that an undue ratio of clients in child guidance clinics are from homes in which one parent has left (Young & Ruth, 1984; Wallerstein, 1984a). Thus, many desperate custodial parents are bringing their offspring to therapists for discipline, motivation, companionship, and love. In effect, the child's worker becomes a surrogate for an absent or a beleaguered parent. A colleague told us of her dismay when she realized that her duties at a family agency consisted of relieving pressure on custodial parents who could or would not parent and who saw their function as making sure that their troubled child got to a professional for nurture unavailable at home. It is dangerous to draw inferences about the general population from the sample of behavior seen at a mental health facility, but it is equally dangerous not to draw inferences from what disproportionate numbers of divorced parents and their children are showing us by filling up caseloads at our family clinics. As Maslow (1971) noted about such raw data, "Facts often point in a direction, i.e., they are vectorial. Facts . . . don't just lie there like pancakes, just doing nothing; they are to a certain extent signposts which tell you what to do. . . . [They] have demand character" (p. 27).

THE "THERAPEUTIC SOCIETY"

The progressive movement champions shifts in divorce mores such as a "Why can't they be civilized?" approach, pathologizing of jealousy, rights of access, joint custody, and preparing children for family breakup by changing their literature. As the ultimate fail-safe, psychotherapy will assist recalcitrant cases to recover from badly handled separations. But all this is not enough, for there are still calls to refashion the culture itself, so that in the "right" society, divorce is accepted "with equanimity."

In this respect, Tessman (1978) is a representative advocate of how society must be revamped in order to make divorce nontraumatic for adults and children alike. As a child psychologist who has treated many children of divorce, Tessman declared that she was neither for nor against divorce. But her view was that "in almost all cases seen, the particular divorce was a step in the right direction for the individuals involved, although it caused pain and did not in itself solve the problems in their lives" (1978, p. viii). She regarded herself more or less as a technician who tried to correct the problems that sadly beset children as a by-product of parental conflict in breakup. Her role was not that of a culture critic.

But in fact Tessman *was* a culture-critic. In a discussion of the indispensable nature of support networks for parting parents, she took note of a major problem in social reactions to divorce:

> The most extreme cases of "social shunning" . . . are those in which a woman has lost custody of her children, or has decided . . . to leave her home and children. This kind of shunning . . . has an aura of the dread of contact within it. It is not clear whether the avoidance by . . . previous friends revolves around a fear of contagion; i.e., that at moments they, too, might be tempted to leave their children, or arises from unresolved feelings over their own childhood dread of abandonment, which makes them feel ambivalent toward any parent who would carry out this act. In effect, this type of shunning creates a rent in the . . . support network which opens the way for a disastrous fall in self-esteem for the parent. (p. 39)

Tessman wanted the self-esteem of a mother who gives up her children protected, as if this act were as respectable as any other. She does not accept that society, in the persons of the "previous friends," deliberately inflicts a rent in self-esteem to a mother who does not mother—that is, by shunning her, the social order affirms the inviolability of the mother–child bond. Tessman went so far as to suggest that the disapproving reactions were not only heartless, but neurotic in origin. But if society upholds a certain moral value, then certain behaviors become prohibited and people who commit these behaviors are punished, stigmatized, or ostracized in order that society safeguard its observance of that value. A society with values is not a universal therapeutic agency that wishes well even to those who violate its norms. Of course, there is an injustice in the fact that a mother is shunned for an action for which a father might encounter, at most, mild disapproval, but this unfairness also reflects society's viewpoint that the mother–child bond is more significant than the father–child bond.

Tessman wanted a "therapeutic society" in which everybody acts along therapeutic lines, forebearing to pass moral judgment. *Tout comprendre c'est tout pardonner.* Her point was that there is so much pain in divorce that society must be supportive, almost no matter what was done. Despite being a clinician ministering to the youthful casualties of divorce, she never protested on behalf of children the cultural ambience in which she operates and is sorely needed. In short, clinicians like Tessman bring up the therapeutic rear in the adjustment of the child of divorce—an army doctor tending to the wounded without uttering a word about the horror of war.

CONCLUSION: NEW HYPOCRISY TO REPLACE OLD

Jacobson and Jacobson (1987) noted that many children of divorce suffer "time lost," but there is no consensus within the divorce therapy field as to the cause of the problem. We have come to the conclusion that the child of divorce generally sustains a twofold injury: one from loss of the intact family unit (the traditional view) and another from how separation is handled (the progressive view). Yet, true to the American credo that anything can be fixed, our culture counts on technology, formulas, and reassurances to save children from harm by divorce. For divorce we shall have! Bernard (1971) depicted the current public attitude as favorable toward divorce, even when children are involved: "The whole trend in current social life is in the direction of *laissez faire* in personal relationships. . . . The idea of forcing people to remain together is repugnant to the present world view" (p. 25). In agreement, but putting a very different spin on this trend, Francke (1983) pointed out that "now divorce is so common that its very normality may have anesthetized us to our children's pain" (p. 23). Epstein (1974) too was concerned that adults are no longer abjured to love each other as best they can, among other reasons "for the sake of the kids"; instead, if they are unhappy, they are urged to head out the door as quickly as possible. He noted that we are now even assured that children will emerge from a divorce/remarriage scenario all the stronger for it, quoting a psychiatrist who said, "I've discovered that people who grow up in these situations cope better with the ambiguities of life" (p. 256). If this psychiatrist is correct, divorce is needed to shape up a youngster! Epstein then assailed the modern view that divorce frees adults and children trapped in a "bad" family system from unnecessary misery:

> What a country America is! Where else does one find optimism running so rampant? To speak of divorce in terms of success at all, let alone as being creative, accruing to the benefit of all involved, is optimism running right down the road to madness. Society . . . does not, strictly speaking, actually punish a divorcing couple. They can usually be relied on to punish each other sufficiently . . . to make any form of state or social punishment seem superfluous. One might learn something . . . from having gone through a divorce, but it is finally a defeat which cannot be turned into a victory. However urgent it might be that a husband and wife break up their marriage, few divorces can be claimed successful and none where young children are involved. (p. 256)

As we see it, breezy progressive cant matches the foregoing hypocrisy of the traditional era, but common sense should tell us that neither extreme can be optimal for children. At least let us acknowledge that unloving parents will cause problems for their offspring. Neither staying in or disbanding a marriage solves this dilemma, and it is a new hypocrisy to think otherwise. Elkin (1994) contrasted the vanishing but still revered "modern nuclear family" with its successor, the "postmodern permeable family" that now mirrors the openness, complexity, and diversity of contemporary society. Nuclear families were meant to be a haven—sacrifices were expected on behalf of the unit. However, the weakness of that system was the relegation of women to a domestic role and its idealization of a rather narrow life style. As for the postmodern permeable family, each member "is empowered to place his or her needs for self-realization and self-fulfill-ment before the needs of the family as a unit" (p. 63). Although relieving parents from the constraints of the nuclear family, as well as giving children an opportunity to develop new competencies, its weakness is that youngsters may be overwhelmed by new demands for autonomy and self-reliance, shifting much of the responsibility for their care from family and society to themselves. Elkin viewed both nuclear and permeable families as unbalanced systems; he urged that society do much more for children by way of programs to make up the imbalance.

Although we certainly agree that America should do more for its children—for example, more accessible day care, more flexible work hours for parents—we wonder whether Elkin's recommendation will be honored. After all, what can be hoped for from a society that does not love children enough to spare them from fairy tale divorce?

❧ V

Resolution of the Breakup: Letting Go versus Reconciling

Introduction

Uncoupling is not a compelling journey that, once embarked
upon, allows no turning back. Granted . . . each phase closes yet
another door. Yet the process may be interrupted at any point.
Even after separation or divorce, a couple may reconcile. . . .
[But] reconciliation is not simply a return to what used to be. It
is yet another transition, with its own costs [and] sometimes . . .
turns out to be temporary.
—VAUGHAN (1986, pp. 184–185)

One frequently hears after breakup that someone "should be over it
by now," as if letting go had a set time line. Yet no one agrees on how
long it should take, except that it usually seems to take too long. There
may even be insinuations that characterological weakness is the problem, as if letting go were accomplished by will power.

But letting go is seldom a linear disengagement over time; it is
rather a sine curve with a downward trend. The vicissitudes occur
because resistance to letting go reflects an internal ambivalence caused
by lingering attachment to the ex-mate versus what has been learned
about the flaws of this person. Moreover, every separation has an
experimental aspect. It is unclear for a time whether both parties will
finally agree to part, or whether the idea of reunion carried by one can
at last win over the other.

Letting go runs its course during the process of breakup and has
a normal progression that each person accomplishes at h/h own pace.
The sequential stages described in Chapter 16 allow ex-mates to
measure their personal standing within the letting-go continuum,
anticipate future directions, and endure backsliding. If letting go can
be worked through, the two parties can move on to a new relationship

without remaining unduly bound to the dead letter of the past marriage. But although letting go is essential in order to achieve truly independent lives, paradoxical as it seems, it is equally essential for setting a stage for successful reunion.

This paradox is explained in Chapter 17, where reconciliation is considered as an alternative to final parting of the ways. Most breakups include reconciliations, but some commentators have been so struck by the regularity with which getting back together fails as to declare that reconciliations don't work. But some do work. Why these and not others? And is it worth the work?

We will argue that many second-chance unions are doomed to failure because they are born of desperation, not aspiration. Thus, rather than being based on a new-found appreciation of the old partner, they tend to be entered into as respites from the strains of separation. The countersymbiant typically goes back only after discovering that breakup was inopportune for some unforeseen reason, and the symbiant typically takes back a tarnished lover to soothe wounded pride as well as to resume h/h unfinished project of caretaking and reforming. In neither case is the motivation love for a real partner, and the reunion is likely to collapse, in the end falling victim to the same old problems and, with another breakup, the same old solution. Hence, those reunions that are successful must be dialectically preceded by letting go so that reunion is based on a fresh look at a somewhat different partner rather than on a return to prior interpersonal patterns.

∾ 16

Love's Labor Lost
Letting Go

[A Zen Problem]
To think I am not going
To think of you anymore
Is still thinking of you.
Let me then try not to think
That I am not going to think of you.
　　　　　—WATZLAWICK (1976, p. 15)

EASIER SAID THAN DONE

This culture fosters the expectation that it is possible to overcome any lingering attachment and regain essentially undamaged ego-functioning soon after a relationship is over. Some practitioners in the mental health field have even offered assurances that detachment can be relatively swift and uncomplicated if the proper attitude or technique is cultivated—the title of Wanderer and Cabot's (1978) *Letting Go: A Twelve Week Personal Action Program to Overcome a Broken Heart* speaks for itself. Nevertheless, unwavering acceptance of the end of a love relationship usually entails much more time. Trafford (1992) estimated a duration of at least one turbulent year after breakup. She called this period "crazy time" but regarded unusual behavior as a normal response to separation.

Disengagement is obviously a problem for symbiants (Baumeister & Wotman, 1992; Tennov, 1979). However, ambivalent enmeshment can also be discerned in countersymbiants; as Kitson (1992) observed, "It is often hard for a divorcing individual to understand that he or she can simultaneously be glad to be out of a relationship and yet still

327

feel tugs back to that person. . . . In fact, the dislocations of the divorce can disconcertingly make [one] want the old familiar partner back to assuage the distress" (p. 347). Nostalgia for the former relationship was evident in both partners in a longitudinal study of postdivorce adjustment by Hetherington, Cox, and Cox (1976). After 2 months of separation, 17% of husbands helped with home repairs, 8% baby-sat while their ex-wives went out on a date, and 13% of the couples had sexual intercourse. About two-thirds said the estranged spouse was the first person they would contact in a personal crisis and that breakup was either a mistake or they should have tried harder to resolve their differences. Two years later, these signs of continued attachment had declined, although about a quarter of this sample still expressed regret about the breakup. Framo (1978) commented on the shock of attorneys when they discover that, in the midst of a legal battle, their clients are having sex. Francke (1983) cited data that 16% of hostile couples still had intercourse after breakup, but a similar rate of sexual contact also occurred in a less combative sample of couples 12–18 months after breakup. Gray, Koopman, and Hunt (1991) found that the most significant variable in letting go was length of time elapsed since separation; although the active agent in the breakup had a less intense grief reaction than the resistant mate, they reached equal disengagement in about 5 years. Kahn (1990) stated that many of her female clients were still emotionally tied to their ex-husbands years after breakup by "the bondage of caring" or "the bondage of bitterness." Weiss (1979b) noted a universal persistence of bonds, but Spanier and Casto (1979) saw this in "only" 70% of separations.

Neither separation nor legal divorce is tantamount to letting go; such external facts cannot impose affective detachment. Differentiating between "psychic" and "legal" divorce, Kressel and Deutsch (1977) observed that litigants who have not yet achieved emotional separation utilize the legal settlement for romantic–passionate purposes; they seem more enmeshed with each other during divorce proceedings than they ever were in marriage. These authors concluded that no matter where a couple stands legally, only after both sides have faced up to breakup can psychic divorce occur.

In short, however much roles and personalities differ, spouses in breakup must muster resources to deal with the new reality that they are now on their own—two individuals alone in this world. To survive, each must adopt Sartre's (1943/1977) existential dictum, "I am the project of the recovery of my being" (p. 340). Putting this in psychological terms, Vaughan (1986) considered that "uncoupling" was complete only when "the participants define themselves and are defined by others as separate and independent of each other—when being partners is no longer a major source of their identity" (p. 173). Each party in the dismantlement of a committed union has to do the work of letting go *autonomously*, without assistance from the reciprocal and sometimes over the vehement protests, enticements, or manipulations of the ex. The reciprocal can certainly make letting go easier or harder, but it is ultimately one's own psychic task, an accomplishment that is not contingent upon the other's reactions or availability. Once former spouses have reached a point where they can write *finis* to their relationship, two things can happen: they can pursue independent lives, or they can proceed to a serious reconciliation. This latter outcome will seem strange in that disengagement does not logically lead to recommitment; but we will detail in the next chapter how and why this surprising end result can ever occur. However, the usual course of letting go is toward increasing alienation and definitive breakup, and this is the topic of the present chapter.

STAGES IN LETTING GO

Breakup is best conceptualized as a process rather than a discrete life event (Pledge, 1992); thus, various models have been proposed in the professional literature that describe phases in readjustment following divorce. Weiss (1975) posited a two-step process for both parties—transition and recovery. Gray, Koopman, and Hunt (1991) described three phases; an initial urge to recover the lost object, disorganization, and reorganization. But Wise (1980) cautioned that ambivalence can cause fixation along the way.

Among clinicians, a grief-based model has been popular. An analogy is drawn between object loss in divorce and accommodation to one's own imminent death, as described in Kübler-Ross's (1969) sequence of denial and isolation, anger, bargaining, depression, and acceptance. The five-stage process elucidated by Wiseman (1975)—denial, loss, anger, reorientation, and acceptance—is an acknowledged adaptation of Kübler-Ross's thanatology to marital separation, as is also that of Crosby, Gage, and Raymond (1983).

In criticism of stage models based on mourning, Rice and Rice (1986) argued that this paradigm is not suitable in divorce because the lost object is usually still accessible, the grief is caused by rejection in love, which is more devastating than simple loss, and depression can cause as well as result from breakup. Further, Rossiter (1991) pointed out that such models do not emerge from direct observation but are simply borrowed from preexisting theory. By assuming that adjustment proceeds in orderly steps in which the central issue is grieving, the end result is a clinical service that can "administer the experience" (i.e., mold the individual to the model) instead of honoring the individual's own experience of separation. In her Canadian practice with a group of divorce noninitiators, Rossiter made several key observations: people did not "recover" in the sense of regaining their former selves but, after initial upset, tended to develop in new directions; progress did not occur in successive stages but rather in terms of a gradually more favorable ratio of "good days" to "bad days"; and her clients' core issues seemed to be loss of identity, a temporary need for moral superiority, and financial problems—but not mourning. Rossiter also pointed out that most models currently in use unjustifiably fit initiators and noninitiators alike into a generalized adjustment process. She was not sure that they necessarily followed the same course in recovery, so that separate data were required to lay out the special issues of each party.

Although Rossiter's critique is astute in many respects, we disagree with her view that mourning is not a core issue in readjustment. Most contributors to the field agree that recurrent emotional involvement with the lost object is the pivotal problem in the postseparation period (e.g., Weiss, 1975; Spanier & Thompson, 1984). Given this premise, it seems sensible to think about stages in a process, albeit such stages will perforce be somewhat arbitrary, overlapping, and irregular. We too have drafted a model based on the Kübler-Ross sequence, reformatting progressive detachment in the context of dying into the divorce experience. However, Rossiter's point is well taken that separate models are needed for initiators and noninitiators; indeed, Hill, Rubin, and Peplau (1976) had already noted that for this crucial variable, the two groups should be studied independently. We have therefore attempted to provide two parallel but distinct paradigms.

For the countersymbiant, we regard the relevant five stages as alienation, breakup, the love entitlement quest, looking back/mourning, and disentanglement. For this party, the letting go process starts early, in the disappointments and disillusion of the working marriage, reaching crisis proportions at breakup, and then still requires attention long after parting of the ways has been accomplished, and sometimes even after the ex-mate has disengaged. For the symbiant, a corresponding but different progression can be described: shock, grief/rage, courting the rejector, distancing, and indifference. Although each stage represents successive steps toward letting go for the symbiant, the most crucial movement away from the ex-partner occurs in distancing. The preceding three stages merely serve to prepare the way, and the succeeding one seals work already done. Because letting go tends to be relatively more complicated, diffuse, and protracted for the countersymbiant, we will first look at the more concentrated process of recovery in the symbiant, whose grief work usually starts in the crisis of breakup.

THE SYMBIANT IN SEPARATION: TOWARD A NEW IDENTITY

Where letting go is concerned, a forsaken mate is legendary for recalcitrance, frailty, and folly. A jilted man threatened to kill his wife, or her lawyer, if the word "divorce" was so much as mentioned. Another man preserved his estranged wife's clothing in the closet, sending them out to be cleaned in expectation of her return. A woman rebuffed a long-awaited bid to reunite—and then fainted in her ex-husband's arms. Another woman invited the man who left the family unit to dinner once a week "at the old house"—she has now followed this ritual for 10 years. So long as the grim fact of breakup is subjectively resisted, a symbiant is susceptible to fruitlessly waiting for, or being "dangled" by, a disengaging partner who may not really intend to ever rejoin the marriage or who returns only momentarily. Hard as it is, and for as long as it takes, a forsaken symbiant has to stop using the relationship to define h/h identity, predicating nearly every action on how it might hypothetically impinge on the lost partner. Strategies for reconciliation or retaliation run counter to the need for self-development. In practical terms, the symbiant must learn "to reject one's rejector" (Baumeister & Wotman, 1992, p. 95). In psychic terms, the self-image of a "rejected" has to be rejected. But this program needs working through, as the stage model shows.

Shock

The typical initial reaction to the announcement or discovery that the relationship is ending is psychic numbing. An incredulous calm often follows upon hearing the news or seeing the evidence—it seems so preposterous. In addition, disbelief mingles with a dissociated sense of being a spectator at a play—this could not possibly be happening to me! In some people, physical reactions such as palpitations or nausea belie the surface calm. Shock is especially pronounced if breakup is a sudden or unexpected event, but a symbiant's psychological defenses are often ill suited to permit processing the information, no matter how obvious, overdue, or inevitable the breakup may seem to the partner. For the moment, life continues by inertia as if it were "as usual;" to keep the patina of sameness there is often a determination not to let others know about this turn of events, particularly the family of origin. At the same time there is an uncanny ability to discuss breakup in ultrarational fashion with the partner. An example is seen in Gillis's (1986) account of her own divorce. Her husband suddenly informed her that he was leaving the marriage; indeed, he had already rented an apartment, ordered new furniture, and was moving in that night. He then matter-of-factly added he would be living with their next-door neighbor, and this woman was simultaneously telling her husband of the new couple's plans. Gillis sat silently, unable to react to what he was saying. "Since you are taking the news like a lady," her husband then said, "we can go over a few details in preparation for the separation" (p. 15). He proceeded to outline a temporary financial settlement until she could get a job, proposed joint custody for their son, and asked for a letter from her stating that she had no hard feelings toward her neighbor, now to be his new mate. Stunned, Gillis complied with everything, somehow expecting he would soon change his mind and they would reconcile. For 3 months she attempted to maintain a calm and cooperative bearing, which only gave way to grief/rage when—contrary to their temporary agreement—he cut off payments for her heat during a blizzard in order to force her to sign a final legal document he had drafted.

Grief/Rage

The realization of "being left" hits home soon enough, and an intense mourning process begins. All the symptoms associated with traumatic depression occur; preoccupied despair, appetite and sleep disturbance, psychophysiological complications, impairment in functioning, and so on. Unable to face life without the partner and barely imagining survival in the immediate days ahead, some symbiants withdraw from all social contact whereas others cannot stand to be without company. Often, a bereft symbiant hovers around the telephone, not daring to leave home for fear of missing a call. As with all depression, much of the grief comes from repression of rage. In order for the symbiant to preserve the beloved as such, the partner's leaving tends to be excused or rationalized away, with some faith that h/s will return once it is realized that a mistake was made. Meanwhile, in the workings of "anger turned inward," the plainly "unlovable" self becomes the scapegoat, so that loss of self-esteem, melancholia, and masochism are dramatic hallmarks of this period.

But the rage aroused by breakup is too powerful to be entirely throttled by depressive symptoms. Hostile feelings will eventually erupt, leading to episodes of stormy confrontation or destructive acting out. By precipitating mayhem, the symbiant echoes the remark composer Arnold Schoenberg made about his atonal contribution to music that while he may not have added much, he certainly took a lot away! (Rosen, 1975). In spite of the self-accusations inherent in depression, an impressive list of self-righteous complaints will be compiled, not least of which is that the out-of-love partner is just that. At this point, a symbiant typically assumes the badge of "victim," with the reciprocal cast in the role of "villain."

The interplay of fervent love and hate feelings can be more upsetting than the separation itself. The symbiant is caught in a welter of contradictory emotions: one moment madly in love, the next moment seething in fury; one day jubilant because of a ray of hope for reunion, the next day despairing and plotting revenge. During the first 6 months or so, functioning is often volatile, inadequate, and self- destructive. The symbiant feels unstable and may lose control to the point of extreme reactions or desperate maneuvers. But a symbiant bereft of a partner is blindly searching within a maze for an avenue to love and be loved. The search is frantic, and the only way for things to come right in h/h mind is to annul a separation that has inflicted so much ego damage. Not only is reconciliation urgently sought to repair self-esteem, but it is also needed to restore meaning and belonging to a familiar social niche (Hancock, 1980). The symbiant tends to cling, or even beg for a few reassurances or attentions from the disengaging partner; this is sometimes done with humiliating loss of dignity, as in the case of a husband who fell on his knees in a session of divorce therapy, "whining and crying and pleading with his wife not to leave him," despite the therapist urging him to stand up (Framo, 1978, p. 100).

Courting the Rejector

Given dire narcissistic injury, it is understandable that a forsaken symbiant is looking for validation as a worthy sexual–romantic mate. The trouble is that, as first choice, h/s avidly pursues the estranged partner on the theory that *this* lover is the most logical one to remove self-doubts engendered by rejection. After regaining some composure, the symbiant is prone to plan ways to woo back the disaffiliated partner. Chances for reunion are deemed to depend on how skillfully one's cards are played, so that startling innovations in appearance, sexuality, and life style may occur. Wanting above all to be with the partner to work on their relationship, the symbiant places special emphasis on creating some ardent form of sexual contact to show what was lost or how splendid things could become. Even if achieved, however, most of these contacts prove to be unproductive because they do not resolve the anguish of separation for long, given that the partner will shortly depart again and resume a separate life (Trafford, 1992).

While cultivated seduction is the major method used to "court the rejector," an incidental avenue apt to be tried is involvement with someone else. Whereas "carrying a torch" in the grief/rage stage tends to convey a steadfast devotion, now—despite still feeling "married"—a paramour may be introduced as bait to snare an ex who is perhaps not prepared to be supplanted. Yet even as dating activities begin, separated symbiants may hardly be able to be with someone new without talking at length about the ex-partner. They want sympathy and reassurance, wishing to hear that they are good lovers and the former partner was "crazy to let you go." The symbiant may even ask the date for assistance in custom-designing stratagems to recapture the ex. As a result, a current companion soon gathers that a serious relationship is not possible. Some will not mind, but others will feel used and leave for more promising pastures. Such new losses do not have much impact on the symbiant, except insofar as they recapitulate the prime separation trauma and thus momentarily increase abandonment depression.

As can be seen, this phase is still bleak. The rewards of mingling in the singles scene do not make up for departure of the partner and family disruption. For symbiants, sexual experience at this point in separation feels fraudulent. Comments by some envious acquaintances, to the effect that they are lucky to have such an array of opportunities, seem ludicrous because it was never their choice to be a "swinging bachelor" or a "gay divorcée." As one man said, "I've had seven good days that still add up to a bad week."

All told, a more sexy bearing, occasional trysts between ex-spouses, and "infidelity" to make the significant other jealous seldom avail to rekindle interest in the countersymbiant. No matter how perfect a suitor or clever a tactician a forsaken symbiant becomes, the ex-partner remains elusive, at most flitting in and out of the relationship at whim. At best, when the ex is somewhat responsive, h/s will more and more be seen as a double-dealing opportunist, so that courting accordingly alternates with fighting. Courting the rejector—a period of strategies to influence the disengaging partner to return—ends when a symbiant appreciates that it does not really matter whether h/s is nice or nasty, suave or jealous, magnanimous or vindictive, seductive or aloof. The separation goes on. The length of time needed to work through this stage can be prolonged by months and years if the ex encourages the symbiant to hang on, but it also depends on how quickly the futility of chasing after the countersymbiant's love is learned.

Distancing

Sooner or later it becomes painfully evident that any version of carrying a torch is not worth the candle. Negative outcomes to efforts at rapprochement finally become seen as an affront: this love object no longer deserves my emotional investment. Henceforward, the symbiant struggles against internal needs to love or be loved by the former partner, pushing h/h away in order to push away these internal needs. The disengaging partner is now apt to be seen as a predator who selfishly impedes the symbiant's progress in escaping from a masochistic orbit. The cry of the symbiant at this point echoes the prior cry of the countersymbiant: "Why can't you just leave me alone?" Outrage at the disengaging partner's repeated refusals to be turned around by courtship now finally gives energy to break free; anger is mobilized in the service of severing now-unwelcome bonds. Emotional distancing is to be achieved by studied coldness, shunning, and even rudeness and callousness—whatever it takes to expel the disengaging partner from one's life space. The goal of letting go has become acceptable at last; indeed, it has become a matter of pride. But during this stage it can not truly be said that the symbiant has stopped caring about the disengaging partner. Rather, the symbiant is distancing because h/s has the dangerous misfortune to still care. This can be seen when the symbiant becomes involved with someone with whom a new committed union is possible. The question is then internally asked, "What if my ex should suddenly want to reconcile—with whom would I want to be?" But asking the question already indicates an ambivalent attachment that the new partner has not been able to fully sever. At least, however, the symbiant is "in circulation."

In this phase, the power equation between the two protagonists has shifted. They are now more nearly matched in autonomy, whereas previously the countersymbiant was in control. No longer will the symbiant court the rejector, and unless the disengaging partner makes a last-minute effort to save the relationship, it is doomed. The countersymbiant is finally forced to recognize that charm can not be turned on to come back whenever h/s pleases, so that nothing is lost by staying away. In short, reconciliation can no longer be taken for granted, just for the asking. However, given the proper approach in terms of time, labor, and penitence by the erstwhile rejector, a resumption of the committed union is still possible.

Indifference

If the disengaging partner does not compensate for the symbiant's distancing to restore a homeostatic balance, growing alienation eventually turns into indifference as the last letting-go stage becomes operative. The preceding distancing was marked by an effort to counteract an existing emotional involvement with the disengaging partner, but still-smoldering passion could conceivably ignite were a resolute ex to fan the flames. However, in this final phase, emotional disengagement will be sought for its own sake; letting go is now relief and even emancipation. The countersymbiant's motives can at this point be accepted as valid needs, despite the fact that they destroyed the marriage. These needs have no further relevance to a symbiant who is no longer playing that role, and the former partner is experienced as alien, perhaps even dull, foolish, or unsavory as a person. The once-forsaken mate will often even wonder how it was possible to be so taken with this person and will exercise sovereign will: *Our relationship is no longer wanted by me.* The rejection has been overcome. It will not make a difference what the formerly beloved does in respect to reconciliation. It is too late, the passion is gone, the identity of someone "rejected in love" has been shed, and there has been reconstitution along new lines. The ex-partner usually becomes "someone I used to know"—words conveying an attitude ranging between disinterest and distaste. Revenge, that rash emotional reaction that once affirmed indissoluble ties despite separation, may at last have been satisfied by living well without the rejector, or at least adapting better than the rejector. Once this point is reached, it is sometimes possible to be friendly with the ex despite a stormy period of separation. Abelsohn (1992) afforded a clinical illustration in the case of a man left by his wife who transcended his original bitterness of the first year by helping his ex emotionally and financially after her lover suddenly departed. This man insisted that he was not seeking reunion but, rather, a mutually respectful relationship after an unhappy marriage together. The point Abelsohn made in presenting this case was to show that divorce could be "civilized." Yes, but it must also be said that such an outcome is possible only after the letting go process has been sufficiently worked through by the two parties, especially the symbiant. In addition, can it be that this man found satisfaction, even revenge, in demonstrating his own new-found strength by *not* offering to take his ex-wife back when she was desperate and would have returned?

DISTANCING IS THE ONLY WAY TO CHANGE THE SYSTEM

Why does it take so long for a forsaken symbiant to catch on to how fruitless it is to pursue the countersymbiant? As we have seen, the symbiant worries that it would be tantamount to giving up on the relationship not to pursue, justifying such clinging on the grounds that it is usually possible to discern in the object some ambivalent wish for contact. Presumably, if the symbiant no longer tries to keep the union alive, the disengaging partner will no longer try either—and the relationship is too important to be thus ended by default. However, "no longer trying" is exactly what is called for. For the symbiant, sooner or later a firm decision has to be made to stop chasing and see what happens. The refusal to chase, amounting to reactive distancing in stage four of our paradigm, requires an active, disciplined stance and is anything but the defeatist "giving up" a symbiant fears it to be.

Fogarty (1976) has written a classic paper about emotional pursuit and distance in marital crisis. Using his terminology in the context of breakup, the "pursuer" is our symbiant, and the "distancer" is our countersymbiant:

> When problems arise, the pursuer tends to blame, accuse, and attack and the distancer to defend. The pursuer can be taken for granted, since he is always moving towards his spouse. A pursuer has to be taught the operating principle, Never pursue a distancer. The more anyone goes after a distancer, the more he will distance. . . . In effect, the pursuer must learn to get from himself many of the things he is hoping to get from his mate. In other words, the pursuer must learn to distance. (p. 326)

We agree that "Never pursue a distancer" is the formula that gives a forsaken symbiant the only way out of a maze. Such refusal to court the rejector has to be authentic, not a ploy that the disengaging partner will always intuitively sense as a trick. Indeed, "never pursue a distancer" defines the psychic mechanism whereby letting go is accomplished—not only obtaining eventual autonomy for the symbiant but also imposing it on the countersymbiant. It is hard work to learn to let the disengaging partner fend on h/h own, but Fogarty insisted that the pursuing mate must not give in to h/h panic but must instead shift the burden of dealing with the panic of loss onto the distancer:

> The distancer must come in under his own steam. Eventually, he must learn that distancing is a useful way to get his head together, but that it never solves a problem. When the distancer sees that nobody is chasing him, he will get in touch with his own loneliness and his fears of losing his spouse. (p. 328)

Thus, reactive distancing by the symbiant, based on the realization that you can't beat a dead horse, may yet lead that horse to turn around. Without a mate in hot pursuit, the countersymbiant is forced into an existential choice: either h/s has to explore reunion (cast now in the role of pursuer) or else by default allow collapse of the relationship. Just how the disengaging partner chooses is an issue that will be determined by what has been learned during separation about alternative sexual–romantic objects, new appreciation of the old mate, and personal traits. If the disengaging partner still does not return in the stark circumstances that reactive distancing presents, it is hard to conceive that return would occur under any circumstances. However, by no longer courting the rejector, a forsaken symbiant is protected in any event. The countersymbiant has to confront aloneness and may possibly sue for reconciliation, but if h/s responds by making no compensatory effort to keep the relationship from lapsing, the symbiant accelerates distancing, taking more and more control of h/h end of the separation process.

Nearly all forsaken symbiants need considerable time to get reorganized as an "I" not searching after the bygone "we." Yet learning to detach will yield major dividends in terms of renewed self-esteem when finally accomplished. Although it will take time, the sooner "courting the rejector" can be stopped, the better off the forsaken symbiant will be. The next two cases illustrate the benefits of distancing from—rather than pursuing—a distancer.

> J and his wife, K, had two children, one of whom was newborn. J decided to leave and went to live with a girlfriend. However, that relationship soon ended, and J went through a series of affairs. He was filled with guilt at his decision to exit the marriage, and he was also the recipient of much criticism from his own family because, with two very small children, K could not work and was a woman in a desperate financial and psychological position. J was not quite sure he wanted a divorce, but he knew he could not live with his wife at that point. However, he did see her whenever he visited his children, and they went through passionate scenes of love making, recriminations, and abrupt farewells. K was distraught and could not perform her motherly duties well. She was at times suicidal. She developed ulcers. J sent as much of his income as he could to his family and even borrowed more than he could afford, gradually finding himself seriously in debt. He began to discuss with K the need to arrive at a more manageable figure for monthly support. On this issue, given her own financial situation, K became implacably antagonistic—and all the more so in that, for her, the obvious solution to each one's economic problems would have been reconciliation. J unilaterally now decided to greatly diminish the amount of his customary monthly allotment. Soon after he reduced his payments, J arrived at his former home to visit as scheduled and found the place vacant, his wife and children gone with no trace. Foul play was ruled out because the furniture too was gone. For 4 months, he heard nothing. Finally, he received a

telephone call from his wife on the far side of the country. He hastened to see her and immediately offered reconciliation when he arrived. But his wife only wanted to make financial arrangements for divorce, and so his cross-country trek ended in their last fight.

K had pursued her husband for more than a year without any result to speak of. She then mobilized her strength to break material and emotional ties, and implemented a course of action that was also designed to hurt him. Just as he came to withhold money as well as love from her, she came to withhold herself plus the children from him. When she reactively distanced, the outcome was the bid for reunion she had sought all along. In her case, she rejected the bid when it at last came. She shortly remarried and had her third child.

L was asked by his wife, M, to move out when their children were ages 11 and 6. Heartbroken, he did so. In spite of jealousy over a series of new men in his estranged wife's life, he nevertheless made every effort to win her back by courting and being useful. Thus, he would drop everything and rush to make repairs when she complained of malfunction in a household appliance or her car. He gave her extra cash on several occasions with which to go on vacation. He took care of her when she was sick. He also visited one time at her request to help her take a boyfriend to the hospital for emergency psychiatric care. L took his children overnight every Friday, Saturday, and Sunday, as M wanted this arrangement because her professional obligations were on weekends. L seemed to have no concept of his own needs for weekend free time, based on his work schedule. He justified his compliance with the existing custody arrangement as follows: he needed the presence of the children to deal with his own loneliness, and he worried that M would demand much more money if he did not do as she insisted. The separation went on in this manner for 3 years, while he carried a banner for reunion by fulfilling nearly every request she made. Finally, L met a new woman who pressed him to spend less time with the children and more with her. L told M that he would not take the children any longer on Sundays, but would return them Saturday afternoon. M reacted to this news with calm acceptance, but she continued to stay out overnight with a lover on Saturday evenings (as she had been doing before), even though the children were now presumably home "with her" instead of with him. After hearing that the kids were left alone, the guilt-stricken L needed all the support he could get from his girlfriend to keep him from telling them to come over to his place if that happened again (as M was perhaps counting on). L then began to decline to rush in to solve M's problems, even finding some satisfaction in actually opposing her demands, especially when she cited Sunday "emergencies." But L still had fantasies that M would reunite with him as soon as she heard he had become serious about another woman. However, as he became more detached, M still did not initiate any overtures. L finally had to acknowledge that she was not alarmed at the prospect of losing him. Five years after breakup he filed for divorce and married his girl-friend. Although this man had great difficulties in learning how to reactively distance, he did ultimately work through an incremental disengagement.

As can be seen, letting go is a long-term process requiring intra-psychic work to the point where the love object is no longer necessarily wanted, even if available. The key is building the ego strength to reactively distance—not pursuing as soon as the ex-partner flashes urgent needs or erotic interest. Such displays by an out-of-love partner are almost always fleeting; grasping at them amounts to continued participation in an essentially unrewarding relationship. But it must be remembered that letting go must run its psychological course and cannot be abbreviated by treating the process as just a matter of will power in the face of reality. If only it were as simple as Wanderer and Cabot (1978) appear to think:

> Your obsessive thoughts about your ex are due to the withdrawal symptoms of having your love connection taken away. . . . You dream about your loved one, imagining them returning to you. You think about it all the time. . . . You have become addicted to your loved one, and certain things trigger your urge for the addictive substance (contact with the ex). In treating any addict, the first thing to do is to remove the triggers. If someone . . . is a food addict, you take . . . sweets away. (pp. 65–66)

The problem here is that recovery requires not only taking the sweets away, but the *wish* for the sweets away—an internal process requiring the development of mastery. If one were to give advice to the lovelorn, it would be that distancing is the method to learn this mastery, culminating in rejecting the rejector, which will ultimately force change in the postseparation relationship.

THE COUNTERSYMBIANT'S SEPARATION: LETTING GO AS UNFINISHED BUSINESS

Some people can leave their committed relationship and never look back—they accomplish total letting go before they exit the marriage. However, this is not the rule. It is ironic that letting-go is still such a major problem for most disengaging partners; it has ostensibly already occurred, yet their enmeshment goes on after breakup. Based on his own experience, Krantzler (1975) observed:

Unforseen emotional pushes and pulls . . . continue to dominate the lives of those who separated of their own volition. In many cases their divorce was an agonizing act of will which followed months or even years of indecision and misery. Having finally taken the step they thought would resolve things once and for all, they are shaken to discover that their feelings are still in thrall to the past. In fact, they find they are devoting *more* thought, *more* energy, *more* emotional juices to their old relationship now than they did during the many years of the marriage itself. (p. 53)

While it is the symbiant who tries to save the relationship, it is often the countersymbiant who exhibits the greater reluctance when it comes to bringing the relationship to a truly decisive end. Thus, if a symbiant calls a halt to postseparation contact between the two (feeling driven to it by the behavior of the ex), it may be over the countersymbiant's strident objections. Thus, many countersymbiants leave, insisting that they must be out of the committed union, yet still attempt to avert the loss entailed in the symbiant's letting go. We see such confusing ambivalence around disengagement in the following vignettes.

One man twice left his wife for another woman; when she would having nothing further to do with him, he complained that she did not try hard enough! Was this a message that he was relying on her to carry *his* wish to keep the relationship open as a permanent option? He definitely was asking her to wait around to be possibly found (and possibly left) yet a third time. Another out-of-love man walked out of his home and later requested that his wife move to the vicinity where he now lived so he could retain daily contact with her. Then there is the gentleman who successfully pleaded in court during divorce proceedings for time to leave his girlfriend in order to reconcile with his wife; the next day he moved his girlfriend into his apartment—a deed he defended to his wife as the fastest way to get rid of his girlfriend! A woman wanted a "friendly divorce" and so annually invited the husband she expelled from the home to go on summer vacation with the family, causing the children much perplexity, and the ex-husband as well.

Perhaps residuals of love contribute to the ambivalence about any conclusive parting of the ways, which in itself may have long delayed the decision to leave the marriage. But what cannot be disputed here is that in many cases the symbiant is still needed in some way after being rejected. The withdrawal of the rejected mate may be something such disengaging partners are still not ready to allow, so that when the symbiant finally attempts to distance, it can be the countersymbiant who clings to aspects of the marriage, at times with duplicitous intimations that the committed union might ultimately be reinstated. Like the forsaken symbiant, most countersymbiants will need to traverse a process of several years' duration to accomplish a letting go free of dependent and perhaps even exploitative motives. However, unlike forsaken symbiants, nearly all countersymbiants have had considerable time to prepare for the forthcoming separation. We have tried to indicate in our stage model just how torturous the course of most countersymbiants will be toward emotional disengagement.

Alienation

In Chapter 3, we observed that the letting-go process starts long before actual severing of the relationship by an emotionally disengaging partner. A complex transformation is involved, which Kayser (1993) conceptualized in three substages—disappointment, transition, and disaffection. Thus, suffering during the relationship and growing disenchantment can coalesce into a wish to leave, which has to be weighed against reasons for staying (first substage). If initial ambivalence swings more and more to negative assessment of the marriage, temptation to leave becomes intention (second substage); however, if the ambivalence remains in rough balance, an outside adjustment may be instituted that renders the union at least temporarily tolerable. In either case, a transitioning partner has already given thought to such matters as where to go, how to manage financially, life style changes, and so forth, and thus is somewhat ready for breakup, whenever or however it occurs. As a transitioning spouse gradually turns into an alienated partner who is past the point of no return (third substage), h/s seldom leaves frivolously, such as occurs in a spat in which there is anger around a single key demand that the mate will not grant. In a spat, the party who storms out can return when the mate relents. In this situation, a point has been made and after a brief lapse the relationship resumes. In marked contrast, a partner at the substage of alienation typically leaves only after a long incubation period for festering unhappiness. When breakup finally takes place, departure will not be subject to negotiation or compromise. The alienated partner is quite sure at the moment that h/s must be out of the committed union *now or very soon,* and is fortified to the fact of losing the mate. On the eve of separation, most are more resolute and unequivocal about terminating the marriage than at any other time prior to completing their letting-go process.

Breakup

Whereas separation is a subjective decision in the preceding stage of emotional alienation, a countersymbiant still has to face the objective reality of the mate's reaction when the decision is conveyed. Even anticipation of such a reaction will already cause the planned format of the breakup to change. The countersymbiant may well have to scrap, delay, or modify plans, and will finally exit in whatever fashion is expedient (see Chapter 5). Further, as a result of having to suppress feelings, in particular, anxiety about the future, h/s may counterphobically leave as a "free spirit," unmindful of long-range practical consequences, as well as determined to burn h/h bridges. In the long run, the method of departure is deemed not to matter much—just getting out is what counts. At this juncture, letting go is regarded as accomplished simply by having achieved a separation.

The Love Entitlement Quest

During the stage of the love entitlement quest (which will somewhat overlap the preceding stages when there is a lover waiting in the wings), the disengaging partner's attention is fixed on developing h/h vision of a suitable sexual–romantic life after breaking marital bonds. This is where nearly all energy is invested, and the goal provides the rationale for h/h life course. Nothing will be allowed to stand in the way of this dream, so long yearned for and for the sake of which so much was sacrificed. Time, money, and affection tend to be lavished on a new, more exciting mate, other long-delayed gratifications, or both.

Insofar as the lesser issue of ties to the former mate is concerned, it is often seen as necessary to ward off feelings that signify persistent involvement with a failed relationship so as to concentrate on new, more exciting experiences. Having escaped from a "bad" marriage, a countersymbiant must resist the symbiant's inducements to return to it. H/s may still "dangle" the ex-mate or provoke the symbiant into various crises of enmeshment, but these behaviors are usually seen as temporary setbacks or passing weaknesses in what may have to be an intricate and prolonged extrication from the marriage. However, in leaving, there are often many facets of the divorce experience with which disengaging partners may not be in touch. For example, it is not unusual to encounter countersymbiants who have neither accepted any internal need to mourn the actual loss of the marriage nor looked at their own role in what went wrong. Moreover, the emotional devastation of the ex-mate is often only an abstract idea, for the countersymbiant tends to flee from any direct perception of it. H/s may even be astonished at the bitterness of the ex and children and may offer the implausible excuse of not knowing that so much pain was unleashed by the breakup. Rather than dealing with the havoc, a disengaging partner may even prefer to think that members of the family left behind are faring well, that h/s is the object of everybody's love, and that h/s still loves everybody! This dynamic may contribute to the willingness of so many countersymbiants for sexual contact with the ex, for not only is it flattering to be courted, but it also fits in with a new self-image of being a consummate dispenser of love, liberated from ordinary restraints and prejudices.

Looking Back/Mourning

After the disengaging partner has had a large enough sample of what separation means, including some inevitable hardships and disillusionments, h/s will begin to see the symbiant from a slightly different perspective. Even if the countersymbiant has been relatively happy in separation, some sympathy and nostalgia may be developed over time for the forsaken symbiant—without, however, any concomitant wish to reunite. But if the world outside does not live up to hopes and expectations, the disengaging partner finds either that being alone is not easy, or when involved in a new committed union, that all relationships have problems. Hence, h/s may then commence to feel that the ex-mate was comparatively not so bad after all and may also begin to miss and mourn some facets of the old life. These factors will raise doubts about the wisdom of the prior breakup and prompt a second look at the ex-mate. Reconciliation can become a possibility to be explored, so that the disengaging partner may suddenly seek contact after a long absence. Of course, some level of looking back and regret over the loss of the marriage does not necessarily lead to reconciliation, because the countersymbiant may decide this is still not a viable person as a mate, or the symbiant may no longer be interested in reunion.

Disentanglement

Only when the countersymbiant has taken a fresh look at the old relationship can the final, and perhaps most painful, part of the letting-go process be inaugurated: coming to terms with the self (Vaughan, 1986). H/s will acknowledge personal faults, which every mate, new or old, has had difficulty handling. If the countersymbiant can tolerate the process of self-evaluation, identifying the mote in h/h own eye, no longer will the failure of the old relationship be totally blamed on the mate. Before letting go is complete, the countersymbiant has to make peace with the notion that h/s chose a particular mate to meet preexisting needs that the mate did not create, was unable to satisfy, and cannot change. It is sad for the mate as well as for the self. Each is a different person, with good and bad features, and both were unable to make the necessary accommodations and reacted to failure with passions and judgments beyond their control. In the final account, the countersymbiant may see the impact of the decision to separate on each member of the family and have the integrity to live with the consequences, including letting the ex-mate disengage in accord with that person's self-interest, while the countersymbiant in the meantime emotionally disentangles from the relationships and proceeds on h/h fallible own.

THE COUNTERSYMBIANT SURVEYS THE WRECKAGE

The task of letting go can take longer for countersymbiants than for symbiants because the former's defenses shield them for a period of time from self-confrontation and owning up (although this is not to say that their reciprocals do not struggle with such issues too). Some disengaging partners cannot do this psychological work, thus cannot learn, and thus repeat the rejecting scenario with new mates while continuing to be enmeshed with old mates. Such disengaging partners do not reach the disentanglement stage and even do precious little looking back or mourning. We will address this pattern of incomplete letting go after we discuss the achievements of those who can do the psychological work.

For the disengaging partner who ultimately comes to grips with the last two stages of the letting-go process, it is hard at times to figure out one's bearings, but clarity will begin to emerge as disturbing questions of the "wrong mistake" type are dealt with. One woman surveyed the damage to her family unit, wondering, "How did I get here? Do I want to be here?" In posing these crucial questions, she had at last become the responsible agent for her fate *in her own consciousness* (as she had always been in reality). Gradually, she could admit that she was as unhappy in separation as she had been in her marriage, but the marriage was no better than what she had made of it. She had let everybody down, especially herself. This is no easy admission to make, even in the privacy of one's own mind. The results of such introspection are not always full of regrets, but a countersymbiant will often have events to take under review and possibly a few things to reconsider.

No human being can come to an understanding of the darker side to h/h personality without a wrenching struggle that threatens to unhinge self-esteem. For the countersymbiant, the hardest issue to examine is that the deprivation experienced within the marriage may have derived from excessive narcissistic entitlement. If this is what the countersymbiant concludes was the case, h/s then can dispense with much of the previous blaming and freely admit to being a coequal producer of the success or failure of any committed union in which h/s partakes. If the countersymbiant was dissatisfied in the marriage, it no longer follows that the mate was neglectful or inadequate. Unmet needs are inherent in every relationship; the mate was not necessarily "bad" for not sparing the partner this problem. To a great extent, happiness arises as a function of our own resources—for example, personal input, standards, and evaluations. It comes as much from within as from without. The countersymbiant has been alerted to the fundamental existential fact that no one else can be charged as keeper of h/h happiness.

Now we pass to those countersymbiants who cannot deal with their own internal dynamics, preferring to pursue the chimera of finding a mate who will "let" them be the person they want to be. A therapist told the story of a man who married seven times, in the end realizing that his first marriage was far and away the best. When a listener commented that this man had divorced "unnecessarily," the therapist pointed out that his patient could not have appreciated his first marriage without having made the other six.

There are no shortcuts, no action programs. To recover from loss, one has to go through the process of mourning loss.

THE DEATH OF LOVE

A subtle aspect of letting go, often underestimated, is accepting the death of one's love for the partner. Fromm (1956) has suggested that behind the fear of not being loved lies the dread of not loving. The wish to invest in another is one of the paramount impulses in life. Loving is a way to subordinate self to a higher purpose; it lends meaning and organization to one's existence. When it seems we no longer love, we feel diminished as human beings. We wonder if we are capable of love and fear that we will never love again. We question what love is. We worry that we, as unloving individuals, are not worthy of love in return. Dealing with not loving and not being loved is surely one of the most poignant of human anxieties.

The reasons for letting go are very different for the two parties to a breakup. For the countersymbiant, letting go is necessary because keeping the symbiant around for security prevents being on one's own, accepting the consequences of decisions, and avoiding exploitation of a vulnerable other. It is a matter of character building. For the symbiant, letting go is necessary because getting beyond the emotional reach of the out-of-love partner is critical to restoring self-esteem. It is a matter of survival. Both must undertake letting go to gain self-reliance. However, for the symbiant this is starkly evident from the instant of breakup, whereas for the countersymbiant the realization that there could be problems in handling independence may come as a belated surprise. The symbiant whose love is unrequited must begin to consider h/h own interest *solely* and make plans for a future that no longer includes the former partner. In contrast, the countersymbiant has to consider the impact of h/h behavior on significant others, as well as the fact that, in getting the separation against stiff opposition, h/s now has to live with it.

Both parties have to go through various rites of passage: the wrenching process of separating, the relinquishing of previous claims on one another, the establishment of autonomy, and the ultimate placing in perspective of former partner and relationship. This means accepting one's own share of responsibility for the demise of the marriage; it is not accomplished when blame is totally placed on the reciprocal. An example of an ex-spouse who has not been able to do this was provided by Bennett (1991). She maintained that a committed relationship can shatter because of the problems of one person, going on to state that her own 25-year marriage ended because of some amorphous "disturbance" in her husband after his business failed, leading to his becoming involved with someone else. Other than his presumed psychopathology, which she attempted to diagnose from a reading of various mental health manuals, she did not see any reason that he should have left her. Not only did Bennett eschew any responsibility for her part in the breakup, but her book demonstrates a continued enmeshment with her ex-husband as if she were now his therapist instead of his wife.

Letting go done with firmness, compassion, and integrity is the only constructive path to release from the bondage of the past. It makes possible the growth of a fresh love, whether with a new partner or a newly appreciated old one. The existential emptiness, leading to an urgent love quest outside the union by one partner, and an equally urgent love quest within the defunct union by the mate, has a natural resolution. This involves the distillation of an identity as the responsible principal in a universe rich in options, yet often devoid of guidelines. Sartre (1943/1977) said, "The one who realizes in anguish his condition as being thrown into a responsibility which extends to his very abandonment no longer has either remorse or regret or excuses; [his] freedom perfectly reveals itself and [his] being resides in this very revelation" (p. 556). In the final analysis, my life is of my own creating.

Letting go is more doing than it is undoing. It is like death, but it is not death. It is metamorphosis.

∽ 17

Reconciliation

On the whole, I'd rather be in Philadelphia
—W. C. FIELDS
(Inscription on his tombstone)

REST IN PEACE

In view of his many scathing references to his native city, this epitaph written by W. C. Fields is probably the highest compliment he ever paid Philadelphia. Was the incorrigible comedian repenting of his many caustic disparagements of a hometown he obviously loved? Or was he insulting Philadelphia yet one more time by disclosing (after due deliberation and the most dire of choices) that the city was just barely preferable to a cemetery?

RECONCILIATION: THE COUNTERSYMBIANT'S PERSPECTIVE

If postseparation experiences prove dismal, a countersymbiant tends to wonder whether there has been a miscalculation: on the whole, is it with the former mate where h/s would rather be? Perhaps reconciliation needs exploring:

> I was talking to my wife today and all of a sudden she said, "Do you want to sit down and talk about what went wrong?" So I said, "Why not, but why?" And she said, "Well, I just thought that we ought to talk about if we did the right thing." And I said, "Well, okay, let's talk about it . . . but how come this is just coming up?" And she started crying a

348

little bit and said, "Well, I'm really lonely. I just have nobody." (Weiss, 1975, pp. 120–121)

This woman has undergone a shift in attitude based on untoward developments in separation—the man she now approaches is the very same man she left. He is interested in discussing reunion with her but is puzzled by why she is suddenly reversing her previous rejection. What he learns can hardly be flattering. She does not hide that he is reevaluated as a mate only after she has had to reconsider her prospects of attracting a higher-grade replacement. Thus, she indicates that reconciliation is the lesser of two evils—he is better than nobody. Philadelphia over Death. She does not say that she is now in love with him, and even if she did, such a statement would be implausible. Still more implausible would be for her to say that she never stopped loving him, despite rejection of him. In effect, what the man is hearing from her is a new-found willingness to *settle for him as a spouse.* Because her life apart is not going well, in retrospect his flaws as a mate no longer seem to her quite so intolerable as they did in the marriage. This woman is swallowing her pride after bitter defeat as a single woman.

It is not clear from this vignette whether her disillusion in breakup has led to far-reaching shifts in her personality that would permit a fresh appreciation of her ex-husband as a mate. After all, perceptions of another are governed in part by one's state of being at the time; as the poet Rilke (1910/1940) declared about a statue of Apollo in a museum, to really see this bust, "you must change your life" (pp. 92–93). Based on the blunt but subtly insulting approach with which this woman opens the question of reconciliation with her ex, it seems she has not changed but rather has badly underestimated the problems of separation. Now alone, she turns to him as a refuge. In her eyes, he is a human resource to be pushed away or pulled back in accord with her needs.

Not all reconciliations are the sort in which a rejecting partner makes what appears to be an abrupt, possibly expedient decision to reconvene the marriage that h/s had disbanded not long before. Yet it is precisely this type of reunion that is most common and also offers the most flimsy chances for success, with a second separation as its most usual outcome. Even if the couple manages to stay together without another split, the marriage is in danger of having been compromised in essential areas—for instance, one party or the other may not feel secure enough in a renewed relationship to make some key concession. The despair of a countersymbiant over the failures of postseparation existence sets a stage for potential reunion, but this hardly eliminates the marital problems that caused breakup in the first place. All told, the unhappiness of a countersymbiant in separation is a necessary but not sufficient condition for successful reconciliation.

The timing of a seemingly "sudden" bid for reconciliation is typically precipitated either by problems with a new partner or by the downfall of financial or other plans. The countersymbiant then sets up a meeting, hinting at h/h availability and waiting for the ex-mate to take the initiative to pull things back together. In general, only if the forsaken symbiant resists the idea of reconciliation does the countersymbiant assume the risk and responsibility of making a direct offer. However, when the ex-mate is unwilling to even consider reunion, a bid for another chance may present as an incongruous mixture of *desperation to get back* and *entitlement to this option*. The following cases illustrate a narcissistic dynamic in which the stance of a countersymbiant unhappy in separation vis-à-vis the ex-mate is: "I need you to take care of me"—evidence that symbiotic attachment persists despite the instituted breakup.

A man left his wife for another woman but was shortly kicked out by his new girlfriend. He immediately called his ex-wife and asked to come home. When she refused, he threatened to return anyway because she had no right to keep him from his children and off his property. Another man gambled away his savings, credit, and business. When destitute, he turned to his ex-wife and teenage children by positioning himself at the family's doorstep, letting them know that he was without a penny in his pocket or a place to go. A woman left her child in the care of her husband so that she could live with her lover. This new man turned out to be brutal, so she called her former mate and insisted she had to return home right away because she could not stand further abuse where she was.

These examples show countersymbiants forced to reverse course when separation proved to be disastrous in some way, but this is, of course, hardly the typical outcome of a breakup. Rather, so long as the countersymbiant's new relationship or life style is functioning well, h/s has little motivation to reverse the decision to break up the family unit and tends to be vehemently uninterested in return; a well-situated countersymbiant will rarely rush back no matter what difficulties ex-mate or children may be encountering. Thus, only if personal troubles get out of hand does a countersymbiant seriously reconsider the decision to leave. When this happens, the countersymbiant (now suffering too) becomes more empathic, and the ex-mate is finally perceived as having endured much in the crisis of separation. The countersymbiant can also convey all the remorse, caring, and missing of the ex h/s may have suppressed in order to leave. At this juncture, rejoining the family circle is the chief priority of a prodigal countersymbiant. The family is a sanctuary, and apologies may now be made for having violated its integrity.

Thus far we have developed the thesis that it is not the belated discovery of love feelings that is the usual impetus for a countersymbiant's second look at the ex-mate, but instead the smashing of h/h dreams in the crucible of separation. In most reunions, the countersymbiant goes back not in a spirit of hope and love, but rather with a sense of frustration and failure. Wolfe (1975) made this point as she described the fate of women in current fiction who left their marriages to pursue "adulterous" relationships, only to be compelled to return by a combination of romantic disenchantment, social pressure, and concern for children:

> The return to the marriage may be the new fictional convention of retribution, as suicide was in nineteenth century novels. . . . Ann Birstein [stated that in her novels], "The heroines' marriages are their retribution. Although they don't walk into the sea, they're treading water while living. Although they don't die, something in them is dead because of the death of their aspirations." (p. 58)

Such reconciliations are clearly experienced as tantamount to punishment in the wake of a wife's failed attempt at independence. The return only reinstates the antecedent marital regime, including the fatal flaws which prompted the wife to leave. Because the "why" of a reunion in these circumstances concerns a woman's inability to develop a viable alternative to marriage, one can expect that the newly reconstructed but same old relationship will founder all over again. At the end of the novel *Fear of Flying* (Jong, 1973), a wife returns after a ruinous affair, enters her husband's place and is taking a bath when he arrives, and the two later hardly discuss her absence; they resume their marital routines almost as if there had been no interruption. The superficiality of such a reunion is shown in the sequel, *How to Save Your Own Life* (Jong, 1977). They conduct parallel lives as before the split—he drawing comfort from his psychoanalysis and she from numerous lovers—until the wife forces a final breakup. As Santayana (1905, p. 284) noted, those who learn nothing from history are doomed to repeat it.

The plight of women forced by adverse circumstances to return may differ in some respects from that of men. For men, the compelling factor in seeking a humiliating reunion may be an inability to manage without a female to either provide a home or contain irresponsible behavior. In one example, a business that supported a man's extravagant life style during separation went into decline because of his neglect, leading to insolvency and the man's return to his wife. Although this case points to economic problems as the motive for reconciliation, it speaks even more to a need for discipline afforded by the marriage. The man's wife had functioned as a source of financial control, so that the same reason that the husband had left (to be free of such control) also brought him back (to be taken in hand). But he did not have to love the parentified spouse upon whom he depended to keep his nose to the grindstone—this man's ambivalence about dependent needs could be expected to resume as soon as he went back, implying a poor prognosis for such a reunion. The more things change, the more they stay the same.

The costly and sometimes destructive quest for autonomy, love, and happiness at the expense of existing commitments does not make countersymbiants who jettison their marriages pillars of emotional stability, but their romantic quest elicits a degree of universal identification inasmuch as such goals are unquenchable human aspirations. Even a forsaken symbiant hopeful of reconciliation will acknowledge the importance of these goals for the ex-partner, despite the belief that failure to attain them in separation and consequent return to the relationship—sadder but presumably wiser—would provide the most suitable ending to unrealistic yearnings. The return is seen as an admission that the countersymbiant, *qua* free spirit, has had wings clipped and finally has feet on the ground. However, in the view of the countersymbiant, reunion can have a different meaning: return to the marriage is the fate of a noble figure in spiritual defeat. For the moment, h/s has lost the struggle for higher ideals in a prosaic world. Tamed for now, it is necessary for h/h to begin again.

THE FORSAKEN SYMBIANT
AND RECONCILIATION: REJECTED NO MORE

Reconciliation is usually a symbiant's most fervid desire, beginning with the very day of breakup. This desire may seem irrational in a person dealing with a partner who departed with the utmost ruthlessness. It is also irrational to consider ways to force the partner back, as if such reunion could possibly work. Still, a forsaken symbiant has much at stake in wanting reunion—not only restoration of the marriage but also psychological benefits such as nullification of rejection, recovery of prior investment in the relationship, and gratification of h/h hypergiving "need to be needed." In general, symbiants do not seek personality change as an avenue to reclaiming the partner, preferring to dream of reforming the partner. Indeed, a symbiant is prone to perceive in reunion an implicit confession that the ex has made a horrible mistake that must be corrected. The reconciliation thus means that the previously unacceptable and therefore forsaken mate was falsely accused of the charge of love failure, now affirming that h/s is—and perhaps always was—a worthy principal in the relationship (Baumeister & Wotman, 1992).

Long after breakup a symbiant is apt to accept an opportunity for reconciliation on almost any terms. Wounded self-esteem demands it, not to mention that the partner may be sorely missed. Such a symbiant has scarcely any doubt that reunion would prove to be a success this time around; h/s wants the relationship so badly and will work hard on behalf of what it ought to be. If an actual bid for reunion comes before substantial letting go has occurred, the offer can barely be examined, let alone refused. On one hand, reconciliation will seem a miraculous outcome, but on the other hand, it is no more than the coming true of vividly held fantasies.

But fantasies shift as psychic needs change. Although reunion long remains a dominating theme, a symbiant tends to elaborate two distinct scenarios in h/h imagination whereby the countersymbiant appears at the door in dire straits and begs to be restored to good graces. Variation A is *Reconciliation–Reject!* In the mind's eye, the countersymbiant is rebuffed, cast out, and left to the mercy of h/h own vices—good riddance to bad rubbish. Here a paradoxical revenge is being subjectively enacted; mastery of the rejection calls for paying back the countersymbiant in h/h own coin. Note, however, that even if reconciliation itself is repudiated, the countersymbiant's bid is the centerpiece of the fantasized plot, so that ambivalent enmeshment is obvious. In this mode of wish fulfillment, the ex-partner is now designated to become the carrier of the relationship, allowing the symbiant to be safely vindictive.

Variation B is *Reconciliation–Accept!* wherein a chastened countersymbiant is taken back and magnanimously invited to resume the previous status of loyal consort (Wymard, 1994). The message is a sublime "turn the other cheek" instead of the more talionic "eye for an eye, tooth for a tooth" of variation A. Subjectively, anger at rejection has been transcended and a future projected based on the transformative power of love. However, the latent side of this altruistic script is that the ex must pay for rejection by becoming a slave to the symbiant's goodness ever after.

The reveries of a forsaken mate serve as rehearsed responses to a possible invitation to reconcile. Variations A and B alternate at first, as if each were tried on to see how it fits. At certain points, one or the other gains ascendancy, expressing whichever side of the ambivalence is predominant—revenge or hypergiving. Until letting go resolves the issue, any actual overture from the countersymbiant simply sets in motion an already existent plan worked out in the symbiant's mind. The reply will be partly determined by the content of the real offer but also by the internalized script of the time. In this manner, reconciliation can be accepted or refused, without much effort to scrutinize the offer or consider the consequences. Thus, when an offer of reunion finally gives scope to the symbiant to make h/h fantasies come true, it is tempting to use this power to reject the erstwhile rejector if only out of spite. But it is usually even more tempting to use this power to reunite, in spite of common sense—a marriage can seldom be safely reconstituted based on an assumption that the ex must have learned h/h lesson.

The receipt of a reconciliation bid, which the countersymbiant makes for h/h own reasons and at a time of h/h choosing, will solve many problems for the symbiant, but it creates new ones as well. Before the offer, the question was how to engineer a reunion; but once an offer has been made, the situation changes. The overture soothes the self-doubt engendered by rejection, but only now can the symbiant tell whether it is actually the partner that was missed, or whether behind the wish for reconciliation there lurked a more urgent need to have hurt pride healed. When a clear-cut proposal to renew the ties is given, a no-longer-forsaken symbiant may discover just how little h/s wants to become reinvolved. It may be that what was most injurious in rejection (and which is now remedied) was the fact of rejection per se. Hence, even the most avidly sought reunion may seem superfluous once the countersymbiant has finally asked for it!

Moreover, the trauma imposed by breakup is still blamed mainly on the countersymbiant, and indeed h/h character will be seen in a far more critical light as a result of the separation's exposure of previously undetected flaws. Therefore, the imminent possibility of resumption of the relationship brings to pass an ironic dilemma: the partner may be emotionally welcomed back, while simultaneously not forgiven for being the sort of person who could have left. Now, just when a reconciliation might be forged, a symbiant is suddenly flooded with aversive reactions because something is brought to awareness largely avoided in previous thinking about reunion—the feeling of regretfully settling for a very imperfect mate.

Nevertheless, if the opportunity arrives, most symbiants jump at the chance to reconcile, particularly in the earlier stages of separation. They tend to brush aside pride, anger, and judgment because their overriding concern frequently is to make a new–old relationship work in order to cancel out the damage to self-esteem caused by the partner's defection. However, they may find that the cure is worse than the disease, for a symbiant may have been better off developing autonomous sources of a sense of worth rather than seeking a short-cut through grasping at the approval implicit in the partner's return to the marriage. Indeed, the decision to accept reunion in order to overcome the pain associated with rejection can prove to be masochistic because it so frequently invites another, and perhaps more devastating, rejection later on.

ON-AGAIN, OFF-AGAIN RELATIONSHIPS

In summary thus far, most reconciliations occur when (1) a countersymbiant is urgently seeking a haven from the hardships of separation by returning to the security of the union; and (2) a symbiant is urgently seeking restoration of a damaged pride system through recapturing the partner. But mutual urgency does not a remarriage make. Both parties may be denying the abyss between them because they feel abandoned or defeated apart. Each wrestles with the issue as to why h/s is getting involved anew with an obviously disappointing other, so that reentry into the committed union is fraught with doubts and trepidation. In reunion, the two parties may be giving and getting far less than they bargained for the first time around—and it was not enough then.

Based on data from Popenoe (1938), Weiss (1975) estimated that 50% of parting couples attempt reconciliation, with 50% of these couples parting again within a span of 1 year. Nevertheless, he suggested that reconciliations are worthwhile because the welfare of children may make the profits of success outweigh the debits of failure. He also pointed out that the odds for success are only slightly worse than those for second marriages to new partners, so that couples who reconcile can create a union "as reliable as any others in these days of marital instability" (p. 121). Should they establish a lasting union, he stated that in hindsight, the breakup will be merely "an incident in their lifelong marriage" (p. 121).

Weiss can hardly be accused of painting a sanguine picture, forecasting that half of separating couples will never reconcile, another quarter will make a futile attempt, and only the remaining quarter will overcome the rift of breakup. But inauspicious as are his estimates, they still err on the side of optimism. Hunt and Hunt (1977) found that ex-partners often think about reunion, but that their actual attempts typically are perfunctory, lasting no more than weeks or months, and generally "serve as final proof that the marriage cannot work" (p. 196). Lawyers are particularly skeptical about successful reunion: Reingold

(1976) quoted one attorney who insisted "you cannot knock a bent nail into the wall straight" (p. 119); he mentioned another who refused to explore reconciliation in matrimonial litigation after a woman he urged to try again with her husband was back in his office 2 years later, this time with an infant in her arms to complicate divorce proceedings. And, of course, statistics on rates of success must go beyond a 1-year follow-up study.

Weiss also greatly underestimated the lasting impact of a marital separation—breakup cannot be just "a passing episode" in a couple's history. Thus, assessment of reconciliation success must take into account quality, not merely duration, as seen in several case examples:

A woman invited her husband to return to the family after he "hassled" her so with jealousy and implorations to try again that she determined to teach him it was not healthy for him to remain in love with her. She also could not tolerate her children's criticism of her decision to put their father out, so that her intention in reconciling was to change their attitude as well. Thus, her husband returned to a wife who was aloof and surly, refused to have sex with him, and came and went without explanation. She was wishing that this time it would be he who would make the decision to end the marriage, thereby incurring the guilt she had been tagged with in the prior breakup. She was also punishing him for "forcing" her to resume the marriage. Two years later, the man admitted this was no marriage and took responsibility for its second demise, with the children now accepting the necessity for divorce. Another man went back to his ex-wife after a fight with his girlfriend; he was using the ex to keep his current lover under control. The reunion technically lasted more than a year, but, in reality, throughout this time the man went back and forth between the two women, at length opting to be with his girlfriend. A woman moved her mother into her home to help with the children after she had asked her husband to leave. When the couple reunited, she refused to move her mother out even though mother and husband had never been able to get along, and 2 years later she and her mother put her husband out again. It is now 3 years since a man came back to the wife he left; he did this immediately after his sister informed him that he could no longer stay in her apartment, leaving him no financial alternative to reconciliation.

As can be seen from such cases, a reconciliation can sometimes be no more than an opportunity designed to validate the disengaging partner's original judgment that the marriage cannot work, or just an opportunistic attempt to use the marriage as shelter in a storm. Thus, from both a quantitative and qualitative viewpoint, prospects for successful reunion must be considered clouded. But, in terms of consolation, even failed attempts are valuable insofar as they aid the couple to conclude that they did their best to salvage their union.

However, just as reconciliation does not prove the marriage is now workable, neither does a second breakup prove the marriage is now unworkable. Caught in ambivalence, some couples develop a cycle of separation and reunion, always seemingly on the verge of either resolving conjugal problems or definitively parting company. Thus, Weiss' figures could be extended to encompass an ongoing process: second separations are followed by second reconciliations half the time, to be succeeded in turn by a third separation half the time, and so on. Kitson (1992, pp. 95–96) offers supporting data for this extrapolation. In her divorce sample, 44% had a separation previous to the one for which they enrolled in her study, 10% had separated 5 or more times, and the mean number per respondent was 2.3 separations. Thus, her respondents at the point of divorce had undergone multiple prior breakups and reunions. Yet even these data understated the extent of indefinite cycles. People who elected to stay together after prior separations would not have volunteered to be subjects in Kitson's study, or could have reconciled *after* volunteering for her study. In general, a series of marital vicissitudes may have to occur before it comes to pass that either divorce or reconciliation is finally chosen by a given couple.

A man left his wife four times to pursue other relationships; each time he met troubles with his new lady, while his wife appeared to be doing comparatively better in her romantic life. He entered therapy and emerged with the conviction that he might just as well stay home and work things out with his wife inasmuch as he had intimacy problems in every relationship. As he phrased it, he had "grown up at last" and was prepared "to stop chasing fantasies." Another man also left four times, feeling he could always go back to his family if he had to. However, he got an increasingly cold shoulder from wife and children, and eventually he was able to return only after proving that he could give up his lady companions for his wife's sake and live alone. In these cases, the wives had become adept at living apart from their husbands and demanded a higher level of commitment from them with each reunion. At last report, both these rocky marriages were settling down after years of turmoil.

But there may also be a quite different outcome. A woman left her husband three times, but could not go on to a new relationship, continued to sleep only with her estranged husband, and at last gave in to his insistent demands for reconciliation. The fourth time she left, she moved away, forced herself to be sexually intimate with a lover, and cut off all contact with her husband. She had concluded that she could not "make it" in that marriage no matter how hard she tried. Another woman reconciled twice after her husband walked out on her, sacrificing her pride because "her kids need their father"; however, when the youngsters came of age, true to her silent vow, she walked out on him in favor of another man.

The on-again, off-again marriage is like a roulette wheel: "Around and around she goes, and where she stops, nobody knows."

DOES RECONCILIATION EVER BECOME AN IMPOSSIBILITY?

The more time elapsing after breakup, the less likely a couple is to reconcile. Yet "there is no point at which the possibility of a reconciliation totally disappears" (Weiss, 1975, p. 124). Both clinical and empirical data support this point. Weiner-Davis (1987) stated she had saved many "irreparably" damaged marriages in family therapy, arguing that there is a chance to salvage a relationship "as long as either partner has the slightest desire and/or hope of keeping a marriage alive. . . . Numerous visits to attorneys prior to treatment do not deter me, nor do separate living quarters" (p. 53). With or without therapy, one out of eight couples drop divorce petitions when they finally get to court (Hunt & Hunt, 1977).

Smith and Smith (1978) stated that there were 10,000 remarriages to the same person per year in the United States. In an article entitled "Will You Marry Me—Again?" Byron (1986) described several such cases—for example, the couple with children who remarried 2 years after their divorce, mainly to allay their children's suffering. Kitson (1992) reviewed pertinent empirical studies: Glick estimated that 4% of divorced individuals remarry their ex-spouses, Briscoe et al. reported 3% of their sample had remarried the same person within 2 years of divorce, and Kitson herself found that 3% of her respondents had remarried the person from whom they were divorced 3 years earlier and another 1.5% were living with a former spouse.

Despite the possibility over time that an estranged couple will reconcile (with or without legal remarriage), this still becomes more improbable with each passing year. Moreover, an effective point of no return will eventually be reached in any relationship, by choice of either partner. Some countersymbiants demonstrate determination never to return by the spirit in which they leave, having done the work of letting go before departure. Similarly, a symbiant in separation can reach a decisive judgment whereby the countersymbiant can no longer be considered a viable partner. Further, even if an estranged couple are tempted to try again, they may realize that they cannot reconstruct a relationship that has been irretrievably damaged by their conduct of the breakup. In the final analysis, experiences in separation tend to pull the partners farther and farther apart until they have almost no common ground to meet or share, not to mention that commitments may have been made to new mates that can largely preclude their ever getting back together.

Most reconciliations that do occur after many years apart have some mutual bond—usually minor children—that keeps the couple in contact and provides a rationale for another go at the marriage. However, it seems obvious that after a lapse of 5 or more years (sufficient time for letting go), it becomes remote in a statistical sense to think in terms of reconciliation, although it remains theoretically possible. To demonstrate that reunion remains an option no matter how much time has passed, Weiss cited a case in which reunion took place after a decade of separation. After divorce, two ex-spouses remarried new partners, but both second spouses eventually died. Thus, the former couple could date again, and they soon remarried each other. Weiss did not comment on the fact that such a belated reconciliation required two unanticipated providential intercessions to bring about this couple's reunion.

SUCCESSFUL VERSUS UNSUCCESSFUL RECONCILIATIONS

Ahrons (1994) observed that many couples reconcile right after one party states a definite plan to leave or does leave; at times, the result is a probing of problems that brings about an improved marriage. However, Ahrons believed that in most instances a quick reconciliation is "a surface illusion, prompted by fear" (p. 106). Although some couples took a trip to Europe, bought a new house, or had a baby, the fundamental issues that divided them were not resolved, shortly emerging to cause a second breakup. For example, when one woman was begged to return, she went back to a husband who was now highly affectionate and took her on a 2-week vacation, but 4 weeks later the woman decided nothing had changed and she left once again, this time for good. Ahrons concluded that when one party seeks separation, "the announcement indicates that all was not well; that deep problems exist; and that communication, attention to facts, and reorganization must now occur. Superficial changes, no matter how spectacular, only delay the pain" (p. 107).

Some reconciliations occur after a long separation and are more considered than the hasty ones described by Ahrons. Yet these too may be put together with deceptive simplicity. An earnest talk is arranged in which the couple express their disappointments and current needs.

They explain why they did certain hurtful things and apologize. They look with questioning and longing at each other, disclosing their loneliness, their nostalgia for aspects of the old union, and their continued caring. They then draw up an informal contract for changes in what had been the prior structure of their relationship. Plans are made for the transition from separate lives back to a working partnership. A schedule is established for the winding up of personal business before reconciliation, including third-party involvements; this timetable also gives the couple time to test their renovated union in the interim. As the couple parts, this fateful encounter has the aura of a surreal event—reunion was precisely the outcome excluded from the realm of possibility when they split up, but it is now the outcome after all.

But complications surface soon enough. For the symbiant, it feels as if the prodigal has had an epiphany and come penitently home. However, that satisfaction is counterbalanced by the manifest necessity to forgive and forget. Forgive, maybe—forget, never! By assenting to the reunion, the symbiant has to allow the ex-partner to kiss away the tears the latter caused to flow. To tolerate this, a symbiant must see the countersymbiant as a changed person: more mature, engaged, and empathic. Such changes are counted on to heal the wounds of breakup. Yet despite an almost blind faith in the restorative powers of reconciliation, a deep-seated distrust remains. Is this partner someone to love and trust again? Will h/s walk out again? Has h/s really learned the error of past ways? Have ties to a third party been cut forever? Does h/s love me?

For the countersymbiant, once reconciliation is imminent, it feels as if what was a bed of thorns may turn out to be a little bit rosy after all (or perhaps just less thorny). The ex-mate can now be affectionately reembraced in a rediscovery of the familiar warmth of hearth and home. Life seems more orderly and sane, the future less solitary. The faults of the mate have been identified and even punished by the clear behavioral statement of quitting the relationship, so the mate now stands forewarned of the consequences of continued neglect of the countersymbiant's vital needs—breakup has at least served that purpose. Such are the positive aspects of reconciling, but the countersymbiant too has a sense of something amiss. Can happiness be found in a relationship that was a proven failure? Has the mate learned the error of past ways? How much autonomy will have to be surrendered in order to regain trust? Will breakup be brought up in every fight? Is all this trouble worth it?

The marital reconciliation takes place in a very different atmosphere than did the original wedding. There may be a degree of honeymoon excitement, but there is also a measured wariness—a suspicion of the process—that accompanies the renewal. Each party is deliberately accepting a spouse who has certain traits not to be abided. Both keenly realize that the potential of the relationship has a definite upper limit. Although failure is surely a realistic concern, an even stronger dread is that success of the reunion will have to be struggled for on a daily basis. As in the Greek myth of Sisyphus, the great stone has to be forever rolled uphill; rest can jeopardize the fruit of preceding labors. In short, reunions that succeed require sustained commitment to intimate relating.

This point has been made by many clinicians. Jagers (1989), a pastoral counselor, held that a committed union can be put back together better than it was before if there is open communication, mutual forgiving, and commitment to a religious ideal of marriage. Similarly, Larson (1993), a divorce mediator, has suggested that there is potential for reconciliation despite separation strife whenever breakup "acts as a catalyst in forcing individuals to come to terms with themselves. . . . Reconciliation becomes possible when the old childhood dramas/traumas are acknowledged as an internal struggle and when their projections as an external struggle with the ex-spouse ends" (p. 96). The common denominator here is that enhanced communication and intimacy, plus taking responsibility for one's own deficits instead of blaming the partner, will bring about a better marriage than the one that was destroyed by the breakup.

The respective attitudes of the two principals are crucial, especially in the first year, for neither can expect to simply pick up where h/s left off. Fights can be deferred for only so long and eventually a quarrel will erupt, so that the problems that drove them apart come up yet again. In these disputes, there is a temptation on both sides to give up and get out. In addition, there are new issues, including redistribution of domestic tasks, each spouse's desire to preserve gains made in separation, and the relinquishing of third-party involvements. In respect to the latter, a spouse may now have trouble giving up a lover who has come to personify an insurance policy against failure of the reconciliation. Jealousy too can become a major issue, either because former lovers are in fact not given up, or because the jealous suspicions of one mate become insupportable to the other. These problems must somehow be addressed, and usually only recall of past anguish in separation can prevent one spouse or the other from walking out the door.

All good reconciliations—and indeed all good marriages—have gone through stressful periods before they can reach a plateau where two very different people who happen to be married to each other can live together in relative harmony. However, unlike the original wedding, a reconciliation does not allow either party to project a blissful future in fantasy—indeed, *reconciliation may be defined as a committed partnership carrying on in the absence of romantic illusions.* The members of the couple know that their match was not made in heaven. They have to admit that they have hurt each other and may at times do so again. Much work has to be done to maintain the relationship; the false intimacy they had in the past has to be replaced by true intimacy in the present. The couple's rewards are the closeness they forge, the intactness of the family unit, and a sense of life honorably (though fallibly) lived. It is like Moses being sent to the Promised Land: it does not matter whether it is garden or desert—one belongs there and one gratefully makes the best of it. All things considered, the couple's equivalent of W. C. Fields's Philadelphia is where they would rather be.

VI

Psychological and Social Adjustment

Introduction

> The final stage is come when Man has obtained full control over himself [and conquered human nature]. But the power of Man to make himself what he pleases means . . . the power of some men to make other men what *they* please. . . . [The conditioners] are emancipated [but not] bad men. They are, rather, not men (in the old sense) at all. [Rather] they have sacrificed their own share in traditional humanity in order to devote themselves to the task of deciding what "humanity" shall henceforth mean. . . . Nor are their subjects necessarily unhappy men. They are not men at all: they are artifacts. Man's final conquest [of human nature] has proved to be the abolition of Man.
> —C. S. LEWIS (1947, pp. 72–77)

Our concluding topic is "adjustment"—a conception of mental health that is double-edged. On one hand, all psychological theories assume that every human being has the task of adjustment to the culture in which h/s was born and so must incorporate its worldview, learn its skills, and accept its values. On the other hand, adaptation can also be evaluated negatively, interpreted to mean that a person conforms to a culture even if its predominant mores conflict with humanistic concerns or miscalculates physical or social reality. Thus, adjustment is necessary for both individual and collective survival, but we are always left with *a critique of the culture itself* as the key to any assessment of its viability.

Insofar as contemporary society impinges on divorce, people tend to be viewed these days as highly adaptable where intimate relationships are concerned. Lifton (1971) has postulated that "protean man" follows cultural patterns so that no fixed human nature exists and all social change is possible. In behavioral psychology (Skinner, 1972), the scientific suggestion is put forth that almost any aspect of behavior can be shaped to comply with social design. Cognitive approaches to psychotherapy assert that clients can bring their feelings into line with a rational appraisal of their situation (Ellis, 1975). Thus, what had always been seen as limitations in human capacity to deal with separation trauma now tend to be replaced by social inculcation, rationality, and will power as governing psychological functioning. Applied to divorce, this thinking takes the form of a concept of adjustment that expects people to ride the rails of object loss with virtual equanimity, no matter what the destination might be. In effect, the modern approach categorically rejects the idea that emotion—including disturbance—is an innate biological mechanism whereby human beings express how well or poorly their essential needs are being met. Rather than basing social norms for committed unions on the principle that folks must not be pushed beyond what they can psychologically bear, proponents of *dispassionate divorce* legislate the withering away of passion as a reaction. Such an ideology spells out an imminent disintegration for any cohesive society and could only arise in a society that is already seriously unglued.

Chapter 18 is written for fellow clinicians. It attempts to detail emerging trends in psychotherapy, some of which reflect anti-psychological attitudes toward human behavior in problematic love relationships and thus are damaging not only to clients but also to the integrity of the field itself. We try to indicate what seems to us more realistic guidelines for individual and family therapists working with clients undergoing marital separation.

Breakup today is also greatly affected by a change in moral climate. Chapter 19 assesses the contemporary status of *guilt,* which once was a major tie holding a restless countersymbiant into a tenuous marriage. The rise of a new standard of morality—now deriving from entitlement instead of responsibility—is surely consequential beyond divorce. The present mores of divorce must obviously be derived from, and consonant with, the overall social values of our culture, but the ramifications of divorce in turn contribute to the setting of community ethical standards. We will show that guilt, along with all the passions of enmeshment, is now expected to be conditioned out of the human psyche in order to make breakup easier. Nevertheless, the survival of guilt in an age that idealizes dispassionate divorce attests to the impossibility of abolishing troubling aspects of human nature without recreating such aspects in more insidious, pathological forms.

This book concludes by examining the stance of the mental health field, which has, by and large, taken a neutral view when commitments are broken inasmuch as ethics lies outside our competence. This position effectively denies the interpersonal and social meaning of behavior and suggests that our society, insofar as represented by these therapists, has lost its moral bearings.

Our own position is that guilt reactions are appropriate and inevitable in breaking a commitment, but that guilt need not preclude one from leaving what is experienced as a bad marriage. Rather, when an unsatisfying marriage is left, the conscience of the individual still requires that responsibility be accepted, a measure of empathic concern shown to those hurt by this action (spouse and children), and acknowledgement made that community standards upholding the institution of the family have been weakened. The individual may resist at these superego demands, but doubts about the course of action taken and underlying character can never be completely suppressed, even by a reassuring course of therapy. Whether consciously admitted or unconsciously acted out, guilt is a part of the price to be paid in opting for divorce.

Furthermore, there are few breakups in which one can "just leave" without family members evaluating the morality of this decision. The violation of profound imperatives inherent in the symbiotic structure of a family unit conveys its own sense of what is right and wrong, taking the form of acrimonious reactions, adverse judgments, and psychological disturbance in ex-mate or children. Thus, the family too forces confrontation with ethical issues.

All told, despite narcissistic trends in the mental health field and society in general that attempt to negate any sense of guilt in the quest for a better life through unilateral dissolution of a committed union, a moral dimension cannot really be eliminated from the phenomenon of divorce (or from social life overall). Even if the culture dictates the abolition of guilt, man as a "social animal" must submit to innate homeostatic mechanisms that regulate personal, family, and communal life, or else pursue the chimera of transformation of the human species as we know it.

~~ 18

The Psychotherapy of Marital Breakups

The fact that so many clinicians are committed to the
preservation of marriage and the nuclear family can play havoc
with their treatment of couples contemplating divorce. . . .
[They] help people settle for mediocre marriages . . . rather than
help them find the courage to achieve a . . . constructive
separation. . . . We can only guess at how often this kind of
thing happens, but we can take a clue from the expressed
attitudes of many professionals toward the evils of divorce. It is
tragic that when people find it impossible to live together, they
are so often directed back to unhappy marital situations by . . .
therapists.

> —GETTLEMAN AND MARKOWITZ (1974, pp. 70–71)

Compounding the [marital crisis was] that counseling itself
pulled us further apart. The very core of what . . . the counseling
profession preaches is the enshrinement of self, at the expense
of marital union and compromise. [When my wife said], "Do
you realize how much pain and effort it would take to work out
this goddamn mess?" [the counselor did not] suggest it was
worth it. . . . I remember telling myself that a marriage
counselor was in the business of saving marriages . . . [but] the
counselor told me: "That isn't true. We are in the business of
saving individuals, not marriages." I am an individual; my
children are individuals; who cared about saving us? Marriage
counseling can't continue to follow the unreal premise that you
treat married persons the same way you treat individuals who
have no connections, no relationships, no responsibilities.

> —MARTIN (1975, pp. 273–274)

PSYCHOPATHOLOGY AND DIVORCE

A marital crisis challenges a person's functioning as a stable, rational,
and loving human being, thereby greatly increasing risk factors for
psychopathology and loading clinical practices with divorce-related
cases (Charlton, 1980). Research has long shown that adult depres-

sion most often occurs in a context of marital tension or separation (Paykel, Myers, Dienelt, Klerman, Lindenthal, & Pepper, 1969), with more than one-quarter of people involved in breakup entering psychotherapy (Gurin, Veroff, & Feld, 1960). As for children, more than twice as many from divorced as compared with intact families were in treatment (Solomon, 1989). Furthermore, up to 80% of cases in child guidance clinics involve minors from single-parent homes—a statistic far exceeding their ratio within the general population (Wallerstein, 1984a).

Instead of regarding divorce trauma as causing such widespread psychopathology, some clinicians argue that those who divorce are apt to be people who already had psychological problems that made them unable to live intimately with a spouse, thus accounting for why their marriages failed and why they—and their children—need therapy. This view has been called "selectivity theory" (Kitson, 1992), according to which such people either never marry or are divorce-prone personalities. The apostle here is Bergler (1948), a psychoanalyst who insisted that divorce is a neurotic solution chosen by neurotic persons, leading to further marriages and divorces: "The futility of divorce can be established clinically; the second, third, and nth marriages are but repetitions of previous experiences" (p. xiv). As for empirical data, Nelson (1994) found higher rates of psychiatric conditions in divorced as contrasted with married people, considering psychiatric disorder as more cause than effect of divorce. In an Ohio sample, Kitson (1992) found that hospitalization for psychological problems, and reports of partners having such problems, were higher for divorced subjects than in a married control group, but—unlike Nelson—she was unsure whether such psychopathology existed before breakup or developed after it. Rice and Rice (1986) summarized the literature, finding that compared with married controls, divorced individuals are more likely to be diagnosed with alcoholism, senility, completed suicides, car accidents, and psychiatric admissions; the divorced population also adjusts less well than the widowed. But, given the usually severe stress of divorce, plus recovery from acute symptoms within 6–12 months, Rice and Rice concluded that in most instances a natural adjustment reaction rather than character disorder accounts for psychopathology after breakup. Moreover, Kressel (1980) pointed out that there tends to be overdiagnosis during the initial postseparation phase in the treatment of patients undergoing divorce.

Distress has been shown to be greater according to degree of attachment to the former spouse (Brown, Felton, Whiteman, & Manela, 1980), but this finding too has been differently interpreted within the divorce literature. On one hand, the ability to mourn may be seen as critical to the ability to love (Bak, 1973). As Vaillant (1985) stated: "Separation from and loss of those we love do not cause psychopathology. Rather, failure to internalize those whom we have loved—or never having loved at all—causes psychopathology" (p. 59). He suggested that loss can be seen as a metaphor for attachment (without which it cannot occur as a psychic experience); symptoms manifested around loss are thus ordinary human adaptive mechanisms that speak to basic psychological health, not disorder.

In contrast, overwhelming grief reactions are seen by some clinicians as a sign of emotional imbalance. Tennov (1979) pointed out that many facets of normal behavior by unrequited lovers are stigmatized by certain theorists as personality defects, regarded as neurotic obsession, addiction, erotomania, morbid dependency, masochism, and so on. She reviewed four books whose authors pathologized romantic unhappiness caused by a relationship's demise: Bohannon (1969) held that passions are used as an excuse when people want to be irresponsible; Bach and Deutsch (1971) described "lovesickness" as a neurotic barrier that impedes getting on with one's life; Rimmer (1973) saw pining in love as "game playing"; and Peele and Brodsky (1975) labeled ongoing attachment an "addiction." Tennov commented that these writers regard the suffering of romantic heartbreak as "willful wrongheadedness" (p. 181), complaining that too many therapists were currently operating out of a frame of reference ill suited for a condition they are often called upon to treat.

Although all divorce therapists agree on the typical postdivorce clinical picture, it is apparent that disagreement abounds as to what is the meaning of psychopathology and which partner has it. To hear Vaillant, it is the partner who never loved or does not miss a mate of many years; to hear Tennov's authors, it is the spouse who vehemently resists divorce and readjustment. In short, corresponding to the divergent positions of a parting couple, the field of divorce therapy has two ideological camps, adherence to which turns out to be more important a factor in treatment than the type of therapy offered or the therapist's theoretical training.

THE EMERGING SPECIALTY OF DIVORCE THERAPY

The clinical involvement of mental health professionals with parting couples has not yet signified the appearance of any general theory on the management of such treatment. There is no training program and licensure for divorce therapy. It is neither a distinct discipline nor a technique, but rather a hybrid enterprise that at times utilizes such modalities as crisis intervention, family therapy, marriage counseling, divorce mediation, support groups, and services for children (Kaslow, 1981). In addition, academic training seldom explicitly addresses love relationships, romantic breakups, and custody dispositions: practitioners must rely mainly on their own personal knowledge and experience about the divorce process (Everett & Volgy, 1991). But the most vexing issue is the fact that there is not a common base of values on which clinicians can agree. For example, Walsh (1991) has insisted that new models of "family" are needed in a society that continues to define the intact nuclear family as the norm, pointing out that for children the most dysfunctional units are nominally intact, but in which the parents are unhappily married. Yet, despite acceptance of this view, ambiguity still abounds as to whether a therapist should attempt to save a particular "bad" marriage (Crosby, 1989).

But even with so much lack of uniformity, there are still commonalities and areas of consensus across the many brands of divorce therapy. Everett and Volgy (1991) based the need for divorce therapy on the impairment of the viability and organization of the family process, so that both emotional and behavioral restructuring for all family members is required. Rice and Rice (1986) made a distinction between *marital therapy* focused on the rehabilitative potential of the union and *divorce therapy* focused on disengagement of the partners—couples can start out with marital therapy but later shift to divorce therapy. Isaacs et al. (1986) saw the protection of children as a primary concern in work with parting parents. Kaslow (1981) set forth the principle that in therapy during the predivorce decision-making phase, the question of breakup is regarded as a joint responsibility rather than a result of "his" or "her" problems. Kressel (1980) stated that in therapy during the postseparation phase, addressing the economic and legal concerns of clients is both legitimate and necessary, without the therapist's having to be a lawyer or an accountant. As for divorce mediation, the field tends to prefer this service to an adversarial legal process, but divorce mediation is not therapy per se, nor is the mediator necessarily a trained therapist.

PRESCRIPTION FOR A PARADOX: THE "HEALTHY" DIVORCE

Earlier in this book, we dealt with the friendly divorce, the no-fault divorce, and the creative divorce; we must now also address the "healthy" divorce. One wonders what is it about divorce that so attracts affirmative qualifiers? The issue goes beyond mere propaganda to enhance the public image of divorce; there is a genuine need within our culture to ameliorate the antisocial aspects of divorce, so that rules of conduct must be applied to restrain its worst excesses. The same restraining process is evident when modern people confront the savagery of warfare; in consequence, we have developed codes of chivalry, military law, the Geneva Convention, concepts of "war crimes," and so forth. To be acceptable to the modern conscience, divorce too must be contained in order to avert such destructive behaviors as vendettas, crimes of passion, and vindictive litigation. Even though the term "healthy divorce" is misleading in the sense that it promises a sanitary manner to sever marital ties, it does convey the need to set limits on the acrimony of the parting couple who must cooperate so as not to ruin their own or their children's lives. Hence, society has turned to therapists to supervise the divorce dynamic—a task that, not by coincidence, helps safeguard the institution of divorce itself.

For the therapist, the most immediate concern in divorce is that parents and children should surmount its travail, emerging as unscathed as possible. Beyond that, in the absence of a common value base in divorce, every therapist is thrown back onto personal preconceptions. If h/s turns to the literature, the "Prescription for a Healthy Divorce" by Cassius and Koonce (1974) is representative of this genre and will do as well as any for a start. These authors list 11 elements, without any set order of priority:

1. Avoid destructive outlets for anger by refusing to act toward your ex the way h/s has treated you.
2. See a lawyer.
3. Make provision for your children.
4. Consider seeing a therapist.
5. Develop new aspirations within your reach.
6. Work on a good self-concept.
7. Eliminate fears that you can't manage on your own.
8. Own the failure of divorce and still be OK; own social opprobrium and still be OK.
9. Sacrifice for the benefit of kids.
10. Help your kids to see that they are not responsible for their parents' separation.
11. Avoid marital reentry with a carbon copy of your ex, or with one who mirrors your own problems.

Cassius and Koonce key healthy divorce to the transactional analysis formula "I'm OK; you're OK," but emphasize "I'm OK." One merely follows the formula so that separation is healthy for each partner; with aid from lawyer or therapist, life soon gets back on track. But there is a moral problem in the tendency to make unjust or grievous situations not intrinsically OK appear to be otherwise (Schwartz, 1985–1986). As for logic, the problem with taking "healthy" divorce too literally is that, were its implementation truly feasible, the couple's separation would be superfluous—if they could work out their divorce as prescribed, they would have already worked out their marital issues, or if apart, they could proceed to reconciliation. In reality, a separation has occurred because two spouses have not been able to come anywhere close to seeing self and partner as OK, restraining anger, sacrificing for children, avoiding neurotic patterns, and so forth. We cannot hope to set standards in breakup that are higher than those that obtained in marriage. It seems naive to expect a couple in breakup to now get along after they have parted company because they could not get along.

However, as noted earlier, "healthy divorce" does not have to be taken so literally; it can be more modestly understood to refer to ways to get apart despite destructive enmeshment. Everett and Everett (1994) offered such an appraisal in *Healthy Divorce*. They specified three major tasks: letting go, developing new social ties, and redefining parental roles. As experienced divorce therapists, they did not expect acrimony to be averted, recognized that considerable time is needed for both parties to adapt, and were aware that trauma and disillusion could befall the children. Yet, although much sensible advice is dispensed, their outlook is often *too* sensible—as if human beings were ahistorical, ignoring past wounds by making only rational, pragmatic choices in the present. Worse yet, their title is apt to be misunderstood by the public and hence will contribute to glossing over the more somber aspects of the divorce reality.

The title of Ahrons's (1994) *The Good Divorce* is subject to equivalent criticism, because it implies that divorce is generally beneficial to the family. Its author would not be upset by this objection inasmuch as her message is that one can achieve a divorce "in which both the couple and the children emerge at least as well emotionally as they were before the divorce" (p. 2). In her view, everybody can profit, providing breakup is well conducted. Ahrons argued that parting couples will arrive at a friendly or, at the minimum, a cooperative divorce if they do such things as consider each other's feelings, maintain lines of communication, give priority to the welfare of children and remember that the co-parent remains part of one's extended family. In her sample of binuclear Wisconsin families, she found that about half the former couples, most now remarried, were able to attain this degree of civil dealings, demonstrating that divorce need not be as "bad" as often advertised. But her optimism raises some serious questions.

First, it is not clear whether this glass is half full or half empty, in that only 50% of her sample achieved a "good divorce." Moreover, it should be noted that other researchers are much less sanguine about prospects; for example, Arendell (1986, p. 103) tallied only 18% of "good divorce" in her sample.

Second, it appears that even the half who did meet Ahrons's criteria still went through turmoil before getting to this point, including Ahrons herself. In an autobiographical aside, she stated, "I was the one who left, and for two miserable years my husband and I battled constantly over custody, visitation, and child support. There were private detectives, a kidnapping, several lawyers, and two years of legal fees that took me ten years to pay off" (pp. 1–2). Given this history, Ahrons can understandably be proud of finally establishing a working partnership around child care with her ex-husband, along the way gleaning much knowledge about divorce from her own experience. Yet, by the same token, she cannot offer a cheerful view of divorce to readers based on her personal story.

Third, Ahrons emphasized efforts at "getting along," based on the concept that former spouses with children become members of an extended binuclear family. But we wonder whether such an approach is in part manipulative, serving to protect the interests and reputation of the divorce initiator by keeping in check the reciprocal's disapproval and hostility. To the extent that our suspicion is warranted in a given case, it is disingenuous to speak of a "good divorce."

All in all, in evaluating Ahrons's position, we agree that acrimony in the divorce process must be contained, but not that the acrimony will cease if a cooperative course is prescribed for both sides, nor that transforming early acrimony about child care into later civility eliminates the dark side of divorce.

THE ESTRANGED COUPLE AND DIVORCE THERAPY

In the postseparation phase, divorce therapy is a clinical approach that still treats an estranged couple as a functional unit, even if they now have minimal and mostly negative dealings with each other. But in these circumstances, conjoint therapy tends to occur as a result of two forms of external pressure: either a child becomes "disturbed" and the estranged parents are urged to enter treatment together to coordinate child care, or the ex-couple are so embroiled in litigation that they are court-remanded to a divorce mediation service. What this means is that even when there is conjoint divorce therapy, most ex-couples did not ask for it of their own volition. This is to be expected, for no matter how wretched their interactions, one or the other ex-spouse resists the idea of treatment because this might be an open admission that they are still "in relationship." They can also object that it is more logical to end their marriage by having nothing further to do with each other rather than by starting conjoint treatment. Another source of resistance comes from the sense that divorce therapy is like locking the barn door after the horse is gone. It is obvious that divorce therapy is bound to be an unwelcome and quasi-absurd service from the point of view of its intended consumers.

In spite of such reservations, professional intervention may still be required for the ex-couple who have not been able to get safely or sanely apart. *The couple who could not cooperate to live together must now cooperate not to live together.* This task pushes many parting partners toward counseling, perhaps conjointly for the couple or family, but far more commonly for one or both partners in individual treatment. Indeed, in many such individual therapies, an effort was made prior to breakup by the patient or therapist to include the other spouse, but that spouse's refusal to participate often decidedly tilts the treatment into an individualized form of divorce therapy (Willi, 1984; Whitaker & Miller, 1972).

Once treatment is sought, however, the couple's issues will be complicated by the influence of a therapist on their interactions. This therapist has a private life in which issues of marriage and separation also had to be addressed, with implications for the conduct of h/h professional practice. Accordingly, we arrive at the highly complicating factor in divorce therapy of countertransference.

IATROGENIC MARRIAGE AND IATROGENIC DIVORCE

"The operation was a success, but the patient died." This statement epitomizes the human fear that professional intercession in the course of a disease can at times be more detrimental than the disease itself. Such dire outcomes occur when the physician has misdiagnosed the condition, miscalculated the patient's ability to endure a procedure, or used an improper procedure. In medicine we speak of "iatrogenic illness" to characterize damage a physician inadvertently causes when remedies are used that turn out to be ill suited to the patient's condition. If the patient dies, we shake our heads and say, "Doctors bury their mistakes."

Psychotherapy too causes iatrogenic illness—sometimes the remedy proves worse than the disease. Although patients seldom die of psychiatric misjudgments, the quality of their lives is bound to suffer in consequence of therapeutic error. However, when it comes to psychotherapy, it is difficult to judge instances of "unhelpful helpfulness" because, among other problems, treatment goals may be controversial or involve issues beyond symptomatic relief. The outcome of therapy—for good or ill in an observer's eyes—thus can be tied to influence of the therapist's values.

Nearly all clinicians agree on this point: Frank (1973) has argued that therapy is essentially a process of persuasion; Bandura and Walters (1963) considered social modeling the basis of treatment, Kohut (1971) cited idealization of the therapist as a curative factor; and Vardy (1972), Kovel (1981), and Peck (1983) have all stressed from different viewpoints that the ideology of the therapist is crucial. Such a generic perspective on treatment means that divorce therapy, like all psychological interventions, is a value-laden enterprise—the therapist's values predetermine to a certain extent the course of the divorce. Because marital breakup is a debatable life choice, therapists will vary in their formulation of the issues, impose their own ideas on how the process should be managed, and develop identifications and countertransferences. This is true of all therapists. Although the field generally adopts the position that therapists must strive to be neutral concerning preservation of a working marriage, not all clinicians abide by this canon of therapeutic practice and none can completely guard against h/h own unconscious intrusions and superego judgments. Of course, it is standard procedure to consult with the patient as to desired marital outcome and structure the therapy accordingly, but this does not speak to the therapist's own predilections that have a bearing on the work. At best, therapists can be candid with the patient if their preferences and principles threaten the treatment, and then strive to be as neutral as possible or make a referral.

But if a therapist will not or cannot control the imposition of h/h own views on the patient, a line is crossed into the domain of unhelpful helpfulness. When a therapist guides the patient toward breakup of a troubled relationship as a means to validate h/h own personal choices regarding marriage, it is fair to speak of "iatrogenic divorce." As for the opposite therapeutic error, when a therapist denies problems with a mate in h/h own marriage and thus cannot accept divorce as an option, it is equally appropriate to think of a committed union in which a patient has been pressured to remain as an "iatrogenic marriage." We will now go into more depth.

Iatrogenic Divorce

In the novel *Kramer vs. Kramer* (Corman, 1977), after an absence of a year, Mrs. Kramer unexpectedly phoned to request a meeting in a restaurant. Mr. Kramer went with ideas of reconciliation dancing in his head—surely she must have discovered that she at least missed their toddler son, that it was a mistake to leave, and that it was worth the hard work to keep a family intact. He asked Mrs. Kramer about her life in the interim and she replied she had taken a job in California and entered therapy. Mr. Kramer then inquired if she had learned anything in therapy about herself. She responded that she now realized that she never should have married him and why she had no choice but to depart so abruptly.

If this was the "insight" imparted in therapy, it would seem that Mrs. Kramer's counseling had a pro-divorce orientation. Such views are rife in the professional literature. For example, Walder (1978) described his work with a patient who was happy when with her lover but unhappy at home when with her spouse. He framed the situation as follows: she had picked the wrong sort of husband, could be more "herself" with someone else, and was looking for a better relationship to supplant the marriage. This formulation must have been just what the patient wanted to hear, and she soon left her husband—a successful outcome, according to Walder. However, when several other patients resisted similar interpretations of their affairs, Walder would counter that they were "covering up" the misery within their marriages because they were fearful to be on their own (pp. 37–42). When therapists encourage their patients to divorce, externalizing blame for conjugal problems by pointing to a "wrong" mate, one may suspect that the therapist is replaying via the patient's treatment the issues in h/h own marriage(s).

A related form of countertransferential pro-divorce bias has to do with treatment of the forsaken mate: this patient must be "educated" to recognize that h/s has construed the experience of rejection in love pathologically so that, while object loss is real, a traumatic reaction is inappropriate and self-inflicted. After all, this position argues, the loss of a lover does not mean that one is an unworthy mate. Although true, a reassurance of this type is not apt to be helpful at the point of crisis. Indeed, it seems to us a defense mechanism that provides self-reassurance to the therapist that no one will ever matter so much as to hurt the therapist in the same way as the patient has been hurt. Consider the following illustration. Myers (1989) supervised a senior resident in psychiatry who was expressing dismay with a patient whose marriage had just ended: "I can't understand why he's so depressed. He's mired in self-pity. Hell, he's young, he's good-looking, he's got a good job—there're all kinds of women out there if only he'd get off his butt and meet some of them!" (p. 261). Myers thought this resident had much to learn about the magnitude of grief involved in breakup, but his comment may be too charitable in that such an attitude does not necessarily arise from ignorance or inexperience so much as from a characterological defense against attachment.

According to Tennov (1979), Albert Ellis is the prime example of a therapist who uses this characterological defense in clinical practice. Ellis stated that only the "illogical interpretation" of a forsaken lover causes severe distress—if the former partner were not idealized and granted a sexual monopoly, a patient could come through breakup a little bit sad, but never be grief-stricken or lastingly disturbed. Ellis held that the more rational solution is for the forsaken party to go out and find a new partner. His method in fending off heartbreak is to reason (Tennov says "browbeat," p. 184) his patients into taking the cognitive stance that love is neither permanent nor exclusive. Tennov reacted to Ellis' avowed treatment philosophy by wondering whether he had ever been in love. She decided from what she knew about him that he had not and, hence, could not understand what is at stake for his patients.

Although Tennov's critique verges on an *ad hominem* dismissal of Ellis' position, she does indicate how countertransference may induce a therapist to become intolerant of a patient's lovelorn anguish and so push instead for new involvements, even if this promotes pointless promiscuity or "falling in love on the rebound." This tendency is exemplified by Wanderer and Cabot (1978), who recommended an affair or "rebound" relationship by the 11th week after breakup "when you're already tired of being alone" and need "instant memories" by immersion in a new love object (p. 196).

Lubetkin and Oumano (1991) used cognitive–behavioral techniques to apply Ellis's ideas to divorce therapy. They urged those who might hesitate to "bail out" of an unhappy marriage to jump from a crashing airplane for their own sake. The cognitive aspect of their work is based on the view that research has shown that "an irrational cognitive component is the basis of every fear you have" (p. 119) and "fear is the single most common reason why people do not bail out" (p. 119), so standard behavioral treatments for anxiety disorder can be applied. Thus, when a patient is afraid of hurting the mate among other reasons for not leaving, they bring to bear such interventions as relaxation and systematic desensitization, with the aim of "reprogramming" the patient (p. 136). In short, Lubetkin and Oumano treat the many compunctions that complicate, delay, or prevent leaving a marriage as phobic reactions.

In a review of the literature, Rice and Rice (1986) doubted whether behavioral contracting, conflict management, and rational problem solving are effective models for divorce therapy. Such treatments focus on eliminating so-called symptoms while not addressing underlying issues of grief, loss, anger, and revenge. Thus, Rice and Rice complained that "some behavior therapists ignore [collusion] between couples, blame noncompliance with the therapist change-efforts mainly on salient skill deficits, and contend it is the job of the therapist to teach such skills" (pp. 53–54). To reduce therapy in this manner to the eradication of bonding implies a denial of attachment needs on the part of the therapist, so it can be surmised that h/h own conduct in close relationships has been idealized as a paradigm of "mental health" for self and patients.

In the course of this book, we have encountered the work of many therapists who promote iatrogenic divorce. The emphasis these therapists collectively place on such values as self-actualization, the cult of individualism, sexual liberation, and serial marriage poses a threat to the viability of the nuclear family, and they do not blanch at this recognition. Such clinicians could hardly be expected to maintain a nuclear family themselves, and most of them more or less proudly acknowledge this in their writings, while openly inviting their patients to follow in their footsteps.

Iatrogenic Marriage

In the novel *Diary of a Mad Housewife* (Kaufman, 1967) an unhappy woman goes to a male therapist with her marital woes and is told she is resisting her feminine role as wife and mother. This piece of counseling is ridiculed in the movie version through the cinematic device of showing the therapist upside-down while he is delivering these weighty words. In effect, the woman can only experience herself as topsy-turvy in relation to the therapist—he does not know (and does not want to know) what she is troubled about, so his interventions are insensitive and controlling. Perhaps this therapist is protecting his own marriage to a "mad housewife." If so, his blind spot in the treatment would duplicate his blind spot within his own home—that is, wanting a woman to stay at her conjugal post, no matter how stultifying her marriage, in the name of being "mature" and "well-adjusted."

A woman entered therapy when the long-standing problems in her marriage became exacerbated by her husband's continued remoteness and lack of support just at a time when one of their children was in danger of dying from a major illness. Having asked her husband to participate with her in marital counseling and been rebuffed, she sought the aid of a male therapist. In treatment, the therapist agreed that her husband was indeed uncooperative and emotionally lacking, but that he "wasn't such a bad guy" and that he was responding in very much the same way as many men, the therapist included, might have. The therapist went on to say that the patient's problem resided in her being "too competent"—were she able to do less, her husband would do more. Thus, she was to make her husband more responsible by learning to be less responsible, paradoxically becoming a better wife by being a less good wife. For a time, the woman did not organize the family finances or social schedule, but the husband seemed not to notice. She even attempted to reduce her previous level of involvement with the children, but the sick child's need for support, combined with the absence of any signs of her husband rushing in to fill the void, caused her grave doubts regarding this course of action, and—by extension—about the wisdom of the therapist. She decided to seek professional consultation about the therapy. When she informed the therapist of her plan, he replied by stating that she was free to do as she wished, but as far as he was concerned there was no serious trouble with the treatment, and if there were, he himself would have sought consultation from a colleague. Feeling blamed for the treatment impasse, and wondering whether the identification of the therapist with her husband's point of view was merely a technique, the woman finally did seek outside consultation—in fact, she saw two different consultants, each time concealing the name of her therapist. Both times she was advised that the therapy in which she was engaged was damaging and should be ended. The second consultant went on to caution her that there was serious risk to her child in trying to manipulate her husband into being more involved. Both consultants also indicated that her therapy was by now a repetition of her marriage, having become a relationship in which all problems were attributed to her. The woman returned to her therapist to tell him about the consultations. His reaction was to say that if both consultants agreed that her treatment was being mismanaged, she must have been "distorting" what she told them about it. He added that she could leave treatment if she chose, but he thought she had violated the trust in the relationship. He was prepared to continue treatment in spite of what had happened, but he did not offer to consult with a colleague or to amend his formulation of the case in any significant respect. Recognizing the futility of any further attempts to resolve their differences, the woman finally left this treatment. Six months after figuratively divorcing her therapist, she commenced the literal task of divorcing her husband.

Chesler (1972) has shown how many male psychiatrists have kept unhappy housewives "in line" through such treatments as electroshock therapy, anti-depressant drugs, and the use of antiquated Freudian concepts of the subordinate role of women. Some have even been able to bully female patients into staying in an unhappy marriage—certainly, we gain this impression from Bergler's (1948) case reports about his treatment of potential divorcees. He warned women who were contemplating divorce that it was their responsibility to preserve the family unit more so than it was that of the more "infantile" man. Is this self-referential? Can it be that he himself depended on his wife to stay with him, no matter how irascible his own behavior?

Myers (1989) testified on behalf of a woman who complained to the local professional association about her husband's therapist because he felt this colleague was "out of order":

> This therapist berated the woman [on a phone call], a complete stranger to him, first of all for leaving her husband "just after he joined A.A.," and secondly for refusing to let her husband see her. When the woman told the therapist that she was a battered wife who had left her husband many times before, and he never changed, and that she was still very afraid of him, the therapist, as quoted by the woman, said: "I know all of that; your husband told me. . . . Don't you think he deserves a second chance now that he is not drinking? He's pretty desperate. How are you going to feel if he kills himself?" (p. 261)

Although averting suicide is a valid therapeutic concern, laying guilt trips in order to preserve a marriage, as in Myers's story, is intrusive and unethical. Moreover, in an allied iatrogenic maneuver that is equally out of order, some therapists use "scare tactics," depicting divorce as too horrid an option to be considered. In this category we view the work of Medved (1989), who made many valid points about the problems of divorce but never stopped prophesying disaster for those who start down the slippery slope of separation.

Marriage–Divorce Neutrality

We have seen that a therapist is forced to confront situations in h/h work similar to those daily encountered at home, or because of which divorce has occurred. In addition, every therapist has aspirations, a sexual–romantic life, and moral values, all of which become part of a biased participation in any treatment. A never-quite-attainable neutrality in therapy is akin to a never-quite-attainable objectivity in journalism; both are ideals to be striven for in spite of manifest human limitations. However, when it comes to therapy, these same human limitations are the indispensable basis for understanding the patient on an emotional level, inasmuch as we all share a common psychic potential that allows us to know each other. Hence, some sort of balance must be struck between, on one hand, the ideal of neutrality and, on the other hand, application of personal experience, which invests a phenomenon with empathic meaning.

Napier and Whitaker (1978) made a notable effort to achieve this balance. As family therapists, these authors appreciated the issues that divorce raises for adults and children, the continuity of the family system after breakup, and the needs of individuals for self-development within an interdependent field. They devoted a chapter to divorce, "The Terrible Choice," when a couple fail to resolve crucial conflicts in treatment and now face stark alternatives. Once the couple come to the abyss of impending breakup, there are two options. Should they decide to stay together, the task of the therapist is to help them share their feelings, learn to fight for their personal objectives, and recognize that the partner can never supply all their needs. Should they choose to divorce, all parties must grieve, *including the therapist*, after which the therapist's work is to help them get separated without undue panic or acting out, meanwhile providing for their children. Napier and Whitaker made no bones of the fact that their preference was for the marriage to be preserved, as each of them acknowledged that they too have struggled to preserve their own marriages. But the couple may make a choice different from theirs, and then they must maintain treatment of the family through the turmoil of separation. Napier and Whitaker summed up their treatment philosophy in the following passage:

> *IF* they are going to get a meaningful divorce, one that includes psychological as well as legal freedom to leave each other, they will need the same thing that is required in a good marriage: *real* individuation. Whatever they do about marriage, they will need to disentangle . . . massively intertwined thinking processes; they need to create . . . genuine autonomy. "Let us help you with individuation," we offer; "When you have achieved that goal, then decide what to do with the investment in your marriage. If you wait to decide, you will have a sounder basis for making a decision." In this way, we avoid taking sides, and we allow both parties to find hope in the work. We also set ourselves a task that is appropriate for the therapist—psychological change, not decisions about reality. (pp. 225–226)

Another example of therapeutic neutrality—but where the therapist's personal sense is in favor of divorce—is provided by Jones (1987).

He described 13 cases in which the presenting problem was what he called "the ambivalent spouse syndrome": one partner came to treatment, not asking for change in self, but complaining that the other was not sure about remaining in the marriage. Such initiating clients saw themselves as helpless victims; they did not assert themselves with their spouses for fear of losing them, nor did they admit that they may have already lost them. Jones assumed that "one partner appears to express emotional pain and depression on behalf of both, while the other spouse acts out the ambivalence for both" (p. 59). He got five "ambivalent spouses" to attend, but four terminated shortly, and two used the conjoint sessions to announce in his presence that they had decided on divorce. Jones also found that at least eight ambivalent spouses had found new partners by the time therapy was started, so "the spouse is not always as ambivalent as the initiating client would like to believe" (p. 60). Jones gave his clients time to decide whether the marriage could be saved and, when he could, he set up conjoint sessions to work with available ambivalent spouses, not foreclosing any option and recognizing that it was the couple's right to make the ultimate decision. However, he concluded that in cases in which one spouse comes to treatment implicitly asking the therapist to bring in the other to change the latter's mind about breakup, both partners are resisting change. The client coming to his office does not want the marriage to get worse or to end; for the most part, the ambivalent spouse does not want it to get better. The couple may even be more or less comfortable (at least for now) in this discomfort. For Jones, the therapist's job in such cases is to challenge the uneasy equilibrium of this marital system and bring about clarification and resolution of an impasse, which generally means divorce.

CULTURE-BOUND COUNTERTRANSFERENCE: THE MODERN THERAPEUTIC MENTALITY

Beyond differing philosophies of individual practitioners, the mental health field by its very development has unwittingly shifted toward an increasingly pro-divorce stance. A major attack on the "therapeutic mentality" has come from Bellah, Masden, Sullivan, Swidler, and Tipton (1985). They accused mental health professionals of adopting a relativistic "contractual ethic" that makes social relations unstable, because "giving" is judged only in relation to "getting," and commitments can be changed or broken according to pragmatic needs or prospects. This utilitarian approach to modern life puts marriages at risk, because at some point a relationship may not be a good return on the current investment, and there is no longer a moral basis to sustain it once it becomes problematic. In conscquence, with eveiy social commitment reduced to a matter of expedience and negotiation, marriage can seldom survive over time, and Bellah et al. believe this is especially apt to happen *when a partner goes into therapy.*

According to Bellah et al., the problem with therapy is in the narrow way therapists conceive of "self." If the self is defined by its ability to choose its own values, on what grounds are these choices made? Preferences turn out to be arbitrary: each individual self constitutes its own moral universe, with no way to determine what is good in itself. Thus, we must refer only to consequences in order to assess whether our actions are good. A self free of external guidance can keep particular socially defined identities at arms' length and never change its own basic identity, because identity depends only on discovering and pursuing personal wants. Bellah et al. contended that the language of "values" as used by contemporary therapists is no longer about moral choice but instead consists of idiosyncratic rationales for behavior, presuming the existence of an empty, unencumbered, and improvisational self. The end result is a therapeutic contradiction: the basis for action is self-interest, but without social connectedness, there is no self.

Bellah et al. pointed out that therapists worry about lack of "community" in their patients' lives, but the fault partly lies in their own ideas about what constitutes a healthy relationship:

> The ideal . . . relationship seems to be one in which . . . all parties know how they feel and what they want. Any intrusion of "oughts" or "shoulds" into the relationship is rejected as an intrusion of external and coercive authoritarianism. The only morality that is acceptable is the purely contractual agreement of the parties: whatever they agree to is right. . . . The endless scanning of one's own and others' feelings while making moment-by-moment calculations of the shifting cost/benefit balances is so ascetic in its demands as to be unendurable. It is the moral content of relationships that allows marriages, families, and communities to persist with some certainty . . . and that are not subject to incessant renegotiation. (pp. 139–140)

A similar critique of the therapeutic mentality was offered by sociologists Berger and Berger (1983). They too describe a prevalent therapeutic ideology in which the basic issue is what is good for the individual, so that for some clinicians the family can become the villain in a scenario of "liberation." They viewed this as a fundamental mistake, inasmuch as the family is "one of the many freely chosen and freely disposable mechanisms whose purpose is the fostering of the individual's project of self-attainment" (p. 122). The British philosopher

Bertrand Russell (1929) reached exactly the same conclusion. He scoffed at claims that the self is depleted by commitments and countered that those very commitments in work, love, and community are what give substance to the self.

What the aforementioned critics hold in common is a sense that choices based on the selfhood of the individual cannot take commitments as commitments, morality as morality, or culture as culture. Although such generalizations about current tendencies certainly go too far in stigmatizing the whole mental health field, and even the divorce therapy field, current therapeutic premises still tend to support an individualistic conception of the self, and therefore tacitly ally with the patient's self against such limitations on autonomy as commitments and responsibilities. Bartholomew (1990) noted that a paradigm shift was only now just starting to occur: "Recently, theorists have come to recognize that psychology has overemphasized the process of individuation, thereby neglecting the importance of a healthy connection with or dependence on others" (p. 148).

Another tacit aspect of the therapeutic mentality extends past countertransference into what Schafer (1970) called "visions of reality." Using terms borrowed from the theater, he maintained that therapists innately organize their theoretical work in accord with one of four encompassing worldviews: comic, romantic, tragic, and ironic. The "comic" is defined as hopefulness that celebrates the power of positive attitudes. The "romantic" is characterized by heroic quest, glorifying the protagonist who challenges the limits of what is possible or permissible. The "tragic" is manifested in a protagonist's downfall, usually resulting from a singular character flaw. The "ironic" aims at keeping proper perspective: detachment is needed to deflate grandiose expectations and to accept the world as it is. Schafer says that comic and romantic visions tend to go together, just as do tragic and ironic visions.

Applied to divorce therapy, a prototypical comic–romantic view is reflected in this farewell toast between parting mates: "Here's to your continued growth!" (Walder, 1978, p. 263). When therapists are this sanguine about divorce, they promote optimism, disengagement, and readjustment, but at the same time they also deny or distort the tragic–ironic dimension. The metaphor of "growth" is used to suggest that ending a marriage is the "mature" thing to do, whereas negative outcomes within this pseudo-paradigm of human development such as "regression" or "failure to thrive" are never considered.

On the other hand, a prototypical tragic–ironic view could be represented by Bergler's (1946) claim that those who divorce have used the mate to satisfy unconscious needs to suffer—a problem not resolved by changing partners. The harshness of this formulation left one man vainly begging for mercy from Dr. Bergler: "Have a heart and don't make it so difficult for the average person!" (1948, p. 228). Here, the disconsolate patient may be reacting more to his therapist's stern prophecies than to his own actual plight.

Schafer noted that psychoanalysis has taken the tragic–ironic viewpoint throughout its history. Although Freudian doctrine does not inculcate a powerless outlook in treatment of psychopathology, it does insist that personality problems may be unavoidable, given one's childhood, and are soluble only to a degree (Balint, 1968). This is not to say that the comic–romantic vision makes no contribution—it does, in terms of struggle against adversity as well as faith in the future—but not all life's distresses are "fixed" by going to therapy, nor is the test of successful therapy the elimination of unhappiness (Schneiderman, 1987). As Freud noted, the purpose of treatment is to remove symptoms so that a patient can deal with the woes of everyday existence (Breuer & Freud, 1895/1955, p. 305).

The predominant trend in current mental health practice makes each self the arbiter of its own values, which are then linked with comic–romantic visions of a noble quest that forces its own happy ending (Ehrenreich, 1985/1986); Walkup, 1985/1986), so there is a serious tilt toward an iatrogenic divorce countertransference on the part of therapists. The pendulum has undoubtedly swung since Bergler's time. In contrast to the influence he once wielded over the field, therapists nowadays tend to foster an implicit mind-set in their patients that makes marriages ever harder to sustain. This shift in the therapeutic worldview seems to us a major factor in the ongoing "normalization" of divorce as a social phenomenon.

TREATING THE PARTING COUPLE: PRINCIPLES OF DIVORCE THERAPY

After having critiqued the field of divorce therapy, it behooves us to state our own conception of how divorce therapy should be conducted. Although we cannot do more than sketch our own approach, we can indicate our most salient concerns.

Neutrality

As already mentioned, hardly any clinical endeavor is more conflictual for a therapist than treatment of an individual or couple in the process of severing a marriage. In doing this work, personal morality, family values, cultural mores, philosophic convictions, and—most of all—the therapist's own character and experience vis-à-vis committed unions stand as factors to be addressed in order to maintain proper therapeutic neutrality.

In doing any type of divorce therapy, the first priority is to adhere to standard principles of psychotherapy—the establishment of a safe context, as well as a consistent frame for treatment governed by a body of sound theoretical and technical premises. To achieve these aims, it is fundamental that the therapist have the capacity to identify and manage h/h countertransference. When countertransference is not well contained and infiltrates the treatment, adverse and even disastrous outcomes may potentially result, as seen in the two clinical examples that follow.

A recently divorced female therapist undertook treatment of a woman involved in a marriage described as "dead and destructive." The therapist, who viewed her own former marriage in similar terms, failed to recognize that the patient—who was more than 10 years older than she, the mother of four children, a devout Catholic, and untrained for any career—was quite unready to be pushed into divorce. When the therapist insisted that the patient's "growth" was being impeded by staying in the marriage, the patient left treatment. She found another therapist who was able to work with her around issues of communication with her husband, despite his serious limitations in matters of intimacy. Both patient and second therapist recognized that her marital life would always involve some measure of bitter disappointment; nevertheless, her choice to stay in the marriage was one that had to be respected—neither patient nor second therapist could truly say that her life outside the marriage would be happier than the one she was now living.

In another case, a mother of a young boy contemplated divorce from her husband. She was referred to a male therapist who followed Bergler's (1946) credo. He believed that it did not matter who your partner was, because psychological difficulties were located in the self—divorce could not solve such problems. On the face of it, this is the classic psychoanalytic position—that is, changing circumstances do not resolve intrapsychic conflicts—but taken here to the absurd extreme of problem solving only by introspection. However, countertransferential aspects were also involved, as was ultimately shown by the therapist's statement that this woman's leaving her marriage would be like "chopping off your 2-year-old son's legs at the knee." This simile plainly meant that the woman must stay in her marriage for her boy's sake. Overidentified with children of divorce, the therapist lost rapport with his patient, who soon left treatment. But years after divorce, she was still haunted by dreams in which she was trying to bandage back her son's amputated limbs.

Both of these examples represent instances in which therapists failed to recognize an entrenched bias regarding the morality and benefits of being married versus getting divorced, dealing with their patients as extensions of themselves. In each case, some measure of harm accrued to the patient, who then sent a signal in leaving that something was amiss in the treatment—namely, that the attitude of the therapist was a function of h/h own history and personality, so that there was neither flexibility in assessment nor recognition that each marriage is unique.

There are also cases in which a therapist is not locked into a point of view one way or the other, but the wish for a particular couple to remain together or come apart may still develop. This can result from an induced countertransference, a subjective reaction providing insight to the clinician in respect to the existing marital situation. In such a context, there can be great benefits when the therapist's feelings, as well as how they crystallized during the course of the treatment, are used as information to be employed in the work.

On the side of induced countertransference wherein the therapist prefers a divorce, a patient may get the therapist to wish for an end to the marriage because of its apparently insoluble conflicts. It can be that the patient covertly desires the therapist to see that the relationship is hopeless and even to take responsibility for pronouncing it over. When the therapist discusses with the patient what h/s experiences in reaction to the marital problems, the patient may own up to entertaining the same conclusion from the outset and then admit to using the therapy to show that h/s had done everything possible before leaving the marriage. Or, conversely, it may soon be clear that once the patient's ambivalent wish for separation has been induced in the therapist, the patient can then externalize this wish and hold onto the marriage.

In the opposite form of induced countertransference, a patient or couple covertly want the therapist to work on behalf of the marriage. For example, a man was remorseful after a brief, halfhearted, and self-terminated affair, but his wife was hurt and unforgiving, so he was not able to return home. They entered therapy to see whether they could repair their marriage, which both of them feared could not be done because of a long history of problems. Although admitting that an affair is not a good way to deal with distress in the relationship, the man maintained that this was his reaction to the wife's constant criticism of him—to make her see that she could not treat him like "chopped liver" and expect he would do never do anything about it. On her part, the wife reluctantly accepted that she had often been shrewish, but added that her behavior was the result of her frustration with his passive–withdrawn manner, so that nagging, snide remarks, and tantrums were the only ways she knew to get his attention. After many stormy sessions, the therapist came to the recognition that this was a couple who still had strong feelings for each other and did not want to part, but were each afraid to get closer to the other. He shared this perception of the situation with the couple and conveyed his conviction that the marriage was salvageable if they were willing to take advantage of the marital crisis to state their needs frankly and respect those of the other as they never had before. This declaration helped give the couple some hope with which to address their problems together. They ultimately decided to reconcile, and by both their subsequent accounts the reunion has proved to be a much better relationship than the prior marriage.

Protection of the System

Beyond attending to h/h own internal issues regarding marital choices, a therapist must remain alert to circumstances that might cause harm to the system. Primary, of course, is *the prevention of catastrophic reactions*—any situation that could result in actual physical danger to a member of the family or to a collateral. Just how this is done depends on whether the therapist is dealing with a symbiant or a countersymbiant. In treating a symbiant, the feelings that prompt a need for revenge must be validated in treatment, but at the same time actions that could wreak havoc must be contained, if necessary by resort to adjunctive services from police or psychiatric hospitalization. When the therapist is working with a countersymbiant, the task is to tamp down provocations that could trigger a drastic response from a distraught symbiant. Such provocations not only ignore the ex-mate as a person whose needs must be considered for the benefit of the system, but also serve as a destructive way to validate the decision to leave by showing how "disturbed" the other truly is.

Having dealt with the issue of *physical* danger, the therapist must also be aware of the potential for *psychological* harm in the system, especially if there are children. Enormous temptation exists in divorce to triangulate children into adult conflicts, and patient or couple must be apprised of circumstances that violate the boundaries of appropriate care of youngsters. In certain cases, this may mean that therapists make specific recommendations in respect to issues of child support, visitation, and custody. Involvement of the father with children after divorce is also important, and in some cases recommendations may be made that foster this relationship. In all cases, however, the therapeutic needs of the patient must be weighed against the long-term problems inherent in direct intervention in the patient's life.

Finally, in dealing with acrimonious divorces, it is wise for the therapist to keep in mind that the pairbond is a system, so that even when one party (probably the patient's mate or ex) is made to look like a villain, it must be investigated whether the reciprocal in the relationship (the patient) is engaging in some form of behavior that provokes or colludes with mistreatment. In one fairly typical example, a therapist was seeing a woman who had been divorced for several years. The woman bitterly complained about her ex's failure to comply with child support payments and visitation schedules, which held especially true when he was seeing another woman. These patterns were congruent with what the woman saw as the husband's self-serving and withholding behaviors in the marriage, which indeed had led to her divorcing him. Upon further inquiry, however, the therapist discovered that despite her preoccupation with grievances against this man, the patient always gave in—for example, allowing him to come over "to see their child" whenever he pleased, and then making love to her. When her failure to set limits was addressed, the patient admitted that her ex's visits provided a way of clinging to him and not coming to grips with the fact of their separation. When she finally was able to insist on adherence to the terms of their separation, his compliance in respect to child care improved, but she went into a depression. After mourning, she completed her letting go.

Technical Considerations

Clearly, the work of divorce therapy varies, depending on whether the therapist is doing extended or brief treatment, or seeing an individual, a couple, a family, or a troubled child of the marriage. In addition, the therapist must differentiate between intense separation reaction in an essentially normal person, and deeper-seated characterological difficulties in a partner that have been brought to the forefront by the current marital crisis. In every case, the patient's developmental, family, relational, and marital history will constitute needed information for assessing dynamics and anticipating stress points. For example, two patients may present with a relational pattern of distancing in marriage. One has a developmental history of many early losses, so that fear of intimacy can be attributed to separation-trauma, while the other describes a childhood fending off an intrusive parent, so that protection of autonomy is a key factor. Despite similarity in marital problems, each of these patients has distinct issues that call for disparate interventions. Thus, no one formulaic set of thought or treatment will fit every case.

The patient's past history is important, but, as always, the best guide to the patient's dynamics will eventually be found in transference toward the therapist. A patient protesting that h/s wanted closeness in a marriage, but who is often late, or misses sessions, or is unreliable in payments, may be sending strong signals about h/h behavior in relationship. By the same token, a patient who comes in saying that the breakup was "all my fault," but is ultimately considerate and responsible in treatment, is displaying behavior that may lead the therapist to wonder whether the causes of the breakup were far more complicated.

The Wrong Mistake: A Tragic–Ironic Perspective

Our own view made explicit is that we stand within the psychoanalytic tradition, which entails certain premises about human nature. The first, as Schafer (1970) noted, is that it is best always to keep an eye to, but avoid being blinded by, the irrevocably tragic–ironic aspects of human existence. This stance has maximum applicability in the treatment of those engaged in a marital breakup. It seems wise to renounce the classically comic–romantic vision of any therapeutic philosophy that implies divorce will have all parties living happily ever after; we also do not believe that any marriage, be it first, second, or nth, promises love in perpetuity without struggle and sacrifice. Life is a series of existential choices that are essentially trade-offs made under the press of characterological needs, pragmatic considerations, and personal values. However, even given these necessary parameters by which to determine choices, subsequent events may retroactively call such choices into question. In other words, marriage/divorce decisions are stark, fraught with unforeseen outcomes, and offer much scope for later regrets. With so much at stake, it is hard to get one's marital bearings. As a colleague commented, "My European friends are appalled at the way in which Americans take affairs so seriously and divorce so lightly!" But perhaps it is a wrong mistake to take either affairs or divorce lightly.

When it comes to unilateral marital separation with its inevitable anguish, we expect that there will be acrimony and do not expect consistently "civilized" behavior from either side, despite working in therapy toward ideally bringing the ex-couple's interactions to a safe and mutually considerate level. In seeking rapport with both parties to the breakup, we support the right of one party to leave the union, but we also support the right of the other party neither to like it nor to facilitate matters. We do not legislate the feelings of either party, but strive to assist each party to understand the position of the reciprocal as valid for that person. Both parties must proceed with the emotional task of disengaging, but either can be expected to get stuck along the way in terms of lingering attachment, which is only normal and neither a "setback" nor a "weakness."

All in all, our work is perhaps not so different from that of most other clinicians who do this type of therapy; perhaps it is the literature that departs from mainstream practice, inasmuch as it is those with an ideological bent one way or the other who are most apt to publish. But then again, we ourselves are publishing with an ideological message, that has at its root the tragic–ironic spirit. In any event, this culture—with its emphasis on entitlement and freedom—will support the "right to divorce" without sufficiently assessing the cost for all concerned parties. We ourselves do not dispute the social benefits inherent in the right to divorce, and we hold no brief for restriction of this right. That said, however, we still maintain that it must be recognized, by patients and therapists alike, that unilateral divorce nearly always has painful consequences that are unavoidable. To think otherwise is an error akin to presuming that there can be such a thing as a free lunch.

∿ 19

The Issue of Guilt

New No-No's
In American society, [we] wave the banner of emotional
expression: we should not hold back feelings, we should
be "up front" with them. But this by no means leads to
an "equal opportunity law" among feelings—there are
new pariahs: jealousy and guilt. Since "jealousy" . . .
reveals a "possessive attitude" toward the loved one, one
is not supposed to feel it even under extreme
circumstances. Guilt has also been drummed out of the
corps as betraying an insufficient ability to live in the
here-and-now. Young Americans . . . have a rather
touching faith in the plasticity of human emotion. . . .
Their bewilderment and guilt when they feel things they
aren't supposed to is exactly what Victorian women felt
when they were sexually aroused, or what Quakers feel in
the grip of rage. (Although it may be the first time
people have felt guilty for feeling guilty.)
                                    —SLATER (1976, pp. 5–6)

THE "RIGHT" TO DIVORCE

In *Help for Today's Troubled Marriages,* Fisher (1968) conveyed the
message that couples whose marriages were failing could get counseling
that might avert divorce. This book attracted little attention. As for
couples who came to her office for consultation, she found that they
were typically more interested in ending their marriages than working
to restore them. Fisher realized her services were being misdirected, so
instead of "Marriage Counselor," she now refashioned her professional
card to read, "Marriage and Divorce Counselor." She also published a
new book, covering much the same ground as the first, but this time
entitled *Divorce: The New Freedom* (1974). More attuned to the concerns

of the public, her second book was commercially successful. Although not advocating divorce, its title had a trendy thrust, suggesting that divorce was now perfectly proper. It had become a "right."

Also in 1974, Epstein's *Divorced in America* was published, but whereas Fisher strove to deal with changing mores, Epstein upheld an intransigent anti-divorce line. Describing divorce as "the most detestable of all permitted things," Epstein refused to make any concession to the growing national sentiment that it was the remedy for a "bad" marriage. Viewing marriage as sacred, he defended the nuclear family against internal threat of breakup by castigating divorce as an abrogation of responsibilities to mate and children. Nevertheless, Epstein realized his thesis was already outmoded. The argument that personal integrity would be compromised by exiting a problematic marriage could not possibly be welcomed by a public on the way to conviction that ending a committed union is no longer to be judged by moral criteria, with some mental health experts even asserting that such endings could be hailed as morally courageous.

In tandem, these two books speak for a divided culture. The division cuts deeper than whether it is morally justified to break a marital commitment, because disagreement is over the nature of morality itself. Thus, in the typical controversy over right and wrong between parting partners, one party asserts the prerogative to divorce without onus of guilt, invoking an ethos that bases conscience on *universal principles of entitlement,* and the other party insists on interdependence and commitment, espousing moral principles resting on *responsibilities to others.* This debate parallels Gilligan's (1982) dichotomy between ethics that are masculine "justice-based" and feminine "care-based." Yet the adversarial positions in breakup do not necessarily follow gender lines (as Gilligan supposed to be usually the case), but rather play out along lines of the symbiant–countersymbiant distinction.

At a cultural level of the same debate, we are now witnessing the gradual passing of the traditional Western moral worldview that Roheim (1950) has described as founded on guilt instead of shame. Shame stems from actual or anticipated social disapproval for violation of a community norm; guilt is based on adherence to an internalized moral precept and need not involve behavior for which there is social disapproval or even knowledge. Although guilt is often seen as a higher level of ethical functioning than shame, both combine in some mixture as the concerns of the superego. However, guilt based on ethical standards is today being displaced by a "plurality of values," which largely undermines any fixed precepts and thereby forces the superego to rely almost entirely on its own resources in the absence of any moral model outside the self. It is to this phenomenon—a necessary precursor to the rising divorce curve—that we address our final chapter. Is it true that considerations of right and wrong do not apply to the breakup of a marriage? In a culture seeking to achieve greater freedom from guilt, what then becomes society's moral norms applied to family maintenance? Further, why does empirical research so seldom deal with guilt? Walters-Chapman, Price, and Serovich (1995) have shown that guilt as a facet of marital breakup was addressed in only 2 articles over the last 5 years in the *Journal of Divorce* and in none of 85 articles on divorce in the past eight volumes of the *Journal of Marriage and the Family.* Finally, although perhaps more shame must be induced by our society to reinforce social values (Schneiderman, 1995), what changes in *individual conscience* have occurred because the culture now superimposes new moral norms on prior standards for responsible self-regulating behavior?

BANISHING GUILT (BUT NOT THE GUILTY)

In a family therapy seminar for clinicians, an instructor commented that he reassured divorcing couples in treatment with him that "breakup is no one's fault; after all, it is the relationship that failed." This "therapeutic absolution" touched off a fierce debate. Those who agreed with the instructor defended the paradigm that "falling out of love" is mainly a miscarriage of the chemistry of attraction—a lamentable event of which it could be said, with Fritz Perls (1969), "It can't be helped." Those who disagreed insisted that an abstraction such as "relationship" could not fail—this was a formula serving to relieve the partners of responsibility. Rather, it had to be the partners—or even one of them—who fail.

    Psychology at the crossroads. What induces the tendency to direct moral censure toward a concept like "relationship" instead of holding two people accountable for their moral choices? In some respects, this trend can be traced back to Freud. In *Civilization and Its Discontents* (1930/1957), he argued that excessive moral demands, especially in the area of sexuality, generated the rampant neuroses of the Victorian epoch. In order to alleviate the harsh conflict between wishes for gratification and the press of social rules, Freud asserted that modern man could sustain mental health only if he made his ideals more realistic and was prepared to view himself as far from "civilized." Although opposed to lowering moral standards, Freud emphasized that mankind is not infinitely perfectible, given that human development is built up from primitive appetites and egoistic drives. To maintain the current level of moral discipline, Freud held, people must be encouraged to feel less guilty about their impulses and fantasies, but not about their actions.

But some post-Freudians have been so ardent in heeding this admonition that whereas Freud "only sought to soften [the starched collar] of culture—others, using bits and pieces of his genius, would like to take it off" (Rieff, 1966, p. 8). Rieff complained that moral standards have not only been humanized, as Freud wished, but that psychoanalytic doctrine is now perversely being used to question whether moral standards apply at all. He feared a "triumph of the therapeutic"—the cultivation of a mass mentality in which actions are "understood" but never "judged." Thus, the culture becomes unduly permissive as psychodynamics replaces morality.

Once our culture moved in this direction, the term "transgression" came to take on a different meaning such that when an individual violates a moral norm, h/s has the right to demand that others change their attitude to make the behavior in question acceptable. The logic here is that in a democracy of values, one's principles are as valid as anyone else's. The advantage of such a contrary stance is that traditions will be challenged and perhaps refashioned along more inclusive and tolerant lines. The disadvantage is that morality can swiftly deteriorate into customized *ex post facto* rationalizations whereby ultimately no one is accountable to any one; such standards as may still exist then tend to be disregarded as mere "prejudices" or "hang-ups," or, at best, as relativistic and situational.

In *Guilt-Free*, McDonald and McDonald (1977) upheld this vision. In respect to divorce, they concluded that those who quit their marriages do not deserve the guilt they suffer, because society as a whole is to blame. Their belief is that (1) society does not sufficiently prepare us for marriage and parenthood; (2) Americans expect too much from romance; and (3) we live in a divorce-prone environment. These remarks are well taken, but the eradication of standards that give rise to guilt feelings will simply add one more factor to the roster of reasons that society is to be held at fault for the prevalence of divorce. What is really being said here is that those who break marital commitments are entitled to moral respectability on the basis of a blanket *amnesty*—the social system absorbs all blame and thereby pardons those who weaken the family as an institution. In proposing that divorce should be guilt-free, the McDonalds do not actually get rid of guilt—they merely diffuse it upward, shifting its locus from the individual onto an abstract entity (in this instance, "society" instead of "bad relationship"). Further, it never occurs to them that the primary source of guilt (in contrast to shame) stems from violation of *internalized ideals*, whereas they appear to assume that if the individual gains social acceptance, there is nothing left about which to feel guilty.

The McDonalds' book and the instructor's reassurance to a divorcing couple are symptomatic of a newly emerging "metamoral" injunction: *Il est interdit d'interdire* (It is forbidden to forbid). These words were inscribed on the walls of Nanterre University during the 1968 student riots in France (McGrady, 1972, p. 12), but McGrady extended this slogan beyond the politics of anarchy to modern sexual–romantic relationships. He held that pop-psychology "love doctors" were instilling the same message in their professional writings and treatment, so that toleration of any deviation in intimate unions is posited as the only moral position. Thus, when a contemporary clinician points out to h/h patient that guilt is a hindrance to enjoyment of life, it is ignored that guilt has expressly this function! Western civilization relies on an acculturation process that inculcates guilt whenever its norms are trespassed. Freud stated that his intention in writing *Civilization and Its Discontents* was "to represent the sense of guilt as the most important problem in the evolution of culture, and to convey that the price of progress in civilization is paid by forfeiting happiness through heightening of the sense of guilt" (Jones, 1963, pp. 467–468). Without guilt, standards would not be internalized nor impulses and drives civilized. Guilt is a learned signal alerting us to the disharmony of behavior in relation to the moral teachings handed down in the course of cultural evolution. Although Freud quite rightly worried about the noxious psychological effects of excessive or inappropriate guilt, it can only be the folly of a morally impoverished society that aims at abolishing guilt per se.

Lasch's (1979) *The Culture of Narcissism* attempted to explain a current moral transmogrification wherein traditional values are progressively superseded by an ethos of self-glorification and indulgence. He argued that the overabundant production of advanced capitalism contrives to create an insatiable market amenable to conspicuous consumption, planned obsolescence, perennial pursuit of an image of youth and beauty, and so forth. This economic superstructure has made a pathological state—narcissism—adaptive to current social conditions; such personality disorder has come to be considered so "normal" nowadays that only very extreme cases are diagnosed. Lasch foresaw a dire American future in terms of quality of life as masses of narcissistic people search for "identity," "growth," and "love" because of bouts of unsatisfied craving. Driven by feelings of emptiness, they enter relationships to be temporarily filled up, pursuing what they call "healthy" sex in hopes of sanitizing it of messy emotional involvement. Their love life fits what used to be called "promiscuous" or "adulterous" behavior; they sample avidly at new possibilities, ostensibly for fear of missing something but really as a way of soothing deeper anxieties. Experience is rapidly devoured for its own sake, as manifested at times by transient immersion in some person or project, until–sated–they pull back into a more usual state of disengagement. Life styles that "keep one's options open" and feature "cool sex" are in, whereas "commitment" and its bastard sequelae–suffering, jealousy, and guilt–are out. If psychotherapy is sought, Lasch noted, patients now seldom enter therapy with the guilt-ridden "neuroses" of yesteryear, instead seeking a type of treatment that extols individualism, personal happiness, and release from inhibitions, but such treatment alienates them even more from significant others than they were when they initially came for counseling.

Struck by the transformation of depth psychology from its Freudian origins into an apologia for narcissistic entitlement, Lasch attributed the ideology of the "culture of narcissism" to the value systems set forth by post-Freudian theory:

> Therapy constitutes an anti-religion . . . because modern society "has no future" and therefore gives no thought to anything beyond immediate needs. Even when therapists speak of the need for "meaning" and "love," they define love and meaning . . . as the fulfillment of the patient's emotional requirements. It hardly occurs to them . . . to encourage the subject to subordinate his interests to those of others, to someone or some cause or tradition outside himself. "Love" as self-sacrifice or self-abasement, "meaning" as submission to a higher loyalty–these sublimations strike the therapeutic sensibility as intolerably oppressive, offensive to common sense, and injurious to personal health and well-being. (pp. 42–43)

In the final analysis, Lasch described a society verging on the insipid. The "culture of narcissism" is neither doctrinaire nor hypocritical. It is merely a society uninterested in any moral ordering of its priorities or any sacrifices on behalf of them. It stands for almost nothing. To a great extent, the "immoral" might now be defined as whatever impedes gratification.

If valid, Lasch's reading of American post-1960s society as a narcissistic culture explains why pursuit of moral issues goes nowhere, either inside or outside the mental health field. In order to accommodate contemporary conditions, emotions which arise in a context of human interdependence have to be consciously discredited and unconsciously repressed. For example, jealousy and guilt are predicated on social principles of fair play that structure expectations and obligations within given relationships. However, according to a narcissistic world-view, interpersonal problems are caused not by *violating* but rather by *having* such standards! Instead of regulating behavior to avert guilt, a narcissist will challenge the rules that engender guilt. Therefore, in lieu of forgoing outside sex to spare a partner jealousy, a narcissist may insist that mate (and society) forgo monogamous ideals. Problems tend to be ascribed to emotional demands others make, whereas self-esteem can be maintained only if others offer no criticism and stop making trouble through their suffering, dependency, and sanctimony.

As an example of narcissistic dynamics around guilt, consider the case of a man who told his estranged wife that he felt he was bleeding inside every time she paraded before his eyes reminders of her lover's existence. She coldly replied, "Your task is to stop bleeding." She thereby relegated him to the status of a person whose feelings did not matter, or who should not even have such feelings. He was asking her to be more circumspect in relation to his jealous sensitivities, but she saw even this limited request as an affront to her basic sense of goodness and her right to do as she pleased. Granted that she did not need to comply with his wish, we merely note that a more empathic response on her part would have required an admission of having hurt him, which would engender, in turn, a guilt she evidently could or would not bear. In reaction, confronted with the woman's emotional demand that her ex-husband relinquish his emotional demand, the man soon repeatedly slashed his forearm with a knife because—as he none too lucidly explained—he was "starting to lose his sense of pain." We understand this to mean that in spite of the woman's directive, injury was natural in his situation; the cutting served to validate his own suffering. His choice was to experience his pain rather than be the unfeeling person she mandated him to be.

OUT, OUT, DAMNED SPOT!: THE GUILT THAT WON'T WASH AWAY

Does a society that increasingly disregards the moral standard of com-mitment find that its population is still forced to contend with an insidious guilt? If so, Freud would call the symptoms of this guilt "the return of the repressed." We have seen that in proportion to their narcissistic pathology, countersymbiants of the identity-seeking rejector type tend to staunchly disavow any guilt pertaining to breakup because of its devastating implications for self-esteem. However, they are not exempt from the unconscious stirring of conscience, often to be dis-cerned in masochistic patterns that are played out till a bitter end. As we discuss the hidden guilt of identity-seeking rejectors who narcissistically bring about the dissolution of a committed union, we are aware that psychodynamically oriented clinicians would question whether a narcissist is capable of "true guilt"—that is, a guilt encompassing regard for others as separate persons, which includes remorse for violation of their rights or reparation for pain caused. Indeed, case history data indicate that deprived of emotional supplies from significant others, the narcissist's vulnerable, rageful, fragmented, and empty self is exposed, leading to desperate reaching for whatever compensating object is available in order to avoid shame and to reinstate h/h sense of grandiosity. Although expressions of contrition may occur in circumstances of deprivation or loss, such apologies are usually shallow, largely driven by secondary gain (e.g., to win back a needed provider who, for the sake of h/h own psychic survival, had to flee the narcissist).

Thus, we use the word "guilt" in this section not to describe a functional superego, but in an undifferentiated and primordial sense that subsumes "bad self" feelings ranging from conscious self-censure to unconscious, acted-out symptoms of introjected self-hatred. For example, when an identity-seeking rejector demands that there be no criticisms or adverse consequences imposed for leaving the marriage, guilt (in our sense of primitive "bad self" feelings) may still be induced from without, such that implicit chastisement is imposed by pursuit of short-sighted choices, mishandling of reparative opportunities, and exploitation that turns supporters into enemies. The frenetic impulsion to live for NOW appears to have the function of staving off TOMORROW, when the dreaded, avenging future will fall due. This morbid fear of inevitable consequences, defended against by insouciant absorption in the distractions of the moment, allows us to infer from narcissistic behavior an inchoate guilt within a moral outlook ostensibly "beyond right and wrong." Thus, we construe ineluctable themes of masochistic atonement in the relentless course toward ruination upon which many identity-seeking rejectors embark, facing moral accountability—if even then—only *after* life has humbled them. In so doing, identity-seeking rejectors tend to demonstrate very limited insight into their life drama of self-aggrandizement followed by the nemesis of a punitive fate.

Overall, the "bad self" guilt of an identity-seeking rejector tends to lack pragmatic value, for if denied, it cannot be useful as a motivator for change. Often, not until long afterward is harm of the ex-mate appreciated as wrongdoing for which regret can be offered, restitution made, or behavior amended. A countersymbiant who, through pain, has finally arrived at a point where h/s can sincerely say about the breakup, "I'm responsible," is shedding narcissistic defenses. But in the absence of such awareness, a countersymbiant may manipulate or provoke significant others into disengaging as h/h unconscious way of saying it. This perverse way of not experiencing guilt but still setting up self-punishment for transgression is used to force the mate to initiate breakup (the style of the insidious type of rejector) or, (in the style of the identity-seeking rejector) after the forsaken mate eventually rejects any further enmesh- ment. In either case, such an induced outcome is too consciously unavail- able to be a constructive way to repair or compensate for what was done. As one man belatedly lamented, when his ex-wife would finally have no more to do with him, "You had to get away from me; I know I'm no good." No longer pursued by the husband she jilted, a woman said of his decision to divorce her, "You deserve better; all I seem able to do is grab the chicken off the plate and run."

A prime example occurs in Mitchell's (1936/1973) novel *Gone with the Wind*. Rhett Butler, fed up with Scarlett O'Hara's preoccupation with another man, announces he is leaving. Scarlett, the narcissist *par excellence*, begs him not to take this drastic step, saying she could not manage without him. He replies with the immortal words, "Frankly, my dear, I don't give a damn!" (p. 1023; the novel omits the "frankly" of the more familiar movie version). She is shocked, distraught, and yet resigned—as if submitting to a well-merited reprimand. Scarlett would be a tragic figure if it were not that her self-involved treatment of her husband made her ultimate fall from grace seem an act of poetic justice. The story concludes as she pathetically notes that she cannot cope now, but will think about the problem tomorrow. This deliberate deferral is a tacit admission that self-condemnation will be the inescap- able outcome of inquiry—the truth has to be avoided because it is already known.

The hidden guilt of a countersymbiant is revealed by (1) the refusal of the insidious rejector to overtly assume the mantle of "rejector" and h/h shifting responsibility and onus to the mate, or (2) the identity- seeking rejector's pervasive yearning for the mantle of respectability, which we view as partly a reaction formation to cover self-hatred. In regard to this latter point, although the identity-seeking rejector con- sciously insists on the right to live as h/s pleases, no matter what anyone thinks, at the same time h/s typically tries to extract a measure of acceptance from precisely those most injured by h/h departure. Such efforts at civil or even friendly relations with people to whom commitments were broken are offensive enough to incite retaliation in a fashion that echoes the identity-seeking rejector's own unconscious judgment of h/h moral failure. Yet, on a conscious level, the identity- seeking rejector usually receives such retaliations as "puzzling" events, coming from "malice" in that no justification is identified in the prior history of the relationship. Thus, a woman who walked out on her marriage complained to her ex-husband that she had not been invited to holiday dinner by his family; she saw no reason that she should not still be welcome at their table. Similarly, a man asked his ex-wife to arrange his brother's funeral despite the fact that he was living with someone else at the time. His plan was to attend the funeral in the company of his ex-wife like "a good family man" and then return home to his lover. When his intention was thwarted by her refusal to cooperate, he declined to attend the funeral.

The identity-seeking rejector's assertions of respectability include being with the new lover in public. On one hand, this is certainly appropriate, amounting to the couple leading their ordinary lives. On the other hand, however, the new couple may now demand social acceptance even from those quarters in whose eyes their union lacks legitimacy. The new pairbond may seem poised and indeed natural in their dealings with the "old" family, but there is often a grotesque degree of imposition foisted upon others left behind that predictably will have the opposite of its intended "normalizing" effect. Two case vignettes follow.

Just after leaving his wife, a man came to pick his children up, parked in the driveway, and walked up to the house. But this time he brought along the girlfriend for whom he left the marriage and with whom he now lived. Greeted by the children, the two adults entered the home and quickly realized that the ex-wife was in the bathroom taking a shower. While waiting, the man went to the liquor cabinet and poured himself and girlfriend a drink. Wrapped in a towel, the wife soon came out of the bathroom, doing a double take when she saw her "visitors." She steamed at the sight of the two of them making themselves comfortable in her home. The man made a fast introduction and explained that he was familiar with the house and so made himself comfortable while waiting; he even offered to fix his ex-wife her usual martini with a twist! He was indignant when his ex responded by throwing the pair out. As he was leaving, the man protested that the only thing he had done was to be sociable under the circumstances. The message this man was forcing on his forsaken wife was that he and his girlfriend had no need to observe formalities since they had done nothing wrong.

A bridegroom's mother, Mrs. Y, in whose house the wedding reception took place, was feuding with her ex-husband. The man had left her to live with her best friend who, in turn, had broken up her marriage to live with him. As was proper, Mrs. Y invited the father of the groom, Mr. Y, to the reception, but unbeknown to him, she also invited her rival's estranged husband. To be sure, "the other woman" in these two overlapping triangles was *not* invited. Both men arrived, stubbornly managed not to notice each other, and hung on until late into the evening. The missing party—the rival—telephoned at this point. Mrs. Y answered and abruptly slammed down the receiver as soon as she ascertained the identity of the caller; she was so upset that she needed ministrations from all her friends to recover. Mr. Y fumed when he heard his caller was disallowed and immediately stormed out. In this incident—which upstaged the son's wedding—the rival was an absent but pivotal protagonist who found a means to get around extrusion by simply telephoning. In so doing, knowing that the hostess would likely answer, she forced communication after all. The rival thought she had a perfect right to call, like anyone else, and Mr. Y thought so too. If she had been permitted to speak with Mr. Y (presumably to ask what time he was coming home), Mrs. Y would have thereby been validating the legitimacy of their union. This validation, to be most meaningful to the new pairbond, must come specifically from Mrs. Y, for they would then be released from any sense of transgression against her. If Mrs. Y had acquiesced in their self-proclaimed designation as "just another couple," their guilt would be exorcised. But from Mrs. Y's perspective, they were insensitively "rubbing in" their illicit union. Their expectation of normal social amenities—and implicit endorsement from Mrs. Y—was extraordinarily out of touch because this attitude only goaded her to fury. To presume entitlement to usual telephone conveniences was to make the futile statement that Mrs. Y had no reason to be perturbed.

These two vignettes illustrate the identity-seeking rejector's efforts to extract some kind of symbolic acceptance from, of all people, the ex-mate and collaterals. Bound to boomerang, such a plan denies the disdain that likely awaits, but also may be an unconscious maneuver to ensure h/s gets it. So much for living guilt-free.

WAS IT WRONG TO LEAVE?

A divorced man told one of us (A. P.) how restless and dissatisfied he had been in his marriage until he finally resolved to leave his wife and two young children, only to spend his first night away from home cowering under a blanket. Three years later, just as on that first night, he was still not able to cope with the issue of guilt. "Tell me, Al," he asked, "I was unhappy in my marriage, but in leaving, did I do the right thing?" I hesitated to reply, for fear that my opinion might hurt or offend the man—and all the more so because his marriage could not be restored no matter what I said. Further, he seemed so painfully in earnest that my spontaneous impulse was to be reassuring, exculpatory, or compassionate. The man's posing of this question suggested a hope that the moral issue could be laid to rest by virtue of soothing outside feedback. Nevertheless, on second thought, I saw the matter quite differently: the man had made an irrevocable self-defining choice in ending his marriage, but it was not the marriage he was brooding over—it was the image of himself he saw reflected in that decision. In other words, the "moral" issue did not concern whether he had let his family down; it had to do with whether he could maintain unsullied self-esteem. I was being invited, perhaps manipulated, to assure him that he had behaved properly. Probably, he set up his question to draw such support from many people; to see himself as a good person, he needed the world to excuse him. If I complied with the implicit need in his question, I would have been reinforcing escape from a guilt which, notwithstanding, continued to shadow his every move. I elected to be candid: "No, by my values, what you did was wrong." The man sighed with relief, pressed his hand to my shoulder, and thanked me for my honesty. He then added, to my puzzlement, that he would now be able to sleep better. In the past it was said that a good conscience is the best pillow. In this instance the man appeared to be saying that finally owning up to a guilty conscience was his next best cushion. His statement seemed odd, because he was stating that he could now sleep, implying he had achieved moral closure by my simple words, whereas I, in his situation, might have had more difficulty sleeping than before.

I stated to him that I thought it was wrong to leave wife and children but I could have added that he chose to do it anyway. Of course, he had a legal as well as a moral claim these days to do so. But once he came to grips with the human consequences of his action, any discussion of his marital breakup would no longer be tied only to the abstract "rightness" of this decision. Instead, the dialogue would encompass, as its existential domain, *what kind of person has he chosen to be, what kind of social world is he creating?*

If he could take responsibility for a decision that directly inflicted suffering on his significant others, without needing excuses, he and I could have proceeded in our talk on the basis of *divorce without rationalization.* Framing discussion in these frank terms, the two of us could have dispensed with utopian discourse about how breakup can be friendly, healthy, or civilized. I would not have to dispute any contention on his part that it was a "bad" relationship by pointing out to him that it was *prima facie* "bad" because he was in it. He would acknowledge taking his problems with him into separation rather than solving them by getting out of the marriage. We could avoid the casuistry that now proclaims "love is not forever," amounting to a self-fulfilling prophecy. Likewise, there would be no need to clarify the mystification of looking for the meaning of life outside marriage, as if it were not available within marriage. He would not tell me that he had outgrown his wife and children, and now, as superadult, he had turned his children over for single parenting by their mother while he went off with a new mate more on his own "advanced" level of maturity. We could discard the usual obligatory mention that "you can't stay together for the sake of the children", as if children were irrelevant. Or that the youngsters would eventually adjust, or even be better off than in the ruptured marriage—offspring being adaptable small adults. I could be spared hearing that everyone should just be prepared to flow with the vicissitudes of life, and that the mate's desire to preserve the marriage was only based on "possessive" and "dependent" needs. Or that marriage, the nuclear family, and long-term commitments have been rendered archaic, given the advent of more modern ideas under which the cardinal sin seems to be the failure to "live your life." It would not be an exchange in which the hidden agenda was the washing away of guilt through the destruction of community standards governing family stability. No, we could be spared all this—if only he could admit that his decision to leave *hurt* wife, children, and society as a whole, but he chose to do it anyway for his own (presumed) benefit. It would be such a novelty to hear at least one identity-seeking rejector take the full moral weight on h/h own mortal shoulders. The nearest approximation appears to be those who learn the bitter lesson that they hurt themselves by hurting others, in which case it is not the moral argument to which they ultimately attend, but one of self-interest. "Divorce without rationalization" leaves us with the bedrock premise that breaking up a family unit generally imposes monumental disruption and unhappiness on others—and thus entails monumental (but probably denied) guilt.

The man could have immediately taken issue with my view that his decision to leave the marriage was wrong but that he chose to do it anyway. My interlocutor might aptly have rejoindered that he was suffering within the marriage and it was a matter of necessity for him to get out, cost what it may. Moral issues were secondary, because he could not have functioned within the family system as the person he was at the time. Absolutely true! He may indeed have been psychologically impelled to leave; in saying that it was wrong to leave by my values, I was not saying he was obliged to stay—I meant that *he could not hope to leave without paying the price of guilt.* Society has standards to safeguard its vital institutions; in violating them, he was not privileged to expect that society would not only excuse him, but even renounce its own standards. As Baumeister and Wotman (1992) pointed out, in modern Western culture, love is a value base, a fundamental good for its own sake, so that a rejector in a committed union is "vulnerable to being in the position of the enemy of the good" (p. 106). The existence of an ethical code, including the sanctity of commitment and preservation of the family unit, does not preclude transgression against these social values, but violators need not be accommodated when they ask to be told, "It's OK." If this man left, let him accept the guilt. If he cannot deal with it, the guilt is his anyway—life will see to it, through recriminations by others as well as the repressed, convoluted, and transpersonal workings of his own conscience.

NEW FUNCTIONS FOR MODERN CONSCIENCE; THE RISE OF AN ANTI-CONSCIENCE

How is it possible for this man to avoid what would seem to be unavoidable guilt feelings? For such a feat to be accomplished, a sophisticated technology must exist for superego neutralization. We now turn to an examination of how a crisis of conscience can be handled in the modern world, and we start by going outside divorce phenomena to the most extreme historical example imaginable.

Arendt's (1974) *Eichmann in Jerusalem* depicted the ways in which Nazi Germany refined methods for the inuring and nullification of conscience. She reported on the trial in Israel after World War II of the man who arranged the roundup and transport of Europe's Jews to the death camps, although he did not personally kill a single one. But Arendt lets us know that Eichmann was a "normal" man; indeed, as a psychiatrist exclaimed, "More normal at any rate than I am after having examined him!" (p. 25).

Eichmann maintained he had led his life in a moral fashion, in accord with the ethical precepts of the German philosopher Immanuel Kant. When challenged, he was able to correctly render the essence of Kant's categorical imperative: "I meant by my remark about Kant that the principle of my will must always be such that it can become the principle of general laws" (p. 136). In spite of being able to cite this humane standard, Eichmann nonetheless absolved himself of responsibility for his role in genocide on the grounds that he was obeying orders issued by the head of state. Moreover, he observed a manifest lack of resistance to those orders at all levels of German society. Eichmann stated that he had harbored no animosity toward Jews, respected and enjoyed working with Jewish officials with whom he dealt, and would have preferred deportation to Madagascar to mass extermination. Hence, to the charge he had committed "crimes against humanity," Eichmann pleaded "not guilty in the sense of the indictment." As he saw it, the real question of this trial was his integrity, not his life. As a loyal German, he did what he did according to the laws of the land. If his country was in error, he agreed he should hang. But he did not regret anything: "Repentance was for little children" (p. 24).

We can assume that Eichmann, like other Germans, began with a conscience. Therefore, the Nazi leaders had to develop methods to steel their officials and troops for genocide. Their expert was Heinrich Himmler. In order for the individual German soldier to perform his duty in the massacre, Himmler recognized that he would need to account for and glorify the emotional hurt each man would experience. He began by instituting euphemistic "language rules." Nazi documents never made mention of "killing" but instead used prescribed terms such as "a medical matter," "special treatment," or "final solution," and deportation to the death camps became "labor in the East." Arendt suggested that the Nazis, who used the code words even among themselves, were not ignorant of what they were doing but did not want their activities equated with usual definitions of what constituted murder or mendacity.

Himmler next set up new ideals that would make counterclaims on the conscience. The ranks of the SS troops who carried out the "purging" of Jews were combed to weed out sadists and criminals whose behavior might cast discredit on the "historic mission," which Himmler represented to his men as "a page of glory in our history which has never been written and is never to be written" (p. 105). The officers had to have academic degrees because, though everyone involved had his personal qualms, intelligent leaders were needed who would not let emotions overrule their ideals. He indoctrinated his men so that they would be able to subdue the revulsion that instinctively comes as one witnesses—let alone inflicts—human suffering. Himself reputed to be squeamish at the sight of blood, Himmler appreciated the fact that "what we are expecting from you is 'superhuman,' to be 'superhumanly inhuman' " (p. 105).

Himmler's resolution of the crisis of conscience to which SS personnel were vulnerable proved extremely efficacious: *he turned the natural feelings of pity and revulsion to his own ends.* Instead of his troops having to say, "What horrible things I did to people," Himmler trained them to look at it this way: "What horrible things I had to watch in the pursuance of my duties, how heavily the task weighed upon my shoulders!" (p. 106). Pangs of conscience were no longer an empathy-based warning of the violation of human values; they became incorporated into the harsh toll the war exacted of each soldier. Living with a "bad" conscience was heroic—something like being wounded in action. To endure in one's grisly duty, despite a bad conscience, became a martyrdom. It was one's moral obligation to rise above one's moral obligation. An alternative framework for morality was being created: *the anti-conscience.*

The SS man had a *cultural* support system that provided an

ideology to override any qualms about "military operations" against unarmed civilians, as well as an *intrapsychic* support system in which he became a "victim" because he felt the suffering of his victims and so had to bravely bear guilt on behalf of his country. In this perverse setting, normal men could be conditioned to commit genocide in a businesslike manner. Evil became unrecognizable as the anti-conscience subverted the usual functions of conscience.

As Eichmann pointed out at his trial, how could a few thousand Nazis, working mostly in offices, have managed the extermination of millions of scattered Jews without "cooperation" from all parties concerned? They did receive the needed cooperation. The German soldiers obeyed orders. The Christian population of occupied Europe, for the most part, raised little objection to the singling out of Jewish co-citizens for exile, forced labor, and slaughter. As for the victims, Eichmann negotiated with Jewish officials for the delivery of communities for "resettlement," relied on Jewish police to maintain order in the ghettos and prevent escapes, used workers selected from the throngs of the doomed to operate death factories, and at one camp even had a Jewish executioner. Aside from a few incidents like the Warsaw uprising, no party involved in the holocaust—German, Christian, or Jew—seemed able to recognize, and therefore resist, evil as such. When there is complicity on the part of multitudes, evil takes on a benumbed level of "banality" (Arendt's term) so that, in effect, "Whatever is, is right."

HOW THE NAZI METAPHOR APPLIES TO DIVORCE

Any metaphor can be stretched to where it no longer fits a particular case, and our foray into Eichmann's trial may well appear far afield to mental health readers. But we have already said that the Nazi epoch provides the clearest illustration of how a crisis in conscience is handled in the modern world. The Eichmann case can serve as an enlarged print to show how guilt feelings are now dealt with across diverse social areas. Thus, some similarities between the unbridled aggression of Hitler's Germany and the unbridled sexual–romantic individualism leading to divorce in contemporary America offer interesting grounds for comparison. Moreover, such a comparison is not without precedent: Baumeister and Wotman (1992) also used this metaphor to explain how rejectors in love claim "victimization," just as a researcher found that the children of Nazi war criminals saw their parents as "victims of the war," which led to "shouting matches between the interviewer and the subjects in his study!" (pp. 112–113). We confine ourselves to five discrete areas in which the comparison can highlight how a countersymbiant may now retain moral equilibrium in divorce despite a queasy superego.

The Deployment of Code Words

A countersymbiant no longer "abandons" or "breaks up" a family unit—h/s "outgrows" it, needs "space" to seek an "identity," and enters "open-ended commitments" and "serial relationships." A divorce is not the dissolution of a nuclear family, but its "reorganization." Children are "adjusted to the ambiguities of modern life" via divorce. Thus, at a conference, a psychologist sympathetically discussed women who had "liberated themselves from husband and children"—not a word was said in the audience, or an eyebrow raised, in response to such terminology.

Ideological Justification

Hunt (1966) declared that divorce "is painful but necessary, temporarily destructive but finally creative, and not only an act of courage but an affirmation of one's belief in the value and possibility of happy marriage" (p. 150). According to this logic, divorce demonstrates a belief in marriage—perhaps even more of a belief in it than in not divorcing. His ideal is to "do away with the bad marriage" so that "marriage remains as popular as ever" no matter how high the divorce rates go. Ostensibly, marital breakup is for the welfare of the entire family unit, in that everyone can expect to be contaminated by the unhappy partner's resentment should they try to co-exist under one roof. A derivative argument is that a person leaving a marriage in search of happiness elsewhere is really helping everybody, so that one often hears, "It will be better for both our sakes"; "We'll each be happier with someone else"; "By closing this door, we'll open another"; "We deserve the chance to be free of earlier choices when we were different people"; and "The children will benefit in the long run." Under the new ideology, visions of an improved, more honest and loving world are projected as if most marital exits were acts of sacrifice and altruism, instead of what they more commonly are: the outcome of non-love and non-commitment.

Failure in Empathic Identification

An interdependent social–moral order is now understood as a threat to personal autonomy and entitlement. In current thought, *primary moral obligation is to the self.* This is new: morality hitherto existed to regulate relations *between* people, at the expense of self-interest. Thus, the ruling wisdom of today is that one should not be constrained into giving up one's own possibilities to "please" or "protect" others—if they do not like what one does, "that's *their* problem!" This non-empathy is seen in Walder's (1978) advice to would-be divorcers: "Pity, a first cousin of guilt, is a ruse to keep you in your marriage. . . . If you're [compassionate] you'll feel sorry your spouse is suffering. The pain is real. So is a child's pain when a child skins a knee. Feel sorry enough and you'll stick around. . . . [But] who will feel sorry for *you*, for staying in an unhappy marriage?" (p. 181).

To Walder, pity is evoked via a mate's "ruse," whose pain is no more serious than a skinned knee. Empathy is a trap—concern should be for oneself, so compassion is misguided. Has modern man reKanted? In effect, the categorical imperative has been revised to "The principle of my will is that I must never feel bad on your account, which then becomes a beneficial general law for all."

The Anti-Conscience

The anti-conscience represents the psychic usurpation of a "victim" identity to counter inner guilt and outer disgrace. This approach is exemplified in the parable of the child who killed both his parents and then threw himself on the mercy of the court on the grounds that he was an orphan. Under the sway of the anti-conscience, empathy is not available for others inasmuch as such sentiment is always rerouted toward the self. In the end, the objects of aggression are blamed for causing one's guilt: their suffering can be held to be aggression against the self because it diminishes self-esteem. Hence, such suffering tends to be viewed as a narcissistic insult that invites suppressive action. Often, cause and effect are reversed: one's own antecedent aggression is excused based on the object's subsequent reaction. In this vein, a man who left his wife and children in dire straits was indignant at his treatment when he visited, finally complaining he had walked out because nobody loved him. A woman lamented that no one in the family unit seemed to care about what separation had cost her by leaving her marriage. She was criticizing her ex-husband and children for not stepping forward to solace her for walking out, when they should have understood, forgiven, and cooperated to make her plight much less distressing.

The Banality of Evil

Arendt (1974) knew full well that evil is never "banal," but she conveyed by that phrase the idea that evil aspires to the unremarkable and commonplace. Evil wishes to insidiously merge into the mores of the culture, and it does so successfully when there is an unformed public consciousness or collusive silence in its presence. When exposed, evil merely poses a temptation to which one may or may not succumb; however, if it goes unrecognized, nearly everyone succumbs. The breakup of a family unit will be regarded as a social evil only to the extent that organized society is prepared to label and judge it that way. Without consensus that it is wrong, nor social cost to transgressors, then indeed this particular evil achieves the status of the banal. To be sure, social disapproval will not hold dysfunctional marriages together, yet it may hold marginal marriages together. But what happens instead is that many influential voices in the mental health field promote values that push vulnerable people beyond the last vestige of conscience-stricken reluctance to divorce. Whenever some new research suggests that the pandemic dissolution of marriages and disruption of family life has reached the proportions of a national crisis, proponents of the cult of individualism rush forward to criticize such findings as "cry of doom" prophecies (e.g., Hunt & Hunt, 1977, p. 267), as if what is so grossly unpleasant must automatically be "overwrought" or "hyperbole."

Summary of the Preceding Five Points

It may be stated that the culture of narcissism, although far from a Nazi culture, shares with the latter a degradation of superego. With the advent of the anti-conscience, the conscience becomes useless as a signal to any discord in our behavior in relation to moral precepts. Rather, the anti-conscience serves to neutralize judgment, externalize blame, and deflect pity into self-pity. Applied to divorce, under the terms of the new metamorality, the pangs of a guilty conscience are perceived as an injustice inflicted by "disturbed" others who have the temerity to proclaim their own woes and to suffer visibly instead of going away nicely. Consider the following examples.

Bernard (1956), a leading sociologist, wondered whether the sullen attitude of a jilted spouse is a "paranoid reaction" or some other psychopathology that then may cause the failure of an ex-partner's new relationship: "The fact that there are relatively fewer successful marriages reported among the divorced as compared with the widowed may be explained in part by the problems which arise when a former spouse is still alive. Failure in remarriage for some divorced persons may be caused by neuroticism not in the remarried spouse but in the spouse who did not remarry" (pp. 204–205). In other words, failure of a second marriage can be blamed on the neurosis of the inexpediently "still alive" mate from the first marriage.

Thamm (1975) mocked the misery of two ex-wives who "committed matrimony" (as he put it) upon him. Under "Acknowledgements," Thamm wrote, "To Kris Larsen and Vickie White who had the misfor tune to be married to me but the foresight to obtain a divorce, I am indeed grateful." A woman summed up her experience with unwelcome suitors as follows: "It's an imposition on me to make me have to hurt somebody" (Baumeister & Wotman, 1992, p. 59). And then there is Walder (1978)—he blamed the problems of children in divorce on their mothers' suffering: "A minority of children do worse [i.e., remain emotionally disturbed more than a year after their parents' breakup]. The deterioration of the mother–child relationship accounts for the downward trend. To my mind, the 'vulnerable child' has a 'vulnerable parent,' one who has not used the divorce experience to grow and mature" (p. 73). Thus, children would take divorce in stride if only their mothers did—allowing blame of upset mothers for troubles children may have when fathers depart.

According to the anti-conscience, a moral view would be that "if you (the symbiant) are good, you will bear your suffering with equanimity—and not punish me with it." Concomitantly, the anti-conscience avers that "if I am good, I will bear feeling badly about your suffering with fortitude—but I also expect support from you for what I have had to go through in hurting you." *The huge mistake that is being made by our culture is that abolishing guilt is held to be equivalent to abolishing evil.* Just the opposite is true—less guilt leads to more evil. We cannot hope to co-opt the guilty conscience to narcissistic ends, for when one hurts another, the guilt does not conveniently go away. Yet despite its now being forbidden to forbid divorce, too many in the late 20th century pursue the mirage that if guilt should still linger, one can turn to the mental health field for a cognitive technology to make nonrepentance the standard of family morality.

HAVE WE LOST OUR ETHICAL BEARINGS?

This brings us to our final words in this chapter and book. We have attempted to describe an American society in insidious crisis, wherein a trend toward cultural disintegration is well advanced. The current situation resembles Yeats's (1921/1983) "The Second Coming":

> Things fall apart; the centre cannot hold;
> Here anarchy is loosed upon the world,
> The blood-dimmed tide is loosed, and everywhere
> The ceremony of innocence is drowned;
> The best lack all conviction, while the worst
> Are full of passionate intensity. (p. 187)

In this vision, Yeats warned society of anarchy as the emerging ethos, to be resolved only by the eventual coming of a second and perhaps not so benign Messiah. In his panorama of unfolding doom, fanatical factions were tearing the culture apart in pursuit of selfish interests. But at the end, rather than the start, of the 20th century, Yeats is somewhat out of date, for the evil of the "worst" may no longer be seen just in "passionate intensity." It more often takes the form of "dispassionate disengagement" in which moral sensibilities are anesthetized. Consider the attitude of the man who announced to his wife that he was ending their marriage and moving out that very night, revealing that he had just withdrawn most of their funds from a joint bank account to rent and furnish his new apartment: "I am leaving you this way because the law says I can. . . . A no-fault divorce means no one is at fault. There is no penalty to me for leaving." (Gillis, 1986, p. 15). If those who equate "civilized" with good manners have their way, gone from one side of divorce will be moral conflict and guilt over hurting another, and gone as well from the other side (through being driven underground) will be emotions expressing attachment. Such passions as may survive will in future be over "entitlement."

In *A Theory of Justice*, Rawls (1971) outlined the contractual nature of a social sense of fairness:

> In a well-ordered society, each person understands the first principles that govern the whole scheme as it is to be carried out over many generations; and all have a settled intention to adhere to these principles in their plan of life. . . . Everyone's more private life is so to speak a plan within a plan, this superordinate plan being realized in the public institutions of society. . . . The regulative public intention is . . . that the constitutional order should realize the principles of justice. (p. 528)

Rawls did not discuss divorce per se, but the family is included among the social institutions he studied. He would not find the extent of divorce a sign of a "well-ordered society," inasmuch as the "plan within a plan" for private lives is violated. A divorce-prone culture would be consistent neither with a consensus about family "justice" nor with a morally cohesive framework for society.

REQUIEM: A FINAL LOOK BACK

In the end, we return to what we stated at the outset—this is not an anti-divorce book. We accept the necessity of breakups, which are about passion, not rationality or consideration. But this recognition does not make divorce "right"; instead, we insist that separation involves social accountability because the parting couple and their children—a family—are engaged in an interdependent symbiotic union within a community composed of many such families.

However, in today's ideological climate, many prominent mental health practitioners believe that we can dispense with both passion and guilt in divorce, as they promulgate a utopian vision of "civilized" marital dissolution. This vision, as rational and promising as it first seems, may in fact prove dangerous because of what it encourages. When a culture leader like Himmler summoned his troops to detach themselves from their own horror at what they were doing, these "modern men" had the psychic means to conform, once given the requisite social support base. In our own times, relative to divorce, Himmler's ideal is within the reach of all of us, for, as it turns out, the temptation to be "superhumanly inhuman" is all too very human.

References

Abelsohn D (1992). A "good-enough" separation: Some characteristic operations and tasks. *Family Process*, 31:61–83.

Abrahamsen D (1973). *The Murdering Mind*. New York: Harper & Row.

Abrahms S (1983). *Children in the Crossfire: The Tragedy of Parental Kidnapping*. New York: Atheneum.

Ackerman D (1995). *A Natural History of Love*. New York: Random House.

Adler A (1956). *The Individual Psychology of Alfred Adler* (H & R Ansbacher, Eds.). New York: Basic Books.

Ahrons CR (1994). *The Good Divorce*. New York: HarperCollins.

Ahrons CR & Miller RB (1993). The effect of the postdivorce relationship on paternal involvement: A longitudinal analysis. *American Journal of Orthopsychiatry*, 63:441–450.

Ainsworth M, Blehar M, Waters E, & Wall S (1978). *Patterns of Attachment*. Hillsdale, NJ: Erlbaum.

Alexander F (1950). *Psychosomatic Medicine*. New York: Norton.

Alexander F (1968). *Psychosomatic Specificity*, vol. I. Chicago: University of Chicago Press.

Althof SE (1989). Psychogenic impotence: Treatment of men and couples (pp. 237–265). In SR Leiblum & RC Rosen (Eds.), *Principles and Practice of Sex Therapy*, second edition. New York: Guilford Press.

Alvarez A (1972). *The Savage God: A Study of Suicide*. New York: Random House.

Arboleda-Florez J (1979). Amok. *Bulletin of the American Academy of Psychiatry and Law*, 7:286–295.

Ardrey R (1961). *African Genesis*. New York: Atheneum.

Arendell T (1986). *Mothers and Divorce: Legal, Economic, and Social Dilemmas*. Berkeley: University of California Press.

Arendt H (1974). *Eichmann in Jerusalem*. New York: McGraw-Hill.

Arlow JA (1980). Object concept and object choice. *Psychoanalytic Quarterly*, 49:109–133.

Artaud A (1965). *Artaud Anthology* (J Hirschman, Ed.). San Francisco: City Lights Books.

417

Atwater L (1982). *The Extramarital Connection: Sex, Intimacy, and Identity.* New York: Irvington.

Bach G & Deutsch R (1971). *Pairing.* New York: Avon.

Bak RC (1973). Being in love and object loss. *International Journal of Psycho-Analysis,* 54:1–7.

Balint M (1968). *The Basic Fault: Therapeutic Aspects of Regression.* London: Tavistock Publications.

Bancroft J (1989). *Human Sexuality and Its Problems,* second edition. Edinburgh: Churchill Livingstone.

Bandura A & Walters R (1963). *Social Learning and Personality Development.* New York: Holt, Rinehart & Winston.

Bartholomew K (1990). Avoidance of intimacy: An attachment perspective. *Journal of Social and Personal Relationships,* 7:147–178.

Bartholomew K (1994). Assessment of individual differences in adult attachment. *Psychological Inquiry,* 5:23–27.

Bartrop R, Lazarus L, Luckhorst E, Kiloh L, & Penny R (1977). Depressed lymphocyte function after bereavement. *Lancet,* 1:834–836.

Baumeister RF & Wotman SR (1992). *Breaking Hearts: The Two Sides of Unrequited Love.* New York: Guilford Press.

Beauvoir S de (1964, November). The question of fidelity. *Harper's,* pp. 57–64.

Beauvoir S de (1984). *Adieux: A Farewell to Sartre.* New York: Pantheon.

Beck AT, Steer R, Kovacs M, & Garrison B (1985). Hopelessness and eventual suicide: A ten-year prospective study of patients hospitalized with suicidal ideation. *American Journal of Psychiatry,* 142:559–563.

Beigel HG (1951). Romantic love. *American Sociological Review,* 16:326–33.

Beilin RL & Izen MG (1991). Custody disputes in context (pp. 305–324). In CA Everett (Ed.), *The Consequences of Divorce.* New York: Haworth Press.

Bell RR (1975). *Marriage and Family Interaction,* fourth edition. Homewood, IL: Dorsey Press.

Bellah R, Madsen R, Sullivan W, Swidler A, & Tipton S (1985). *Habits of the Heart: Individualism and Commitment in American Life.* Berkeley: University of California Press.

Belsky J & Cassidy J (1994). Attachment and close relationships: An individual-difference perspective. *Psychological Inquiry,* 5:27–30.

Bennett M (1991). *Wife Rejection in Happy Marriages.* New York: William Morrow.

Berger B & Berger P (1983). *The War over the Family: Capturing the Middle Ground.* New York: Anchor Books.

Bergler E (1946). *Unhappy Marriage and Divorce: A Study of Neurotic Change of Marital Partners.* New York: International Universities Press.

Bergler E (1948). *Divorce Won't Help.* New York: Harper & Row.

Bergmann MS (1971). Psychoanalytic observations on the capacity to love (pp. 15–40). In J McDevitt & C Settlage (Eds.), *Separation–Individuation: Essays in Honor of Margaret S. Mahler.* New York: International Universities Press.

Bergmann MS (1980). On the intrapsychic function of falling in love. *Psychoanalytic Quarterly,* 49:56–77.

Bergner R (1977). The marital system of the hysterical individual. *Family Process,* 16:85–95.

Berman WH (1988). The role of attachment in the post-divorce experience. *Journal of Personality and Social Psychology,* 54:496–503.

Bernard J (1956). *Remarriage: A Study of Marriage.* New York: Dryden Press.

Bernard J (1971). No news, but new ideas (pp. 3–25). In P Bohannan (Ed.), *Divorce and After.* Garden City, NY: Anchor Books.

Bernard J (1977). Jealousy and marriage (pp. 141–150). In G Clanton & L Smith (Eds.), *Jealousy.* Englewood Cliffs, NJ: Prentice-Hall.

Bernard ME (1986). *Staying Rational in an Irrational World: Albert Ellis and Rational-Emotive Therapy.* New York: Carol Publishing Group.

Bernhard KF (1986). *Jealousy: Its Nature and Treatment.* Springfield, IL: Charles C Thomas.

Besnard P (1988). The true nature of anomie. *Sociological Theory,* 6:91–95.

Bjorksten O & Stewart T (1984). Contemporary trends in American marriage (pp. 3–59). In C Nadelson & D Polonsky (Eds.), *Marriage and Divorce: A Contemporary Perspective.* New York: Guilford Press.

Blinder M (1985). *Lovers, Killers, Husbands, and Wives: A Court Psychiatrist Looks at Crimes of Passion.* New York: St. Martin's Press.

Block J, Block JH, & Gjerde PF (1988). Parental functioning and the home environment in families of divorce: Prospective and concurrent analysis. *Journal of the American Academy of Child and Adolescent Psychiatry,* 27:207–213.

Blum S (1976, August 29). The re-mating game. *New York Times,* Sunday Magazine Section, pp. 10–22.

Blumstein P & Schwartz P (1983). *American Couples: Money, Work, Sex.* New York: Morrow.

Boesky D (1980). Symposium on object relations theory and love: Introduction. *Psychoanalytic Quarterly,* 49:48–55.

Bohannan P (1969). *Love, Sex, and Being Human.* Garden City, NY: Doubleday.

Bohannon P (1971). *Divorce and After.* Garden City, New York: Anchor Books.

Bottome P (1939). *Alfred Adler: A Biography.* New York: Putnam's Sons.

Bowen M (1978). *Family Therapy in Clinical Practice.* New York: Jason Aronson.

Boszormenyi-Nagy I & Framo J (1965). *Intensive Family Therapy.* New York: Hoeber.

Bowlby J (1979). *The Making and Breaking of Affectional Ties.* London: Tavistock.

Brandwein RA, Brown CA, & Fox EM (1974). Women and children last: The social situation of divorced mothers and their families. *Journal of Marriage and the Family,* 36:498–514.

Breuer J & Freud S (1895/1955). Studies in hysteria. In *The Standard Edition of the Complete Psychological Works of Sigmund Freud,* vol. 2 (J Strachey, Ed. and Trans.). London: Hogarth Press.

Bromberg W (1961). *The Mold of Murder: A Psychiatric Study of Homicide.* New York: Grune & Stratton.

Brown EM (1991). *Patterns of Infidelity and their Treatment.* New York: Brunner/Mazel.

Brown P, Felton B, Whiteman V, & Manela R (1980). Attachment and distress following marital separation. *Journal of Divorce,* 3:303–317.

Brownmiller S (1975). *Against Our Will: Men, Women, and Rape.* New York: Simon & Schuster.

Buchanan CM, Maccoby EE, & Dornbusch SM (1991). Caught between parents: Adolescents' experience in divorced homes. *Child Development,* 62:1008–1029.

Burgess EW & Wallin P (1953). *Engagement and Marriage.* Philadelphia: Lippincott.

Byron E (1986, February). Will you marry me—*again? Redbook,* pp. 90–146.

Calvin DA (1981). Joint custody: As family and social policy (pp. 99–145). In IR Stuart & LE Abt (Eds.), *Children of Separation and Divorce: Management and Treatment.* New York: Van Nostrand Reinhold.

Cannon W (1957). Voodoo death. *Psychosomatic Medicine,* 19:182–190.

Caprio F (1953). *Marital Infidelity.* New York: Citadel Press.

Carr A & Schoenberg B (1970). Object loss and somatic symptom formation (pp. 36–47). In B Schoenberg, A Carr, D Peretz, & A Kutscher (Eds.), *Loss and Grief: Psychological Management in Medical Practice.* New York: Columbia University Press.

Cassius J & Koonce K (1974). Divorce as a final option: A transactional perspective (pp. 140–154). In J Kull & R Hardy (Eds.), *Deciding on Divorce.* Springfield, IL: Charles C Thomas.

Chambers W & Reiser F (1953). Emotional stress in the precipitation of congestive heart failure. *Psychosomatic Medicine,* 15:38–60.

Charlton RS (1980, April). Divorce as a psychological experience. *Psychiatric Annals,* 10:138–144.

Charny I (1972). *Marital Love and Hate.* New York: Macmillan.

Chen E & Cobb S (1960). Family structure in relation to health and disease. *Journal of Chronic Disease,* 12:544–567.

Cherlin A (1978). Remarriage as an incomplete institution. *American Journal of Sociology,* 84:634–650.

Chesler P (1972). *Women and Madness.* New York: Avon.

Chesler P. (1986). *Mothers on Trial: The Battle for Children and Custody.* New York: McGraw-Hill.

Chimbos PD (1978). *Marital Violence: A Study of Interspouse Homicide.* San Francisco: R & E Research Associates.

Clanton G & Smith L (1977). *Jealousy.* Englewood Cliffs, NJ: Prentice-Hall.

Cohen S & Jones FN (1983). Issues of divorce in family therapy (pp. 465–478). In B Wolman & G Stricker (Eds.), *Handbook of Marital and Family Therapy.* New York: Plenum Press.

Comfort A (1974). Sexuality in a zero-growth society. In J Smith & L Smith (Eds.), *Beyond Monogamy.* Baltimore: Johns Hopkins University Press.

Constantine L & Constantine J (1972). Counseling implications of co-marital and multilateral relations (pp. 537–552). In C Sager & H Kaplan (Eds.), *Progress in Group and Family Therapy,* New York: Brunner/Mazel.

Cooper AM (1989). Narcissism and masochism: The narcissistic–masochistic character. *Psychiatric Clinics of North America*, 12:541–552.

Cooper D (1970). *The Death of the Family*. New York: Pantheon.

Corman A (1977). *Kramer vs. Kramer*. New York: Random House.

Cousins N (1984). *The Healing Heart*. New York: Avon.

Crosby J, Gage B, & Raymond M (1983). The grief resolution process in divorce. *Journal of Divorce*, 7:3–18.

Crosby JF (1989). *When One Wants Out and the Other Doesn't: Doing Therapy with Polarized Couples*. New York: Brunner/Mazel.

Crowell JA & Waters E (1994). Bowlby's theory grown up: The role of attachment in adult love relationships. *Psychological Inquiry*, 5:31–34.

Daly M & Wilson M (1988). *Homicide*. New York: Aldine de Gruyter.

Davis K (1936). Jealousy and sexual property. *Social Forces*, 14:395–405.

DeRougemont D (1956). *Love in the Western World*. New York: Pantheon.

Despert JL (1953). *Children of Divorce*. Garden City, NY: Dolphin.

DeWolf R (1970). *The Bonds of Acrimony*. Philadelphia: Lippincott.

Dicks HV (1967). *Marital Tensions: Clinical Studies toward a Psychological Theory of Interaction*. New York: Basic Books.

Dorpat TL (1976). Suicide in murderers (pp. 193–197). In M Wolfgang (Ed.), *Studies in Homicide*. NY: Harper & Row.

Douglas JWB (1970). Broken families and child behaviour. *Journal of the Royal College of Physicians of London*, 4:203–210.

Dreikurs R (1968). Determinants of changing attitudes of marital partners toward each other (pp. 83–103). In S Rosenbaum & I Alger (Eds.), *The Marriage Relationship: Psychoanalytic Perspective*. New York: Society of Medical Psychoanalysis.

Dubos R (1959). *Mirage of Health: Utopias, Progress, and Biological Change*. New York: Harper.

Duck S (1994). Attaching meaning to attachment. *Psychological Inquiry*, 5:34–38.

Dudley JR (1994). Fathers who have infrequent contact with their children (pp. 242–257). In AS Skolnick & JH Skolnick (Eds.), *Family in Transition*, eighth edition. New York: HarperCollins.

Dullea G (1980, February 3). Is joint custody good for children? *New York Times*, Sunday Magazine Section, pp. 32–46.

Dunbar F (1948). *Psychosomatic Diagnosis*. New York: Hoeber.

Durbin K (1977). On sexual jealousy (pp. 36–45). In G Clanton & L Smith (Eds.), *Jealousy*. Englewood Cliffs NJ: Prentice-Hall.

Durkheim E (1897). *Suicide: A Study in Sociology* (originally published in French, J Spaulding & G Simpson, Trans.). New York: Free Press, 1951.

Eckhardt KW (1973). Deviance, visibility, and legal action: The duty to support (pp. 55–64). In C Bryant & J Wells (Eds.), *Deviancy and the Family*. Philadelphia: Davis.

Edwards R (1995, February). Healthy divorces can lead to well-adjusted children. *American Psychological Association, Monitor*, p. 7.

Ehrenreich B (1985, December 28/1986, January 4). The moral bypass. *The Nation*, pp. 717–718.

Elkin D (1994). *Ties That Stress: The New Family Imbalance.* Cambridge: Harvard University Press.

Ellis A (1972). *The Civilized Couple's Guide to Extramarital Adventure.* New York: Wyden.

Ellis A (1975). *A New Guide to Rational Living.* Englewood Cliffs, NJ: Prentice-Hall.

Engel G & Schmale A (1967). Psychoanalytic theory of somatic disorder. *Journal of the American Psychoanalytic Association,* 15:344–365.

English OS (1971). The positive values of the affair (pp. 173–192). In H Otto (Ed.), *The New Sexuality.* Palo Alto, CA: Science & Behavior Books.

Ephron D (1986). *Funny Sauce: Us, the Ex, the Ex's New Mate, the New Mate's Ex, and the Kids.* New York: Viking.

Epstein J (1974). *Divorced in America.* New York: Penguin.

Eskapa S (1984). *Woman versus Woman.* New York: Franklin Watts.

Everett CA & Everett SV (1994). *Healthy Divorce.* San Francisco: Jossey-Bass.

Everett CA & Volgy SS (1991). Treating divorce in family therapy practice (pp. 508–524). In AS Gurman & DP Kniskern (Eds.), *Handbook of Family Therapy,* vol. 2. New York: Brunner/Mazel.

Fairbairn WR (1952). *An Object-Relations Theory of the Personality.* New York: Basic Books.

Fanon F (1966). *The Wretched of the Earth.* New York: Grove.

Feifer G (1995). *Divorce: An Oral Portrait.* New York: The New Press.

Fenichel O (1945). *The Psychoanalytic Theory of Neurosis.* New York: Norton.

Fisher A with Weller S (1993). *My Story.* New York: Pocket Books.

Fisher EO (1968). *Help for Today's Troubled Marriages.* New York: Hawthorne Press.

Fisher EO (1974). *Divorce: The New Freedom.* New York: Harper & Row.

Fogarty T (1976). Marital Crisis (pp. 325–334). In P Guerin (Ed.), *Family Therapy: Theory and Practice.* New York: Gardner.

Forel A (1933). *The Sexual Question.* New York: Physicians & Surgeons Book Co.

Framo JL (1978, February). The friendly divorce. *Psychology Today,* pp. 77–102 passim.

Framo JL (1982). Husbands' reactions to wives' infidelity (pp. 152–160). *Explorations in Marital and Family Therapy: Selected Papers of James L. Framo.* New York: Springer.

Francke LB (1983). *Growing Up Divorced.* New York: Linden.

Frank J (1973). *Persuasion and Healing.* Baltimore: Johns Hopkins University Press.

Freeman MD (1985). Doing his best to sustain the sanctity of marriage. *Sociological Review Monograph,* 31:124–146.

Freud S (1912/1925). On the universal tendency to debasement in the sphere of love (pp. 177–190). In *The Standard Edition of the Complete Psychological Works of Sigmund Freud,* vol. 11 (J Strachey, Ed. and Trans.). London: Hogarth Press.

Freud S (1913/1955). Totem and taboo (pp. 1–161). In *The Standard Edition of the Complete Psychological Works of Sigmund Freud*, vol. 13 (J Strachey, Ed. and Trans.). London: Hogarth Press.

Freud S (1917/1957). Mourning and melancholia (pp. 243–258). In *The Standard Edition of the Complete Psychological Works of Sigmund Freud*, vol. 14 (J Strachey, Ed. and Trans.). London: Hogarth Press.

Freud S (1922/1957). Certain neurotic mechanisms in jealousy, paranoia, and homosexuality (pp. 221–232). In *The Standard Edition of the Complete Psychological Works of Sigmund Freud*, vol. 18 (J Strachey, Ed. and Trans.). London: Hogarth Press.

Freud S (1930/1957). Civilization and its discontents (pp. 59–145). In *The Standard Edition of the Complete Psychological Works of Sigmund Freud*, vol. 21 (J Strachey, Ed. and Trans.). London: Hogarth Press.

Friday N (1985). *Jealousy*. Toronto: Perigord Press.

Friedman A & Rosenman R (1968). Etiology and pathogenesis of coronary arteriosclerosis. *Cardiovascular Disease*. Philadelphia: Davis.

Fromm E (1956). *The Art of Loving*, New York: Harper & Row.

Fuchs V (1974). *Who Shall Live?* New York: Basic Books.

Furstenberg FF & Cherlin AJ (1991). *Divided Families: What Happens to Children When Parents Part*. Cambridge: Harvard University Press.

Furstenberg RR (1994). Good dads—Bad dads: Two faces of fatherhood (pp. 348–368). In AS Skolnick & JH Skolnick (Eds.), *Family in Transition*, eighth edition. New York: HarperCollins.

Gardner R (1976). *Psychotherapy with Children of Divorce*. New York: Jason Aronson.

Garrity CB & Baris MA (1994). *Caught in the Middle: Protecting the Children of High-Conflict Divorce*. New York: Lexington Books.

Gatchel RJ & Blanchard EB (1993). *Psychophysiological Disorders: Research and Clinical Applications*. Washington: American Psychological Association.

Gernsbacher LM (1985). *The Suicide Syndrome*. New York: Human Sciences Press.

Gersick KE (1979). Fathers by choice: Divorced men who receive custody of their children (pp. 307–323). In G Levinger & OC Moles (Eds.), *Divorce and Separation: Context, Causes, and Consequences*. New York: Basic Books.

Gettleman S & Markowitz J (1974). *The Courage to Divorce*. New York: Ballantine.

Gillespie WH (1967). Notes on the analysis of sexual perversions (pp. 26–40). In H Ruitenbeek (Ed.), *The Psychotherapy of Perversions*. New York: Citadel Press.

Gilligan C (1982). *In a Different Voice*. Cambridge, MA: Harvard University Press.

Gillis P (1986). *Days Like This*. New York: McGraw-Hill.

Glick PC (1994). American families: As they are and were (pp. 91–104). In AS Skolnick & JH Skolnick (Eds.), *Family in Transition*, eighth edition. New York: HarperCollins.

Glueck S & Glueck E (1950). *Unraveling Juvenile Delinquency*. New York: Commonwealth Fund.

Glueck S & Glueck E (1962). *Family Environment and Delinquency.* London: Routledge & Kegan Paul.

Godwin J (1978). *Murder USA: The Ways We Kill Each Other.* New York: Ballantine Books.

Goldenberg H & Goldenberg I (1982). Homicide and the family (pp. 199–206). In BL Danto, J Bruhns, & AH Kutscher (Eds.), *The Human Side of Homicide.* New York: Columbia University Press.

Goldner V, Penn P, Sheinberg M, & Walker G (1990). Love and violence: Gender paradoxes in volatile attachments. *Family Process,* 29:343–364.

Goldstein J, Freud A, & Solnit A (1973). *Beyond the Best Interests of the Child.* New York: Free Press.

Goode WJ (1956). *After Divorce.* Glencoe, IL: Free Press.

Goode WJ (1959). The theoretical importance of love. *American Sociological Review,* 24:38–47.

Goode WJ (1964). *The Family.* Englewood Cliffs, NJ: Prentice-Hall.

Gordon E (1962). *Through the Valley of the Kwai.* New York: Harper & Row.

Gottman JM (1994). *Why Marriages Succeed or Fail.* New York: Simon & Schuster.

Grant VW (1976). *Falling in Love: The Psychology of the Romantic Emotion.* New York: Springer.

Gray C, Koopman E, & Hunt J (1991). The emotional phases of marital separation: An empirical investigation. *American Journal of Orthopsychiatry,* 61:138–143.

Greenfield S (1965). Love and marriage in modern America: A functional analysis. *Sociological Quarterly,* 6:361–377.

Grinker RR (1973). *Psychosomatic Concepts.* New York: Jason Aronson.

Grolnick L (1972). A family perspective of psychosomatic factors in illness: A review of the literature. *Family Process,* 11:457–486.

Gurin G, Veroff J, & Feld S (1960). *Americans View Their Mental Health: A Nationwide Survey.* New York: Basic Books.

Guttmacher M (1960). *The Mind of the Murderer.* New York: Farrar, Straus, & Cudahy.

Hacker A (1979, May 3). Divorce a la mode. *New York Review of Books,* 26:23–27.

Hancock E (1980). The dimensions of meaning and belonging in the process of divorce. *American Journal of Orthopsychiatry,* 50:18–27.

Hazan C & Shaver PR (1994a). Attachment as an organizational framework for research on close relationships. *Psychological Inquiry,* 5:1–22.

Hazan C & Shaver PR (1994b). Deeper into attachment theory. *Psychological Inquiry,* 5:68–79.

Heiman JR & Grafton-Becker V (1989). Orgasmic disorders in women (pp. 51–88). In SR Leiblum & RC Rosen (Eds.), *Principles and Practice of Sex Therapy,* second edition. New York: Guilford Press.

Hendin H (1995). *Suicide in America.* New York: Norton.

Hendrick C & Hendrick SS (1994). Attachment theory and close adult relationships. *Psychological Inquiry,* 5:38–41.

Henkin F (1964). Physical illness in disturbed marriages. *Medical Times*, 92:206–208.

Hetherington EM (1979). Divorce: A child's perspective. *American Psychologist*, 34:851–858.

Hetherington EM (1989). Coping with family transitions: Winners, losers, and survivors. *Child Development*, 60:1–14.

Hetherington EM, Cox M, & Cox R (1976). Divorced fathers. *Family Coordinator*, 25:417–428.

Hetherington EM, Law TC, & O'Connor TG (1993). Divorce: Challenges, changes, and new chances (pp. 208–234). In F Walsh (Ed.), *Normal Family Processes*, second edition. New York: Guilford Press.

Hill CT, Rubin Z, & Peplau LA (1976). Breakups before marriage: The end of 103 affairs. *Journal of Social Issues*, 32:147–168.

Hitschmann E (1952). Freud's conception of love. *International Journal of Psycho-Analysis*, 33:421–428.

Hodges WF (1986). *Interventions for Children of Divorce*. New York: Wiley.

Hopkins P (1959). Health and happiness in the family. *British Journal of Clinical Practice*, 13:311–313.

Houts M (1970). *They Asked for Death*. New York: Cowles Book Co.

Hunt M (1966). *The World of the Formerly Married*. New York: McGraw-Hill.

Hunt M (1969). *The Affair*. New York: World Publishing.

Hunt M & Hunt B (1977). *The Divorce Experience*. New York: McGraw-Hill.

Hunter JD (1992). *Culture Wars: The Struggle to Control Family, Art, Education, Law, and Politics in America*. New York: Basic Books.

Hutschnecker A (1951). *The Will to Live*. New York: Cromwell.

Hyde M & Hyde L (1985). *Missing Children*. New York: Franklin Watts.

Imboden J, Canter A, & Cliff L (1963). Separation experiences and health records in a group of normal adults. *Psychosomatic Medicine*, 25:433–440.

Isaacs MB, Montalvo B, & Abelsohn D (1986). *The Difficult Divorce*. New York: Basic Books.

Jackson DD (1965). Family rules and marital quid pro quo. *Archives of General Psychiatry*, 12:588–594.

Jacobs JW (1988). Euripedes' Medea: A psychodynamic model of severe divorce pathology. *American Journal of Psychotherapy*, 42:308–319.

Jacobson GF & Jacobson DS (1987). Impact of marital dissolution on adults and children (pp. 316–344). In J Bloom-Feshbach & S Bloom-Feshbach (Eds.), *The Psychology of Separation and Loss*. San Francisco: Jossey-Bass.

Jagers JL (1989). Putting Humpty-Dumpty together again: Reconciling the post-affair marriage. *Journal of Psychology and Christianity*, 8:63–72.

Johnston JR, Kline M, & Tschann JM (1989). Ongoing postdivorce conflict: Effects on children of joint custody and frequent access. *American Journal of Orthopsychiatry*, 59:576–592.

Jones BW (1987). Dysfunctional marital patterns: The ambivalent spouse syndrome. *Journal of Divorce*, 10:57–67.

Jones E (1963). *The Life and Work of Sigmund Freud,* abridged edition. Garden City, NY: Anchor Books.

Jong E (1973). *Fear of Flying.* New York: Holt, Rinehart & Winston.

Jong E (1977). *How to Save Your Own Life.* New York: Holt, Rinehart & Winston.

Josephson M (1946). *Stendhal, or the Pursuit of Happiness.* Garden City, NY: Doubleday.

Jurich AP (1989). The art of depolarization (pp. 45–65). In JF Crosby (Ed.), *When One Wants Out and the Other Doesn't.* New York: Brunner/Mazel.

Kahn SS (1990). *The Ex-Wife Syndrome: Cutting the Cord and Breaking Free after the Marriage Is Over.* New York: Random House.

Kanner B (1993, August). Love is blind. *Ladies Home Journal,* pp. 56–168 passim.

Kaplan HS (1996). Erotic obsession: Relationship to hypoactive sexual desire disorder and paraphilia. *American Journal of Psychiatry,* July Festschrift Supplement, 153:30–41.

Kaslow FW (1981). Divorce and divorce therapy (pp. 662–696). In AS Gurman & DP Kniskern (Eds.), *Handbook of Family Therapy,* vol. 1. New York: Brunner/Mazel.

Kaufman S (1967). *Diary of a Mad Housewife.* New York: Random House.

Kayser K (1993). *When Love Dies: The Process of Marital Disaffection.* New York: Guilford Press.

Kelly JB (1981). The visiting relationship after divorce: Research findings and clinical implications (pp. 338–361). In IR Stuart & LE Abt (Eds.), *Children of Separation and Divorce: Management and Treatment.* New York: Van Nostrand Reinhold.

Kernberg OF (1980). *Internal World and External Reality.* New York: Jason Aronson.

Kernberg OF (1995). *Love Relations: Normality and Pathology.* New Haven: Yale University Press.

Kiecolt-Glaser JK, Fisher L, Ogrocki P, Stout JC, Speicher CE, & Glaser R (1987). Marital quality, marital disruption, and immune function. *Psychosomatic Medicine,* 49:13–34.

Kiecolt-Glaser JK, Kennedy S, Malkoff S, Fisher L, Speicher CE, & Glaser R (1988). Marital discord and immunity in males. *Psychosomatic Medicine,* 50:213–229.

Kitson GC (1992). *Portrait of Divorce.* New York: Guilford Press.

Knox D (1981). *Death March: The Survivors of Bataan.* San Diego: Harvest.

Kogan E (1980). *Theory and Practice of Hell.* New York: Berkley.

Kohut H (1971). *The Analysis of the Self.* New York: International Universities Press.

Kovel J (1981). *The Age of Desire: Case Histories of a Radical Psychoanalyst.* New York: Pantheon Books.

Kramer PD (1993). *Listening to Prozac: A Psychiatrist Explores Antidepressant Drugs and the Remaking of the Self.* New York: Viking.

Krantzler M (1975). *Creative Divorce: A New Opportunity for Personal Growth.* New York: Signet.

Kreitman N, Sainsbury P, Pearce K, & Costain W (1965). Hypochondriasis and depression in outpatients at a general hospital. *British Journal of Psychiatry,* 111:607–615.

Kressel K (1980). Patterns of coping in divorce and some implications for clinical practice. *Family Relations,* 29:234–240.

Kressel K & Deutsch M (1977). Divorce therapy: An in-depth survey of therapists' views. *Family Process,* 16:413–433.

Kruk E (1991). Discontinuity between pre- and post-divorce father–child relationships: New evidence regarding paternal disengagement (pp. 195–227). In CA Everett (Ed.), *The Consequences of Divorce.* New York: Haworth Press.

Kübler-Ross E (1969). *On Death and Dying.* New York: Macmillan.

Lacey J (1956/1957). The evaluation of autonomic responses: Toward a general solution. *Annals of the New York Academy of Sciences,* 67:125–163.

Lacey J, Bateman D, & Van Lehn R (1952). Autonomic response specificity and Rorschach color responses. *Psychosomatic Medicine,* 14:256–260.

Lacey J, Bateman D, & Van Lehn R (1953). Autonomic response specificity. *Psychosomatic Medicine,* 15:8–21.

Laing RD (1965). Mystification, confusion, and conflict (pp. 343–363). In I Boszormenyi-Nagy & JL Framo (Eds.), *Intensive Family Therapy: Theoretical and Practical Aspects.* New York: Hoeber.

Laing RD (1969). *The Politics of the Family.* New York: Vintage Books.

Larson JM (1993). Exploring reconciliation. *Mediation Quarterly,* 11:95–106.

Lasch C (1977). *Haven in a Heartless World: The Family Besieged.* New York: Basic Books.

Lasch C (1979). *The Culture of Narcissism: American Life in an Age of Diminishing Expectations.* New York: Warner Books.

Lawson A (1988). *Adultery: An Analysis of Love and Betrayal.* New York: Basic Books.

Lehrer T (1981). The masochism tango (pp. 55–59). In *Too Many Songs by Tom Lehrer and Not Enough Drawings by Ronald Searle.* New York: Pantheon.

Leigh W (1985). *The Infidelity Report: An Investigation of Extramarital Affairs.* New York: Morrow.

Lester D (1992). *Why People Kill Themselves: A 1990's Summary of Research Findings on Suicidal Behavior.* Springfield, IL: Charles C Thomas.

Lester D & Lester G (1975). *Crime of Passion: Murder and the Murderer.* Chicago: Nelson-Hall.

Levin J & Fox J (1985). *Mass Murder: America's Growing Menace.* New York: Plenum Press.

Lewis CS (1947). *The Abolition of Man.* London: Centenary Press.

Lewis M (1994). Does attachment imply a relationship or multiple relationships? *Psychological Inquiry,* 5:47–51.

Libby RW (1978). Today's changing sexual mores (pp. 563–576). In J Money & H Musaph (Eds.), *Handbook of Sexology,* vol. 1. New York: Elsevier.

Lief HI (1974). Sexual knowledge, attitudes, and behavior of medical students: Implications for medical practice (pp. 474–494). In DW Abse, EM Nash,

& LM Louden (Eds.), *Marital and Sexual Counseling in Medical Practice,* second edition. New York: Harper & Row.

Lifton RJ (1971). Protean man. *Archives of General Psychiatry,* 24:298–304.

Litman RE (1970a). Suicide as acting out (pp. 293–304). In ES Shneidman, NL Farberow, & RE Litman (Eds.), *The Psychology of Suicide.* New York: Science House.

Litman RE (1970b). Sigmund Freud on suicide (pp. 565–586). In ES Shneidman, NL Farberow, & RE Litman (Eds.), *The Psychology of Suicide.* New York: Science House.

Lobsenz N (1977). Taming the green-eyed monster (pp. 26–34). In G Clanton & L Smith (Eds.), *Jealousy.* Englewood Cliffs, NJ: Prentice-Hall.

Locke S & Hornig-Rohan M (1983). *Mind and Immunity: Behavioral Immunology.* New York: Institute for the Advancement of Health.

Lonsdorf BJ (1991). The role of coercion in affecting women's inferior outcomes in divorce: Implications for researchers and therapists (pp. 69–106). In CA Everett (Ed.), *The Consequences of Divorce.* New York: Haworth Press.

Lubetkin B & Oumano E (1991). *Bailing Out.* New York: Simon & Schuster.

Lynch JJ (1977). *The Broken Heart: The Medical Consequences of Loneliness.* New York: Basic Books.

Maccoby EE & Mnookin RH (1992). *Dividing the Child: Social and Legal Dilemmas of Custody.* Cambridge: Harvard University Press.

Main M & Solomon J (1990). Procedures for identifying infants as disorganized/disoriented during the Ainsworth Strange Situation (pp. 121–160). In MT Greenberg, D Ciccetti, & EM Cummings (Eds.), *Attachment in the Pre-School Years.* Chicago: University of Chicago Press.

Martin A (1975). *One Man, Hurt.* New York: Macmillan.

Maslow AH (1971). *The Farther Reaches of Human Nature.* New York: Viking Press.

Masterson JF (1981). *The Narcissistic and Borderline Disorders.* New York: Brunner/Mazel.

Masterson JF (1993). *The Emerging Self: A Developmental, Self, and Object Relations Approach to the Treatment of the Closet Narcissistic Disorder of the Self.* New York: Brunner/Mazel.

Maugham WS (1915/1963). *Of Human Bondage.* New York: Penguin Books.

May R (1969). *Love and Will.* New York: Norton.

Mayer N (1978). *The Male Mid-Life Crisis.* Garden City, NY: Doubleday.

Mazur R (1973). *The New Intimacy: Open-Ended Marriage and Alternative Lifestyles.* Boston: Beacon.

McCord W & McCord J (1959). *The Origins of Crime.* New York: Columbia University Press.

McDonald J (1961). *The Murderer and His Victim.* Springfield, IL: Thomas.

McDonald J (1968). *Homicidal Threats.* Springfield, IL: Charles C Thomas.

McDonald P & McDonald D (1977). *Guilt-Free.* New York: Ballantine.

McFadden C (1986, October 12). Sharper than lots of serpents' teeth. *New York Times,* Book Review Section, p. 13.

McGoldrick M & Carter B (1989). Forming a remarried family (pp. 402–429). In B Carter & M McGoldrick (Eds.), *The Changing Family Life Cycle*, second edition. Boston: Allyn & Bacon.

McGrady PM (1972). *The Love Doctors.* New York: Macmillan.

Mednick MT (1994). Single mothers: A review and critique of current research (pp. 368–383). In AS Skolnick & JH Skolnick (Eds.), *Family in Transition*, eighth edition. New York: HarperCollins.

Medved D (1989). *The Case against Divorce.* New York: Ivy Books.

Meerloo J (1968). *Suicide and Mass Suicide.* New York: Dutton.

Memmi A (1979/1984). *Dependence* (originally published in French, PA Facey, Trans.). Boston: Beacon Press.

Menninger K (1938). *Man against Himself.* New York: Harcourt, Brace.

Metropolitan Life Insurance Company (1957, February). Mortality lowest in married population. *Statistical Bulletin*, 38:4–7.

Millet K (1971). *Sexual Politics.* New York: Avon Books.

Mitchell M (1936/1973). *Gone with the Wind.* New York: Avon Books.

Monahan T (1958). The changing nature and instability of remarriages. *Eugenics Quarterly*, 5:53–85.

Money J (1980). *Love and Love Sickness.* Baltimore: Johns Hopkins University Press.

Monroe RL (1955). *Schools of Psychoanalytic Thought.* New York: Holt, Rinehart & Winston.

Moreland J, Schwebel AI, Fine MA, & Vess JD (1982). Postdivorce family therapy: Suggestions for professionals. *Professional Psychology*, 13:639–646.

Morris T & Blom-Cooper M (1976). The victim's contribution (pp. 66–71). In M. Wolfgang (Ed.), *Studies in Homicide.* New York: Harper & Row.

Moultrup DJ (1990). *Husbands, Wives, and Lovers: The Emotional System of the Extramarital Affair.* New York: Guilford Press.

Mowat RR (1966). *Morbid Jealousy and Murder.* London: Tavistock Publications.

Moynihan DP (1992). Defining deviancy down. *American Scholar*, 61:17–30.

Mullen J (1981). *Kierkegaard's Philosophy, Self-Deception, and Cowardice in the Present Age.* New York: Mentor.

Mullen PE (1991). Jealousy: The pathology of passion. *British Journal of Psychiatry*, 158:593–601.

Murphy G & Robins E (1967). Social factors in suicide. *Journal of the American Medical Association*, 199:303–308.

Murstein B (1976). *Who Will Marry Whom?* New York: Springer.

Mussen P & Eisenberg-Berg N (1977). *Roots of Caring, Sharing, and Helping: The Development of Prosocial Behavior in Children.* San Francisco: Freeman.

Myers MF (1989). *Men and Divorce.* New York: Guilford Press.

Napier AY (1978). The rejection-intrusion pattern: A central family dynamic. *Journal of Marriage and Family Counseling*, 4:5–12.

Napier AY (1988). *The Fragile Bond: In Search of an Equal, Intimate, and Enduring Marriage.* New York: Harper & Row.

Napier AY & Whitaker C (1978). *The Family Crucible.* New York: Harper & Row.

Nelson G (1994). Emotional well-being of separated and married women: Long-term follow-up study. *American Journal of Orthopsychiatry*, 64:150–160.

Noller P & Feeney JA (1994). Whither attachment theory: Attachment to our caregivers or to our models? *Psychological Inquiry*, 5:51–56.

Nordheimer J (1987, August 2). As tensions grow in divorce proceedings, attacks on court officers mount. *New York Times*, Section I, p. 22.

Norman M (1980, November 23). The new extended family. *New York Times*, Sunday Magazine Section, pp. 26–173 passim.

Norton A & Glick P (1979). Marital instability in America: Past, present, and future (pp. 6–19). In G Levinger & O Moles (Eds.), *Divorce and Separation*. New York: Basic Books.

Offit AK (1995). *Night Thoughts: Reflections of a Sex Therapist*, revised edition. Northvale, NJ: Jason Aronson.

O'Leary A (1990). Stress, emotion, and human immune function. *Psychological Bulletin*, 108:363–382.

O'Neill N & O'Neill G (1972). *Open Marriage: A New Life Style for Couples*. New York: New American Library.

O'Neil WL (1967). *Divorce in the Progressive Era*. New Haven: Yale University Press.

Oppawsky J (1991). The effects of parental divorce on children in West Germany: Emphasis from the view of the children (pp. 291–304). In CA Everett (Ed.), *The Consequences of Divorce*. New York: Haworth Press.

Ottenheimer L (1968). Psychodynamics of the choice of a mate (pp. 59–69). In S Rosenbaum & I Alger (Eds.), *The Marriage Relationship*. New York: Basic Books.

Ovesey L (1969). *Homosexuality and Pseudohomosexuality*. New York: Science House.

Pam A (1990). A critique of the scientific status of biological psychiatry. *Acta Psychiatrica Scandinavica*, 82 (Suppl. 362).

Pam A, Plutchik R, & Conte HR (1975). Love: A psychometric approach. *Psychological Reports*, 37:83–88.

Pam A & Pearson J (1994). The geometry of the eternal triangle. *Family Process*, 33:175–190.

Paykel ES (1980). Recent life events and attempted suicide (pp. 105–115). In R Farmer & S Hirsch (Eds.), *The Suicide Syndrome*. London: Croom Helm.

Paykel E, Myers J, Dienelt M, Klerman G, Lindenthal J, & Pepper M (1969). Life events and depression: A controlled study. *Archives of General Psychiatry*, 21:753–60.

Pearce D (1978). The feminization of poverty: Women, work, and welfare. *Urban and Social Change Review*, 11:28–36.

Peck MS (1983). *People of the Lie: The Hope for Healing Human Evil*. New York: Simon & Schuster.

Peele S & Brodsky A (1975). *Love and Addiction*. New York: Signet.

Perls F (1969). *Gestalt Therapy Verbatim*. Lafayette, CA: Real People Press.

Pittman FS (1987). *Turning Points: Treating Families in Transition and Crisis*. New York: Norton.

Pittman FS (1989). *Private Lies: Infidelity and the Betrayal of Intimacy*. New York: Norton.

Pledge DS (1992). Marital separation/divorce: A review of individual responses to a major life stressor. *Journal of Divorce and Remarriage*, 17:151–181.

Popenoe P (1938). Remarriage of divorcees to each other. *American Sociological Review*, 3:695–699.

Price SJ & McKenry PC (1988). *Divorce*. Newbury Park, CA: Sage Press.

Rachlin S, Milton J, & Pam A (1977). Countersymbiotic suicide. *Archives of General Psychiatry*, 34:965–967.

Rawls J (1971). *A Theory of Justice*. Cambridge: Harvard University Press.

Rees WD & Lutkin SG (1967, October). Mortality of bereavement. *British Medical Journal*, pp. 13–16.

Reik T (1959). *The Compulsion to Confess: On the Psychoanalysis of Crime and Punishment*. New York: Farrar, Straus, & Cudahy.

Reingold CB (1976). *Remarriage*. New York: Harper & Row.

Reiss IL (1978). Changing sociocultural mores (pp. 311–325). In J Money & H Musaph (Eds.), *Handbook of Sexology*, vol. 1. New York: Elsevier.

Rice JK & Rice DG (1986). *Living through Divorce: A Developmental Approach to Divorce Therapy*. New York: Guilford Press.

Richards A & Willis I (1977). *How to Get It Together When Your Parents Are Coming Apart*. New York: Bantam Books.

Richardson L (1985). *The New Other Woman*. New York: Free Press.

Rieff P (1966). *The Triumph of the Therapeutic: Uses of Faith after Freud*. New York: Harper & Row.

Rilke RM (1940). *Selected Poems* (CF MacIntyre, Trans.). Berkeley: University of California Press.

Rimmer R (1973). *Adventures in Loving*. New York: Signet.

Risen CB (1995). A guide to taking a sexual history. *Psychiatric Clinics of North America*, 18:39–52.

Robins E, Murphy G, Wilkinson R, Gassner S, & Kayes J (1959). Some clinical considerations in the prevention of suicide based on a study of 134 successful suicides. *American Journal of Public Health*, 49:888–899.

Robinson K (1994). The divorce debate: Which side are you on? *Family Therapy Networker*, 18:18–30.

Rogers C (1977). *On Personal Power: Inner Strength and Its Revolutionary Impact*. New York: Delta.

Roheim G (1950). *Psychoanalysis and Anthropology*. New York: International Universities Press.

Roman JO (1980). *Exit House*. New York: Seaview Books.

Roman M & Haddad W (1978). *The Disposable Parent*. New York: Holt, Rinehart & Winston.

Rosen C (1975). *Arnold Schoenberg*. New York: Viking.

Rossiter AB (1991). Initiator status and separation adjustment. *Journal of Divorce and Remarriage*, 15:141–155.

Rowe BR (1991). The economics of divorce: Findings from seven states (pp.

5–17). In CA Everett (Ed.), *The Consequences of Divorce.* New York: Haworth Press.

Rowland GA (1989, May). A crime with passion. *Pennsylvania Medicine,* p. 42.

Russell B (1929). *Marriage and Morals.* New York: Liveright.

Russell DEH (1982). *Rape in Marriage.* New York: Macmillan.

Sachs H (1948). *Masks of Love and Life.* Cambridge, MA: Sci-Art.

Sager C & Hunt B (1979). *Intimate Partners: Hidden Patterns in Love Relationships.* New York: McGraw-Hill.

Salovey P & Rodin J (1985). The heart of jealousy. *Psychology Today,* 19:22–29.

Sands M (1978). *The Mistress' Survival Manual.* New York: Berkley Medallion Books.

Sands M (1982). *The Second Wife's Survival Manual.* New York: Berkley Books.

Santayana G (1905). *The Life of Reason: Reason in Common Sense.* New York: Scribner's.

Sartre J-P (1943/1977). *Being and Nothingness* (originally published in French, H Barnes, Trans.). Secaucus NJ: Citadel Press.

Saul L (1950). The distinction between loving and being loved. *Psychoanalytic Quarterly,* 19:412–413.

Saul L (1967). *Fidelity and Infidelity.* Philadelphia: Lippincott.

Scanzoni J (1979). A historical perspective on husband–wife bargaining power and marital dissolution (pp. 20–36). In G Levinger & OC Moles (Eds.), *Divorce and Separation: Context, Causes, and Consequences.* New York: Basic Books.

Schachter D (1986). Amnesia and crime: How much do we really know? *American Psychologist,* 41:286–295.

Schafer R (1970). The psychoanalytic vision of reality. *International Journal of Psycho-Analysis,* 51:279–297.

Schleifer S, Keller S, Camerino M, Thornton J, & Stein M (1983). Suppression of lymphocyte stimulation following bereavement. *Journal of the American Medical Association,* 250:374–377.

Schmale AH (1958). Relationship of separation and depression to disease. *Psychosomatic Medicine,* 20:259–277.

Schneiderman S (1987, November 1). Why novelists are so sane. *New York Times,* Book Review Section, p. 32.

Schneiderman S (1995). *Saving Face: America and the Politics of Shame.* New York: Knopf.

Schwartz LS (1985 December 28/1986, January 4). The moral bypass. *The Nation,* pp. 720–721.

Schwartzer A (1984). *After the Second Sex: Conversations with Simone de Beauvoir.* New York: Pantheon.

Searles HF (1959). The effort to drive the other person crazy—An element in the etiology and psychotherapy of schizophrenia. *British Journal of Medical Psychology,* 32:1–18.

Seinfeld J (1996). *Containing Rage, Terror, and Despair: An Object-Relations Approach to Psychotherapy.* Northvale, NJ: Jason Aronson.

Seligman MEP (1989). *Helplessness.* New York: Freeman.

Seltzer JA (1991). Relationships between fathers and children who live apart: The father's role after separation. *Journal of Marriage and the Family,* 53:79–101.

Selye H (1976). *The Stress of Life.* New York: McGraw-Hill.

Shakespeare W (1598/1937). Love's Labour's Lost (pp. 191–221). In *The Complete Works of William Shakespeare.* New York: Walter J Black.

Shaw GB (1967). *Pygmalion and My Fair Lady* (Adaptation and lyrics by AJ Lerner and music by F Loewe). New York: New American Library.

Sheehy G (1976). *Passages: Predictable Crises of Adult Life.* New York: Dutton.

Shepard M (1975). *Fritz.* New York: Dutton.

Sheresky N & Mannes M (1972). *Uncoupling: The Art of Coming Apart.* New York: Viking Press.

Shneidman ES (1970a). The logic of suicide (pp. 63–71). In ES Shneidman, NL Farberow, & RE Litman (Eds.), *The Psychology of Suicide.* New York: Science House.

Shneidman ES (1970b). A look into the dark: A review of Joost M. Meerloo's *Suicide and Mass Suicide* (pp. 617–620). In ES Shneidman, NL Farberow, & RE Litman (Eds.), *The Psychology of Suicide.* New York: Science House.

Shneidman ES (1970c). A review of D. J. West's *Murder Followed by Suicide* (pp. 635–636). In ES Shneidman, NL Farberow, & RE Litman (Eds.), *The Psychology of Suicide.* New York: Science House.

Simon AW (1964). *Stepchild in the Family: A View of Children in Remarriage.* New York: Odyssey.

Simon P (1975). Fifty ways to leave your lover. From the album *Still Crazy After All these Years.* Columbia Records.

Simpson JA (1990). Influence of attachment styles on romantic relationships. *Journal of Personality and Social Psychology,* 59:971–980.

Skinner BF (1972). *Beyond Freedom and Dignity.* Toronto: Bantam Books.

Slater P (1976). *The Pursuit of Loneliness: American Culture at the Breaking Point.* Boston: Beacon Press.

Smith LG & Smith JR (1978). Divorce and remarriage: Trends and patterns in contemporary society (pp. 551–561). In J Money & H Musaph (Eds.), *Handbook of Sexology,* vol. 1. New York: Elsevier.

Socarides C (1966). On vengeance—The desire to "get even." *Journal of the American Psychoanalytic Association,* 14:356–375.

Sokoloff B (1947). *Jealousy: A Psychiatric Study.* New York: Howell, Soskin.

Solomon MF (1989). *Narcissism and Intimacy: Love and Marriage in an Age of Confusion.* New York: Norton.

South SJ & Lloyd KM (1995). Spousal alternatives and marital dissolution. *American Sociological Review,* 60:21–35.

Spanier GB & Casto RF (1979). Adjustment to separation and divorce: A qualitative analysis (pp. 211–227). In G Levinger & OC Moles (Eds.), *Divorce and Separation: Context, Causes, and Consequences.* New York: Basic Books.

Spanier GB & Thompson L (1984). *Parting: The Aftermath of Separation and Divorce.* Beverly Hills: Sage.

Spencer D (1981). *Love Gone Wrong: The Jean Harris Scarsdale Murder Case*. New York: Signet.

Sperling M (1968). Acting-out behavior and psychosomatic symptoms: Clinical and theoretical aspects. *International Journal of Psycho-Analysis*, 49:250–253.

Spilke FS (1979). *What about the Children? A Divorced Parent's Handbook*. New York: Crown.

Spotnitz H & Freeman L (1964). *The Wandering Husband*. Englewood Cliffs, NJ: Prentice-Hall.

Stainback B (1976). *A Very Different Love Story: Burt and Linda Pugach's Intimate Account of Their Triumph over Tragedy*. New York: Morrow.

Stekel W (1935). *Sadism and Masochism: The Psychology of Hatred and Cruelty*, vol. 1. London: John Lane.

Stendhal HB (1822/1957). *Love* (G & S Sale, Trans.). London: Merlin.

Stengel E (1965). *Concern for Suicide–Before and After*. Baltimore: Penguin.

Stoller R (1975). *Perversion: The Erotic Form of Hatred*. New York: Pantheon Books.

Stoudemire A (1991). Somatothymia. *Psychosomatics*, 32:365–381.

Strean HS (1980). *The Extramarital Affair*. New York: Free Press.

Sullivan HS (1953). *Conceptions of Modern Psychiatry*. New York: Norton.

Sullivan J (1974). *Mama Doesn't Live Here Anymore*. New York: Fields.

Sutherland D & Cressey D (1960). *Principles of Criminology*. Philadelphia: Lippincott.

Szasz T (1973). *The Second Sin*. Garden City, NY: Anchor Books.

Tennov D (1979). *Love and Limerance: The Experience of Being in Love*. New York: Stein & Day.

Tessman LH (1978). *Children of Parting Parents*. New York: Jason Aronson.

Thamm R. (1975). *Beyond Marriage and the Nuclear Family*. San Francisco: Canfield Press.

Time (1980, October 20). Death notice, p. 105.

Toffler A (1970). *Future Shock*. New York: Random House.

Tolstoy L (1878/1965). *Anna Karenina* (originally published in Russian, C Garnett, Trans.). New York: Modern Library.

Trafford A (1992). *Crazy Time: Surviving Divorce and Building a New Life*, revised edition. New York: HarperPerennial.

Travin S & Protter B (1993). *Sexual Perversion: Integrative Approaches for the Clinican*. New York: Plenum Press.

Turow R (1978). *Daddy Doesn't Live Here Anymore*. Garden City, NY: Anchor Books.

Vaillant GE (1985). Loss as a metaphor for attachment. *The American Journal of Psychoanalysis*, 45:59–67.

Vardy M (1972). Role of the mental health professional: Therapist-healer or agent of social change? *Professional Psychology*, 3:277–280.

Vaughan D (1986). *Uncoupling: Turning Points in Intimate Relationships*. New York: Oxford University Press.

Vaughan P (1989). *The Monogamy Myth*. New York: Newmarket Press.

Victor I & Winkler W (1977). *Fathers and Custody*. New York: Hawthorn Books.

Viorst J (1977). Confessions of a jealous wife (pp. 17–24). In G Clanton & L Smith (Eds.), *Jealousy*. Englewood Cliffs, NJ: Prentice-Hall.

Visher EB & Visher JS (1993). Remarriage families and stepparenting (pp. 235–253). In F Walsh (Ed.), *Normal Family Processes*, second edition. New York: Guilford Press.

Von Hentig H (1948). *The Criminal and His Victim*. New Haven: Yale University Press.

Walder E (1978). *How to Get Out of an Unhappy Marriage*. New York: G P Putnam's Sons.

Walkup J (1985, December 28/1986, January 4). The moral bypass. *The Nation*, pp. 722–723.

Wallerstein J (1984a). The impact of divorce on children (pp. 225–239). In C Nadelson & D Polonsky (Eds.), *Marriage and Divorce: A Contemporary Perspective*. New York: Guilford Press.

Wallerstein JS (1984b). Children of divorce: Preliminary report of a ten-year follow-up of young children. *American Journal of Orthopsychiatry*, 54:444–458.

Wallerstein JS (1991). The long-term effect of divorce on children: A review. *Journal of the American Academy of Child and Adolescent Psychiatry*, 30:349–360.

Wallerstein JS & Blakeslee S (1989). *Second Chances: Men, Women, and Children a Decade after Divorce*. New York: Ticknor & Fields.

Wallerstein JS & Kelly JB (1980). *Surviving the Breakup: How Children and Parents Cope with Divorce*. New York: Basic Books.

Walsh F (1991). Promoting healthy functioning in divorced and remarried families (pp. 525–545). In AS Gurman & DP Kniskern (Eds.), *Handbook of Family Therapy*, vol. 2. New York: Brunner/Mazel.

Walsh F (Ed.) (1993). *Normal Family Processes*, second edition. New York: Guilford Press.

Walters-Chapman SF, Price SJ, & Serovich JM (1995). The effects of guilt on divorce adjustment. *Journal of Divorce and Remarriage*, 22:163–177.

Wanderer Z & Cabot T (1978). *Letting Go: A Twelve Week Action Program to Overcome a Broken Heart*. New York: Putnam's Sons.

Warshak RA (1992). *The Custody Revolution: The Father Factor and the Motherhood Mystique*. New York: Poseidon Press.

Watzlawick P (1976). *How Real Is Real?* New York: Random House.

Weiner-Davis M (1987, January/February). Confessions of an unabashed marriage saver. *Family Therapy Networker*, pp. 53–56.

Weiss R (1975). *Marital Separation*. New York: Basic Books.

Weiss R (1979a). *Going It Alone: The Family Life and Social Situation of the Single Parent*. New York: Basic Books.

Weiss R (1979b). The emotional impact of marital separation (pp. 201–210). In G Levinger & OC Moles (Eds.), *Divorce and Separation: Context, Causes, and Consequences*. New York: Basic Books.

Weiss R (1994). Is the attachment system of adults a development of Bowlby's attachment system of childhood? *Psychological Inquiry*, 5:65–67.

Weitzman LJ (1985). *The Divorce Revolution: The Unexpected Consequences for Women and Children in America.* New York: Free Press.

West B & Kissman K (1991). Mothers without custody: Treatment issues (pp. 229–237). In CA Everett (Ed.), *The Consequences of Divorce.* New York: Haworth Press.

West DJ (1965). *Murder Followed by Suicide.* London: Heinemann.

Westoff LA (1977). *The Second Time Around: Remarriage in America.* Hammondsworth, England: Penguin Books.

Whatley MA (1993). For better or worse: The case of marital rape. *Violence and Victims,* 8:29–39.

Wheeler M (1980). *Divided Children: A Legal Guide for Divorcing Parents.* New York: Norton.

Whitaker C & Miller M (1972). A re-evaluation of "psychiatric help" when divorce impends (pp. 521–530). In C Sager & H Kaplan (Eds.), *Progress in Group and Family Therapy.* New York: Brunner/Mazel.

White GL & Mullen PE (1989). *Jealousy: Theory, Research, and Clinical Strategies.* New York: Guilford Press.

Whitehurst RN (1969). Extramarital sex: Alienation or extension of normal behavior? (pp. 129–145). In G Neubeck (Ed.), *Extramarital Relations.* Englewood Cliffs, NJ: Prentice-Hall.

Wilde O (1905/1977). *De Profundis and Other Writings.* Hammondsworth, England: Penguin Books.

Willi J (1984). *Dynamics of Couple Therapy.* New York: Jason Aronson.

Willison M (1980). *Diary of a Divorced Mother.* New York: Wyden.

Winch R (1958). *Mate Selection.* New York: Harper.

Winnick C (1956). *Dictionary of Anthropology.* New York: Philosophical Library.

Winnicott D (1965). *Maturational Process and the Facilitating Environment.* New York: International Universities Press.

Wise MJ (1980). The aftermath of divorce. *The American Journal of Psychoanalysis,* 40:149–158.

Wiseman R (1975). Crisis theory and the process of divorce. *Social Casework,* 56:205–212.

Wolfe L (1975). *Playing Around: Women and Extramarital Sex.* New York: Signet.

Wolfgang M (1958). *Patterns in Criminal Homicide.* Philadelphia: University of Pennsylvania Press.

Wolfgang M (1959). Suicide by means of victim-precipitated homicide. *Journal of Clinical and Experimental Psychopathology,* 20:335–349.

Wolfgang M (1976). Victim-precipitated criminal homicide (pp 72–87). In M Wolfgang (Ed.), *Studies in Homicide.* New York: Harper & Row.

Wolman BB (1988). *Psychosomatic Disorders.* New York: Plenum Medical Book Co.

Wymard E (1994). *Men on Divorce: Conversations with Ex-Husbands.* New York: Hay House.

Wynne LC, Ryckoff IM, Day J, & Hirsch SI (1958). Pseudo-mutuality in the family relations of schizophrenics. *Psychiatry,* 21:205–220.

Yapko M (1997). Stronger medicine. *Family Therapy Networker,* 21:42–47.

Yarvis RM (1991). *Homicide: Causative Factors and Roots.* Lexington, MA: DC Heath.

Yeats WB (1921/1983). The Second Coming (p. 187). In *The Poems.* New York: Macmillan.

Young H & Ruth B (1984). Special treatment problems with the one-parent family (pp. 377–386). In Wolman B & Stricker G (Eds.), *Handbook of Marital and Family Therapy.* New York: Plenum Press.

Index